SICKLE CELL DISEASE - PAIN AND COMMON CHRONIC COMPLICATIONS

Edited by **Baba Psalm Duniya Inusa**

Sickle Cell Disease - Pain and Common Chronic Complications
http://dx.doi.org/10.5772/62012
Edited by Baba Psalm Duniya Inusa

Contributors

Kalpna Gupta, Alvin J Beitz, Anupam Aich, Raffaella Colombatti, Laura Sainati, Maria Montanaro, Israel Israel Afolabi, Anne Greenough, Murtadha Al-Khabori, Mohammed Al-Huneini, Abdulhakeem Al-Rawas, Betty Pace, Charles Quinn, Omar Niss, Ebru Dündar Yenilmez, Stephan Lobitz, Kai Sostmann, Kristina Curtis, Jamie Kawadler, Fenella J. Kirkham, Aravind Yadav, Wilfredo De Jesus Rojas, Ricardo A. Mosquera, Julie Kanter, Caterina Minniti, Aditi Singh, Baba P.D. Inusa

Published by InTech

Janeza Trdine 9, 51000 Rijeka, Croatia

Notice

Statements and opinions expressed in the chapters are these of the individual contributors and not necessarily those of the editors or publisher. No responsibility is accepted for the accuracy of information contained in the published chapters. The publisher assumes no responsibility for any damage or injury to persons or property arising out of the use of any materials, instructions, methods or ideas contained in the book.

Publishing Process Manager Dajana Pemac

Technical Editor SPi Global

Cover InTech Design team

First published November, 2016

Printed in Croatia

Additional hard copies can be obtained from orders@intechopen.com

Sickle Cell Disease - Pain and Common Chronic Complications , Edited by Baba Psalm Duniya Inusa

p. cm.

Print ISBN 978-953-51-2766-6
Online ISBN 978-953-51-2767-3

For EU product safety concerns:
IN TECH d.o.o., Prolaz Marije Krucifikse Kozulić 3, 51000 Rijeka, Croatia,
info@intechopen.com or visit our website at intechopen.com.

Meet the editor

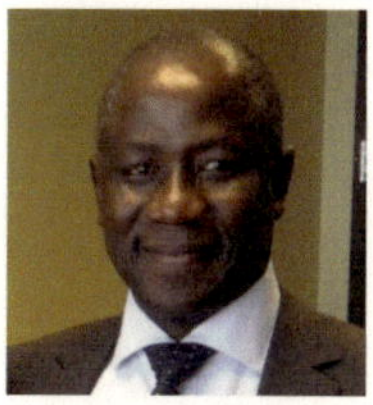

Baba PD Inusa, qualified from Zaria, Nigeria, leads the paediatric haematology at Evelina London and Guy's and St Thomas' NHS Foundation Trust, London, and he is a visiting professor at the Kaduna State University. He is a fellow of the Royal College of Paediatrics and Child Health and American Society of Hematology and a member of the international management committee responsible for global haematology. He is a director at the Academy for Sickle Cell and Thalassaemia (ASCAT) which now is in its 10th anniversary. He founded the sickle cell cohort research (www.score-international.org). His research includes neurological disorders (stroke, neuropsychological studies) and renal impairment in sickle cell disease, and he leads a number of drug trials in the UK and extensive research collaboration in the USA, UK and Africa. He is also a reviewer of over ten high-impact journals and currently editing a book on sickle cell disease.

Contents

Preface

This book aims to provide the reader a good insight into sickle cell disease. The chapters were derived from the themes of the annual meeting which enters its 10th year on October 2016. There is an overview of sickle cell disease addressing the progress made from the first formal description in medical literature in 1910, the molecular basis and early treatment. It also includes description of new therapies and common complications of sickle cell disease.

This book is not intended to cover all the relevant topics as these may be coming in subsequent editions. It attempts to address detailed research findings in pain and the role of therapeutic intervention. Pain as the prototype clinical feature in sickle cell disease is discussed in detail bringing out very useful research themes. There is an overview of sickle cell disease in childhood that addresses newborn screening and regular follow-up from birth through to adulthood. It describes some common assessment tools and pragmatic tests that can be easily undertaken in less developed clinical settings. The fact that over 80% of all patients with sickle cell disease lack access to comprehensive care means that a minimum tool is required to reduce mortality and improve the quality of life.

Every chapter addresses the mechanism of disease and seeks to address common management strategies, a useful guide to researchers and frontline management professionals.

Dr. Baba Psalm Duniya Inusa
Associate Professor of Paediatric Haematology and
Lead Consultant of sickle cell disease and thalassaemia at Evelina London Children's Hospital
and Guy's and St Thomas' NHS Foundation Trust,
London, UK

Section 1

Introduction to Sickle Cell Disease - An Overview

Chapter 1

Introductory Chapter: Introduction to the History, Pathology and Clinical Management of Sickle Cell Disease

Baba Inusa, Maddalena Casale and Nicholas Ward

Additional information is available at the end of the chapter

http://dx.doi.org/10.5772/65648

1. Introduction

Sickle cell disease (SCD) is due to a single point mutation (Glub6Val) that causes polymerisation of the mutant hemoglobin (Hb) S, resulting in sickling of erythrocytes [1]. Inflammation, haemolysis, microvascular obstruction and organ damage characterise the clinical expression of SCD, which is highly variable in individual patients. Environmental and multiple genetic factors modify many aspects of SCD and therefore contribute to the clinical variability [2, 3].

This chronic, complex and monogenetic haematological condition that leads to haemolytic anaemia, severe acute complications and chronic organ damage was formally reported in 1910 [4]. One hundred years after Herrick's initial report, there have been significant advances in the diagnosis and management [5].

Forty years ago only half of children with sickle cell anaemia were expected to reach adulthood [6]. However, advances in the diagnosis and management of SCD have improved the survival and quality of life significantly. Recent figures suggest survival of 53 years for men and 58.5 years for women [7, 8] and over 94% surviving to adulthood [8, 9].

SCD is now one of the most common genetic disorders in the world with high prevalence in sub-Saharan Africa (SSA), the Middle East, the Mediterranean and the Indian subcontinent [1, 10, 11]. In the United States, almost 1 in 10 African Americans has the sickle cell trait, with 1 in 600 being homozygous for the sickle hemoglobin allele [12, 13]. In the UK, it is diagnosed at birth, through routine Newborn screening with incidence of about 1 in every 2000 births [3, 14]. However despite the high prevalence in sub-Saharan Africa (SSA) essential public health programmes have not been implemented due to limited medical resources and infrastructures [10, 11, 15, 16]. As a consequence, infant and childhood mortality due to SCD remains high. It is estimated that without intervention, up to 50-90% of affected infants may die by 5 years of age from SCD [11, 15, 17, 18]. While high regional disease prevalence would be expected to facilitate epidemiologic, translational and clinical research, the majority of SSA countries lack the capacity to provide the comprehensive care for SCD [11].

2. Early description

James Herrick is widely acknowledged as the first physician to describe a case of sickle cell. However, the term 'sickle cell anaemia' was not coined until 1922 [19], when a review of the first four cases of the disease was conducted, including that described by Herrick [20, 21].

However, it is argued that case reports, up to 60 years prior to that by Herrick, may have described sickle cell disease [6, 17]. A post-mortem, performed in 1898, of a patient who died in hospital after being admitted for pains, jaundice and previous leg ulcers shows that these symptoms are suggestive of SCD [22]. It has also been proposed that the clinical illness had been previously recognised in Africa as "cold-season rheumatism" and that the possibility of genetic inheritance of the illness had even been noted [10].

3. Discovery of molecular and genetic basis

It was not until 40 years after the first description of sickle cell anaemia that a homozygous pattern of inheritance was confirmed simultaneously by two separate studies, one a pedigree study in Africa [11, 12]. These studies demonstrated that sickle cell anaemia was inherited in an autosomal recessive pattern. In the late 1940s, Pauling discovered that blood from sickle cell patients had differing mobility during electrophoresis [23, 24]. This indicated that there were chemical differences between the hemoglobin of the different cells. Thus, Pauling and colleagues proposed that sickle cell anaemia was a molecular disease, the first disease of this kind [23].

Vernon Ingram was to be the discoverer of the exact difference between sickle cell and normal adult hemoglobin. Ingram identified that sickle hemoglobin (HbS) was more positively charge hemoglobin A (HbA) [21, 25]. The amino acid sequence of hemoglobin was shown to differ by only one substitution of glutamic acid with valine in the β chain of HbS [26]. As knowledge of the pathophysiology of SCD is a complex phenomenon between vaso-occlusion and hemolysis [27–29].

4. Prophylactic penicillin and pneumococcal vaccination

Studies have shown that infant mortality is particularly high in sickle cell disease. Scott's observations revealed that the number of children reaching adulthood was only approximately 50% [4] in the 1960s. The Cooperative Study of Sickle Cell Disease (CSSD) has shown that the peak incidence of death was between the ages of 1 and 3 [30]. Furthermore, the CSSD showed that the largest killer in SCD was infection, with this being the cause of death in 50% of subjects being followed below the age of 20 [20]. Infection was also shown to be a predominant factor in other studies of mortality [21, 22] with pneumococcal disease being identified as a major killer [19, 20]. It has even been calculated that the risk of developing meningitis from *Streptococcus pneumoniae* is 30 times more likely in the sickle cell population than in the general population [23].

The increased risk of infection may be attributed to many factors, including decreased immunoglobulin function, poor cell-mediated immunity and reduced opsonisations [24–27]. Importantly, there is a decrease in splenic function as a result of microvascular occlusions and infarctions [24]. The decrease in immune function leads to a vulnerability to encapsulated organisms particularly *Streptococcus pneumoniae, Haemophilus influenzae* type B and *Salmonella* [28].

Following the recognition of infection playing a major role in the disease, a study commencing in 1983 showed the benefit of prophylactic penicillin. Gaston and colleagues recruited sickle cell patients under the age of 3 to a randomised control study to determine if daily prophylactic penicillin would be effective at reducing childhood infections. Astonishingly it was found to reduce septicaemia by 84% and the trial was terminated early. The Penicillin Prophylaxis in SCD study (PROPS) therefore recommended that all children should be screened and started on penicillin by the time they reached 4 months of age [31].

In addition to prophylactic antibiotics, pneumococcal vaccination has also become an important part of sickle cell management. Those immunised had lower incidence of pneumococcal septicaemia than the control group [32, 33]. The introduction of new conjugated vaccines against other encapsulated bacteria (13 strains of *Streptococcus pneumoniae; Meningococcus* A, C, W, Y and B and *Haemophilus influenzae*) has reduced the rate of pneumococcal bacteraemia by 93.4% in children aged <5 years to 134 cases per 100,000 person-years, $P<0.001$ [33–35]. Incidence of invasive pneumococcal disease among individuals with sickle cell disease before and after the introduction of the pneumococcal conjugate vaccine [32, 35].

5. Prenatal and Neonatal SCD Screening

SCD is associated with high infant mortality rate; therefore, early preventive intervention is essential in reducing these deaths [14, 36]. A maternal blood screen during or preceding pregnancy seems the most cost-effective method of initiating a screening programme, as if the mother does not carry the sickle allele, then there is no risk of the child having sickle cell disease and additionally this initial screen does not need repetition for future pregnancies. If maternal screening reveals a sickle cell trait or SCD, the father can be invited for investigation [14, 36].

Since 1978 it has been possible to obtain foetal DNA to diagnose sickle cell disease prenatally [18], via amniocentesis or chorionic villus sampling (CVS). CVS offers the advantage that the family is given the choice early in pregnancy. Prior to this it was only possible to diagnose sickle cell disease via direct viewing of foetal blood. In some countries it has been in use for national screening programmes and rates of termination of pregnancy are as high as 74% in Cuba [37–40].

The importance of neonatal identification of SCD is emphasised [36, 41, 42].

By 1994 the majority of United States cities had implemented universal neonatal hemoglobinopathy screening [12, 43]; the UK has only fully implemented its universal sickle cell screening programme in the last few years [14, 44]. In Africa, only Ghana and the Republic of Benin have established selective and pilot Newborn screening programme, respectively [37, 41, 45, 46].

5.1. Pain management

The clinical severity of SCD is variable and usually defies genetic or phenotypic explanation. The cooperative study of the natural history of sickle cell disease showed that about 5% of patients accounted for one-third of hospital days devoted to pain control [19]. Acute VOC and chronic pain syndrome could be disabling to the patient, and studies have demonstrated an association of acute pain syndromes with other complications of SCD, including death [19, 47].

Pain management guidelines and the need to rule out life-threatening comorbidities suggest the need for rapid physician evaluation of patients who present to the emergency department (ED) with complaints related to SCD [47]. The American Pain Society guidelines recommend initial assessment and analgesia within 30 min of arrival [5, 48].

5.2. Hydroxyurea (HU)

From the difficulty in identifying sickle-shaped erythrocytes in neonates, Janet Watson postulated, in 1948, that high fetal hemoglobin leads to a decrease in cells that could sickle and therefore a decrease in sickle hemoglobin in those red blood cells [49]. Several years later it was suggested that by increasing or prolonging the concentration of foetal hemoglobin in erythrocytes, it would be possible to decrease the frequency and severity of the clinical manifestations of SCD [50–52].

HU, an anti-leukaemia agent with the capacity to increase foetal Hb, was introduced to treat sickle cell disease with significant clinical and symptomatic improvement. In 1992 a randomised double-blind study, the Multicentre Study of HU in Sickle Cell Anaemia (MSH), showed that this new drug could decrease episodes of painful crises, acute chest syndrome and the need for transfusion [53, 54]. The study recruited 299 adults with more than three painful crises in the year prior to the start of HU, and the clinical effect was great enough for the trial to terminate 3 months early [54, 55].

The paediatric studies on the use of hydroxyurea reflected the results of the adult trials, with reduced acute complications and with no toxicity or decreased growth, and suggested reduced end organ damage if administered early [56–58].

6. Stroke and stroke prevention

Stroke is an important cause of morbidity and mortality of SCD with an estimated 11% having had a stroke by the age of 20 [59]. Although the treatment of strokes in SCD had been improving, it was a ground breaking trial in the final decade of the twentieth century that changed the way SCD was monitored [60, 61] to prevent stoke in this group of patients.

Landmark's work into the use of transcranial Doppler (TCD) ultrasounds showed that severe sickle cell disease could lead to the narrowing of cerebral blood vessels. These would appear on ultrasonography as increased flow in that region and patients with abnormal flow are at increased risk of stroke [60, 62]. Silent cerebral infarcts are the most common neurologic injury in children with sickle cell anaemia and are associated with the recurrence of an infarct (stroke or silent cerebral infarct), and regular blood transfusion therapy significantly reduced the incidence of the recurrence of cerebral infarct in children with sickle cell anaemia by 58% [63, 64].

7. Pulmonary hypertension

Pulmonary hypertension (PAH) is recognised to be a common complication of SCD and other haemolytic disorders and is associated with increased mortality and morbidity. Retrospective studies suggest a prevalence of PAH ranging from 20 to 40% [65, 66] among adults, and a prospective study showed that prevalence of PAH in paediatric population is 31%, and the two-year mortality rates approach 50% [65, 66].

Chronic hemolysis represents a prominent mechanistic pathway in the pathogenesis of SCD-associated PAH via a nitric oxide (NO) scavenging and abrogation of NO salutatory effects on vascular function. These processes lead to acute and chronic pulmonary vasoconstriction [65]. Many known infectious risk factors for PAH, i.e. human immunodeficiency virus (HIV) infection, chronic hepatitis B and C viral infections and possibly malaria, are hyper endemic in African countries where the prevalence of SCD is very high. Interactions between these infectious complications and SCD-related hemolysis could yield an even higher incidence of PAH among the African SCD patients.

Self-reported history of cardiovascular and renal complications, systolic hypertension, high lactate dehydrogenase levels (index of haemolysis), high level of alkaline phosphatase, low transferrin concentration (indicating iron overload) and priapism in men were found to be independent correlates of PAH [20, 67].

Therapy for SCD-related PAH remains challenging. Treatment with HU at maximum tolerated dose and judicious use of blood transfusion support and iron-chelating agents where indicated is recommended [66]. While HU is a potential NO donor effect, it has not been shown to impact mortality of SCD-related PAH [51]. There is increasing interest in the use of sildenafil in SCD-related PAH. Sildenafil was well tolerated by both male and female patients and it reduced the estimated pulmonary artery systolic pressure and increased the 6-min walk distance [68, 69].

Gene therapy has the potential to correct the underlying defect leading to the clinical manifestations of sickle cell disease. It would reduce the need for many of the preventative treatments and invasive therapies. A few years ago, this may not have seemed possible; however, gene therapy has been proven to be effective in mouse models [1, 2], and there are currently several teams working on phase II trials using viral vectors [70–72].

8. Global perspectives

The World Health Organization has estimated that there may be approximately 216,000 babies born with HbSS disease in Africa each year and that the disease may account for 10–20% of neonatal mortality in West Africa, very little is known about the overall global burden of SCD [68].

Although there have been improvements in the management of SCD in developed countries, much less progress has been made in the developing world in which the disease is common, where it is still an important cause of childhood mortality. In low-income countries, basic facilities for management are lacking, systemic screening is not a common practice, and diagnosis is made late.

Research collaborations between sickle cell research groups in rich and poor countries would be of considerable benefit to the health and well-being of patients with SCD in the developing countries. In particular, interactions of this kind offer an opportunity to improve clinical and diagnostic facilities and hence the management of patients in the developing world. We cannot yet cure SCD, but we have learnt that simple interventions significantly improve morbidity and mortality.

9. Conclusion

Although there has been dramatic improvement in the diagnosis, management and monitoring of sickle cell disease over the last century, bone marrow transplantation (BMT) is currently the only cure for SCD with a curative success rate of approximately 90–93% [68, 69]. Conversely, there are severe risks and complications including rejection, marrow aplasia, neurological disorders, graft-versus-host disease and death, and standard BMT is limited by a requirement for human leukocyte antigen (HLA)-matched sibling donors [70]. Currently transplantation is only considered for those children with HLA-identical siblings and in whom the clinical manifestation of the disease does not respond to standard care.

The past 100 years have shown great accomplishments for SCD including newborn screening, penicillin prophylaxis, primary stroke prevention using blood transfusion, stroke prevention trial in sickle cell anaemia (STOP) and controlled trial of transfusions for silent cerebral infarct in sickle cell anaemia. The role of hydroxyurea therapy in adults and children to reduce pain, hospitalisations and most recently as an alternative for controlling cerebral blood velocity—transcranial Doppler (TCD) with Transfusion Changing to Hydroxyurea (TWiTCH) therapy. Although a risk-free cure has not been found in this last and current century, the following 100 years look to be extremely promising for sickle cell anaemia; stem cell transplantation is now more commonly used in SCD.

Competing interests

The authors declare that they have no competing interests.

Authors' contributions

MC and NW reviewed the literature and wrote the draft of the manuscript, BI designed, reviewed and made the substantial changes the manuscript. All authors discussed, read and approved the manuscript.

Acknowledgements

Dr Serajul Islam contributed to the design, literature review and was initially a co-author but did not review the manuscript following substantial revisions. We appreciated his contribution.

Author details

Baba Inusa[1,2]*, Maddalena Casale[3] and Nicholas Ward[2]

*Address all correspondence to: baba.inusa@gstt.nhs.uk

1 Paediatric Haematology, Guy's and St Thomas' Hospital, London, United Kingdom

2 King's College London, London, United Kingdom

3 The Second University of Naples, Caserta, Naples, Italy

References

[1] Chakravorty S, Williams TN. Sickle cell disease: a neglected chronic disease of increasing global health importance. Arch Dis Child [Internet]. 2014;100(1):48–53. Available from: http://adc.bmj.com/cgi/doi/10.1136/archdischild-2013-303773

[2] Weatherall DJ. The challenge of haemoglobinopathies in resource-poor countries. Br J Haematol. 2011;(July):736–44.

[3] Modell B, Darlison M, Birgens H, Cario H, Faustino P, Giordano PC, et al. Epidemiology of haemoglobin disorders in Europe: an overview. Scand J Clin Lab Invest. 2007;67(1):39–69.

[4] Noel WC, Senn N, Hek L, Murphy JB, Wil DH, Fenger C, et al. The Rest of the ZO0GJDBDOŒ ^ DDLZÛQDDDE. 2016;4354.

[5] Inati A. Recent advances in improving the management of sickle cell disease. Blood Rev [Internet]. 2009;23(Suppl. 1):S9–13. Available from: http://dx.doi.org/10.1016/S0268-960X(09)70004-9

[6] Modell B. Global epidemiology of haemoglobin disorders and derived service indicators. Bull World Health Organ [Internet]. 2008[cited 2012 Nov 12];2008(6):480–7. Available from: http://www.who.int/bulletin/volumes/86/6/06-036673.pdf

[7] Platt O, Brambilla D, Rosse W, Milner P. Mortality in Sickle Cell Disease. N Engl J Med. 1994;330(23):1639–44.

[8] Quinn CT, Rogers ZR, Buchanan GR. Survival of children with sickle cell disease. Blood [Internet]. 2004 [cited 2012 Oct 25];103(11):4023–7. Available from: http://www.pubmedcentral.nih.gov/articlerender.fcgi?artid=1828870&tool=pmcentrez&rendertype=abstract

[9] Telfer P, Coen P, Chakravorty S, Wilkey O, Evans J, Newell H, et al. Clinical outcomes in children with sickle cell disease living in England: a neonatal cohort in East London. Haematologica [Internet]. 2007 [cited 2013 Feb 19];92(7):905–12. Available from: http://www.ncbi.nlm.nih.gov/pubmed/17606440

[10] Piel FB, Patil AP, Howes RE, Nyangiri OA, Gething PW, Dewi M, et al. Global epidemiology of Sickle haemoglobin in neonates: A contemporary geostatistical model-based map and population estimates. Lancet [Internet]. 2013;381(9861):142–51. Available from: http://dx.doi.org/10.1016/S0140-6736(12)61229-X

[11] Grosse SD, Odame I, Atrash HK, Amendah DD, Piel FB, Williams TN. Sickle cell disease in Africa: a neglected cause of early childhood mortality. Am J Prev Med [Internet]. 2011 [cited 2012 Nov 25];41(6 Suppl. 4):S398–405. Available from: http://www.ncbi.nlm.nih.gov/pubmed/22099364

[12] Angastiniotis M, Modell B. Global epidemiology of hemoglobin disorders. Ann N Y Acad Sci. 1998;850:251–69.

[13] Biswas T. Global burden of sickle cell anaemia is set to rise by a third by 2050. Brtish Med J [Internet]. 2013;4676(July 2013):6638. Available from: http://www.bmj.com/content/347/bmj.f4676.pdf+html

[14] Streetly A, Latinovic R, Hall K, Henthorn J. Implementation of universal newborn bloodspot screening for sickle cell disease and other clinically significant haemoglobi nopathies in England: screening results for 2005-7. J Clin Pathol [Internet]. 2009;62(1):26–30. Available from: http://www.pubmedcentral.nih.gov/articlerender.fcgi?artid=2603283&tool=pmcentrez&rendertype=abstract

[15] Williams TN, Weatherall DJ. World distribution, population genetics, and health burden of the hemoglobinopathies. Cold Spring Harb Perspect Med. 2012;2(9):1–14.

[16] Weatherall DJ. The inherited diseases of hemoglobin are an emerging global health burden. [Internet]. Blood. 2010:4331–6. Available from: http://www.pubmedcentral.nih.gov/articlerender.fcgi?artid=2881491&tool=pmcentrez&rendertype=abstract

[17] Fleming AF. The presentation, management and prevention of crisis in sickle cell disease in Africa. Blood Rev. 1989;3(1):18–28.

[18] Odame I, Kulkarni R, Ohene-Frempong K. Concerted global effort to combat sickle cell disease: The first global congress on sickle cell disease in Accra, Ghana. Am J Prev Med [Internet]. 2011;41(6 Suppl. 4):S417–21. Available from: http://dx.doi.org/10.1016/j.amepre.2011.09.019

[19] Ballas SK, Ballas SK. Defining the Phenotypes of Sickle Cell Disease. 2016;269(August).

[20] Rees DC, Williams TN, Gladwin MT. Sickle-cell disease. Lancet [Internet]. 2010;376 (9757):2018–31. Available from: http://dx.doi.org/10.1016/S0140-6736(10)61029-X

[21] Ingram VM. Abnormal human haemoglobins. I. The comparison of normal human and sickle-cell haemoglobins by fingerprinting. Biochim Biophys Acta [Internet]. 1958;28 (28):539–45. Available from: http://www.sciencedirect.com/science/article/pii/000630025890516X

[22] Lanzkron S, Carroll CP, Jr CH. Mortality rates and age at death from sickle cell disease: U.S., 1979–2005. Public Heal reports (Washington, DC 1974). 2013;128(2):110–6.

[23] Strasser BJ. Linus Pauling's "molecular diseases": Between history and memory. 2002;93 (2):83–93.

[24] Eaton WA. Linus Pauling and sickle cell disease. Biophys Chem. 2003;100(1–3):109–16.

[25] Ingram VM. A specific chemical difference between the globins of normal human and sickle-cell anaemia haemoglobin. Nature. 1956;178(4537):792–4.

[26] Riggs MG, Ingram VM. Differences in erythrocyte membrane proteins and glycoproteins in sickle cell disease. Biochem Biophys Res Commun [Internet]. 1977;74(1):191–8. Available from: http://eutils.ncbi.nlm.nih.gov/entrez/eutils/elink.fcgi?dbfrom=pubmed&id=836277&retmode=ref&cmd=prlinks\nfile:///Users/Aniradha/Desktop/Dropbox/Papers2/Library.papers3/Files/FE/FEF819A5-3466-4159-9CF8-8AA03710A3F3.pdf\npapers3://publication/uuid/E0DE2EAB-

[27] Hebbel RP, Osarogiagbon R, Kaul D. The endothelial biology of sickle cell disease: Inflammation and a chronic vasculopathy. Microcirculation [Internet]. 2004 [cited 2013 Jan 27];11(2):129–51. Available from: http://doi.wiley.com/10.1080/10739680490278402

[28] Kato GJ. New insights into sickle cell disease. Curr Opin Hematol [Internet]. 2016;23 (3):224–32. Available from: http://content.wkhealth.com/linkback/openurl?sid=WKPTLP:landingpage&an=00062752-201605000-00007

[29] Minniti CP, Delaney KH, Gorbach AM, Xu D, Lee CR, Malik N, et al. NIH Public Access. 2014;89(1):1–6.

[30] Bonds DR. Three decades of innovation in the management of sickle cell disease: The road to understanding the sickle cell disease clinical phenotype. Blood Rev. 2005;19(2):99–110.

[31] Gaston MH, Verter JI, Woods G, Pegelow C, Kelleher J, Presbury G, et al. Prophylaxis with oral penicillin in children with sickle cell anemia. N Engl J Med. 1986;314 (25):1593–9.

[32] Cober MP, Phelps SJ, Ohio N. Brief review article penicillin prophylaxis in children with sickle cell disease. 2010;15(3).

[33] Affairs P. Penicillin prophylaxis in children with sickle cell disease. 1991;302(May):1205–6.

[34] Preventing infections in sickle cell disease: The unfinished. 2016;63(5):25911.

[35] Booth C, Inusa B, Obaro SK. Infection in sickle cell disease: A review. 2010:2–12.

[36] Pt M, Sd G, Santos B, V DO, Bernardino L, Nj K, et al. A cost-effectiveness analysis of a pilot neonatal screening program for sickle cell anemia in the Republic of Angola. 2015;3476(15):26477868.

[37] McGann PT, Ferris MG, Ramamurthy U, Santos B, de Oliveira V, Bernardino L, et al. A prospective newborn screening and treatment program for sickle cell anemia in Luanda, Angola. Am J Hematol. 2013;88(12):984–9.

[38] Petrou M, Brugiatelli M, Ward RH, Modell B. Factors affecting the uptake of prenatal diagnosis for sickle cell disease. J Med Genet [Internet]. 1992;29(11):820–3. Available from: http://www.pubmedcentral.nih.gov/articlerender.fcgi?artid=1016180&tool=pmcentrez&rendertype=abstract

[39] Loader S, Sutera CJ, Segelman SG, Kozyra A, Rowley PT. Prenatal hemoglobinopathy screening. IV. Follow-up of women at risk for a child with a clinically significant hemoglobinopathy. Am J Hum Genet. 1991;49(6):1292–9.

[40] Rowley PT, Loader S, Sutera CJ, Walden M, Kozyra A. Prenatal screening for hemoglobinopathies. I. A prospective regional trial. Am J Hum Genet [Internet]. 1991;48(3):439–46. Available from: http://www.ncbi.nlm.nih.gov/pmc/articles/PMC1682994/\nhttp://www.pubmedcentral.nih.gov/articlerender.fcgi?artid=1682994&tool=pmcentrez&rendertype=abstract

[41] Inusa BP, Juliana Olufunke YD, John Dada L. Sickle cell disease screening in Northern Nigeria: The co-existence of B-thalassemia inheritance. Pediatr Ther [Internet]. 2015;5 (3):3–6. Available from: http://www.omicsonline.org/open-access/sickle-cell-disease-screening-in-northern-nigeria-the-coexistence-of-thalassemia-inheritance-2161-0665-1000262.php?aid=59622

[42] Modell B. Delivering genetic screening to the community. Ann Med. 1997;29(6):591–9.

[43] Vichinsky E, Lubin BH. Suggested guidelines for the treatment of children with sickle cell anemia. Hematol Oncol Clin North Am. 1987;1(3):483–501.

[44] Henthorn JS, Almeida AM, Davies SC. Neonatal screening for sickle cell disorders. Br J Haematol. 2004;124(3):259–63.

[45] Tshilolo L, Aissi LM, Lukusa D, Kinsiama C, Wembonyama S, Gulbis B, et al. Neonatal screening for sickle cell anaemia in the Democratic Republic of the Congo: Experience from a pioneer project on 31 204 newborns. 2009;(fig 1):35–8.

[46] Ohene-frempong K, Oduro J. Screening newborns for sickle cell disease in ghana submitted by Kwaku Ohene-Frempong suppression of the olivocochlear reflex: A neurotoxic adverse effect of vincristine submitted by Helen Kosmidis transplantation for the treatment of thalassemia: The g. 1993;

[47] Colombatti R, Sainati L. Management of children with sickle cell disease in Europe: Current situation and future perspectives. 2016;(July):129–35.

[48] Melorose J, Perroy R, Careas S. Evidence-based management of sickle cell disease. Expert Panel Report, 2014. US Dep Heal Humand Serv NIH. 2015;1.

[49] Ideguchi H. Congenital hemolytic anemia. Nippon Rinsho Jpn J Clin Med. 2005;63:415–9.

[50] Mpalampa L, Ndugwa CM, Ddungu H, Idro R. Foetal haemoglobin and disease severity in sickle cell anaemia patients in Kampala, Uganda. BMC Blood Disord [Internet]. 2012 [cited 2012 Nov 25];12(1):11. Available from: http://www.ncbi.nlm.nih.gov/pubmed/22958547

[51] Saraf SL, Molokie RE, Nouraie M, Sable CA, Luchtman-Jones L, Ensing GJ, et al. Differences in the clinical and genotypic presentation of sickle cell disease around the world. Paediatr Respir Rev. 2014;15(1):4–12.

[52] Rooks Y, Pack B. A profile of sickle cell disease. Nurs Clin North Am. 1983;18:131–8.

[53] Moore RD, Charache S, Terrin ML, Barton FB. Cost-effectiveness of hydroxyurea in sickle cell anemia. 2000;31(January):26–31.

[54] Charache S, Barton FB, Moore RD, Terrin ML, Steinberg MH, Dover GJ, et al. Hydroxyurea and sickle cell anemia. Clinical utility of a myelosuppressive "switching" agent. The multicenter study of hydroxyurea in sickle cell anemia. Medicine (Baltimore). 1996;75 (6):300–26.

[55] Charache S. Mechanism of action of hydroxyurea in the management of sickle cell anemia in adults. Semin Hematol. 1997;34(3 Suppl 3):15–21.

[56] Wang WC, Ware RE, Miller ST, Iyer R V, Casella JF, Minniti CP, et al. Hydroxycarbamide in very young children with sickle-cell anaemia: a multicentre, randomised, controlled trial (BABY HUG). Lancet [Internet]. 2011 [cited 2012 Nov 25];377(9778):1663–72. Available from: http://www.pubmedcentral.nih.gov/articlerender.fcgi?artid=3133619&tool=pmcentrez&rendertype=abstract

[57] Hankins JS, Ware RE, Rogers ZR, Wynn LW, Lane PA, Scott JP, et al. Long-term hydroxyurea therapy for infants with sickle cell anemia: The HUSOFT extension study. Blood. 2005;106(7):2269–75.

[58] Kinney TR, Helms RW, Branski EEO, Ohene-frempong K, Wang W, Daeschner C, et al. Safety of hydroxyurea in children with sickle cell anemia: Results of the HUG-KIDS study, a phase I/II trial. 1999;1550–4.

[59] Ohene-Frempong K, Weiner SJ, Sleeper L a, Miller ST, Embury S, Moohr JW, et al. Cerebrovascular accidents in sickle cell disease: Rates and risk factors. Blood [Internet]. 1998;91(1):288–94. Available from: http://www.ncbi.nlm.nih.gov/pubmed/9414296

[60] Nichols FT, Jones AM, Adams RJ. Stroke prevention in sickle cell disease (STOP) study guidelines for transcranial Doppler testing. J Neuroimaging [Internet]. 2001 [cited 2013 Feb 19];11(4):354–62. Available from: http://www.ncbi.nlm.nih.gov/pubmed/11677874

[61] Adams R, McKie V, Nichols F. The use of transcranial ultrasonography to predict stroke in sickle cell disease. N Engl J Med [Internet]. 1992 [cited 2013 Feb 10]; Available from: http://www.nejm.org/doi/full/10.1056/NEJM199202273260905

[62] Adams RJ. Big strokes in small persons. Arch Neurol [Internet]. 2007;64(11):1567–74. Available from: http://www.ncbi.nlm.nih.gov/pubmed/17998439

[63] DeBaun MR, Gordon M, McKinstry RC, Noetzel MJ, White DA, Sarnaik SA, et al. Controlled trial of transfusions for silent cerebral infarcts in sickle cell anemia. N Engl J Med [Internet]. 2014;371(8):699–710. Available from: http://www.ncbi.nlm.nih.gov/pubmed/25140956

[64] DeBaun MR, Armstrong FD, McKinstry RC, Ware RE, Vichinsky E, Kirkham FJ. Silent cerebral infarcts: A review on a prevalent and progressive cause of neurologic injury in sickle cell anemia. Blood [Internet]. 2012 [cited 2012 Nov 3];119(20):4587–96. Available from: http://www.ncbi.nlm.nih.gov/pubmed/22354000

[65] Gladwin MT, Ghofrani H. Pulmonary and critical care updates. Update on pulmonary hypertension. 2009;(6).

[66] Ansong D, Akoto AO, Ocloo D, Ohene-frempong K. Sickle cell disease: Management options and challenges in developing countries. 2013.

[67] Kato GJ, McGowan V, Machado RF, Little JA, Taylor J, Morris CR, et al. Lactate dehydrogenase as a biomarker of hemolysis-associated nitric oxide resistance, priapism, leg ulceration, pulmonary hypertension, and death in patients with sickle cell disease. Blood [Internet]. 2006 [cited 2012 Nov 24];107(6):2279–85. Available from: http://www.pubmedcentral.nih.gov/articlerender.fcgi?artid=1895723&tool=pmcentrez&rendertype=abstract

[68] Kato GJ, Hsieh M, Machado R, Vi JT, Little J, Butman JA, et al. NIH Public Access. 2008;81(7):503–10.

[69] Sebastiani P, Nolan VG, Baldwin CT, Abad-grau MM, Wang L, Adewoye AH, et al. Red cells a network model to predict the risk of death in sickle cell disease. Cell. 2007;110(7):2727–35.

[70] Menzel S, Rooks H, Zelenika D, Mtatiro SN, Gnanakulasekaran A, Drasar E, et al. Global genetic architecture of an erythroid quantitative trait locus, HMIP-2. Ann Hum Genet. 2014;434–51.

[71] Mtatiro SN, Makani J, Mmbando B, Thein SL, Menzel S, Cox SE. Genetic variants at HbF-modifier loci moderate anemia and leukocytosis in sickle cell disease in Tanzania. Am J Hematol [Internet]. 2015;90(1):E1–4. Available from: http://doi.wiley.com/10.1002/ajh.23859

[72] National Heart Lung and Blood Institute. Evidence-based management of sickle cell disease: Expert Panel Report (EPR). Guidel Expert Panel Rep. 2014.

Chapter 2

A Global Perspective on Milestones of Care for Children with Sickle Cell Disease

Laura Sainati, Maria Montanaro and Raffaella Colombatti

Additional information is available at the end of the chapter

http://dx.doi.org/10.5772/64656

Abstract

Sickle cell disease (SCD) is one of the most common severe and monogenic disorders worldwide. Acute and chronic complications deeply impact the health of children with SCD. Milestones of treatment include newborn screening, comprehensive care and prevention of cerebrovascular complications.

Keywords: sickle cell disease, children, newborn screening, comprehensive care, stroke

1. Introduction

Sickle cell disease (SCD) is one of the most common severe and monogenic disorders worldwide with an average of 300,000 children born annually with sickle syndromes, the majority in Africa [1, 2]. SCD was initially endemic in areas of malaria disease (Africa, Southern India, Mediterranean countries, Southern Asia), but various waves of migration brought populations from areas of high prevalence of the HbS gene to the Americas and Europe (**Figure 1**). Moreover, the recent migration movements of the past decade have further increased the frequency of SCD in areas where it was generally uncommon. In Europe, SCD has become the paradigm of immigration hematology [3] and is now the most prevalent genetic disease in France [4] and the United Kingdom [5]; its frequency is steadily rising in many other countries of northern, central and southern Europe [6–10] posing a challenge to health systems. In addition, awareness regarding SCD is increasing in India [11] and in many African countries [12] where the prevalence of the disease is high. Although in low-resource settings a great effort in terms of funding, care and research is still mainly destined to infectious diseases, the burden SCD poses on mortality and health systems in Africa is finally starting to be recognized [13–16]. Several African countries have developed dedicated services for children with SCD [17–20], including newborn screening [21–26]. Patients with SCD in many centers are being evaluated in a standardized comprehensive manner both in prospective observational cohorts [17, 19, 27] and randomized clinical trials [28, 29]. Although some experiences are still conceived as pilot programs and have yet to be scaled up at a national level, their results are promising and demonstrate increased commitment to tackle SCD at a global level.

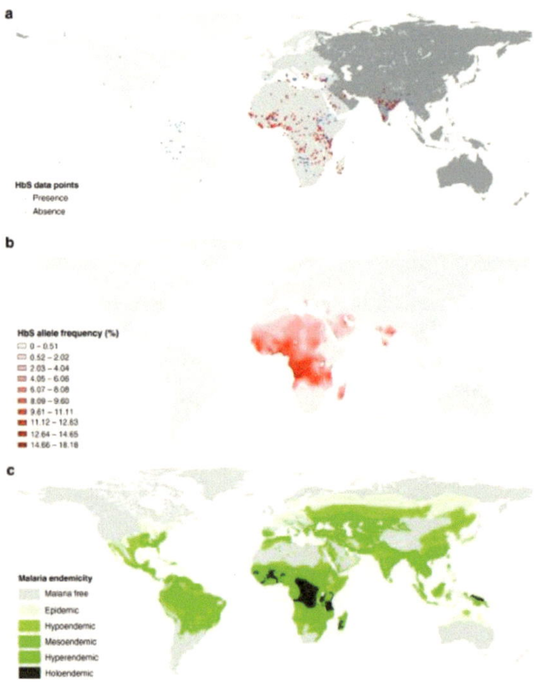

Figure 1. Global distribution of the sickle cell gene. (a) Distribution of the data points. Red dots represent the presence and blue dots the absence of the *HbS* gene. The regional subdivisions were informed by Weatherall and Clegg and are as follows: the Americas (light gray), Africa, including the western part of Saudi Arabia, and Europe (medium gray) and Asia (dark gray); (b) Raster map of HbS allele frequency (posterior median) generated by a Bayesian model-based geostatistical framework. The Jenks optimized classification method was used to define the classes; (c) the historical map of malaria endemicity was digitized from its source using the method outlined in Hay *et al.* The classes are defined by parasite rates (PR_{2-10}, the proportion of 2- up to 10-year-olds with the parasite in their peripheral blood): malaria-free, $PR_{2-10}=0$; epidemic, $PR_{2-10}=0$; hypoendemic, $PR_{2-10}<0.10$; mesoendemic, $PR_{2-10}\geq0.10$ and <0.50; hyperendemic, $PR_{2-10}\geq0.50$ and <0.75; holoendemic, $PR_{0-1}\geq0.75$ (this class was measured in 0- up to 1-year-olds). From Piel et al. Global distribution of the sickle cell gene and geographical confirmation of the malaria hypothesis. Nat Commun. 2010 Nov 2; 1: 104. Published online 2010 Nov 2. doi: 10.1038/ncomms1104. Copyright © 2010, Nature Publishing Group, a division of Macmillan Publishers Limited. All Rights Reserved.

SCD can be defined as a globalized disease, and its presence in so ethnically diverse populations, living in extremely variable environments and in very different socio-cultural societies, is a factor that must be taken into consideration when addressing its management. In fact, although SCD is a monogenic disorder, its phenotype can be highly variable, not only among individuals, but also among ethnic groups and populations [30, 31].

In this chapter, we will review the management of children with SCD from a global perspective focusing on the three milestones of care: newborn screening, comprehensive *prix-en-charge* and cerebrovascular complications.

2. Neonatal screening programs

Newborn screening programs for SCD allow the early identification of patients, with the advantage of starting prophylaxis with penicillin at two months of age, significantly reducing mortality from infections. Moreover, newborn screening allows the early enrollment of patients in specialized programs of care in reference centers, thereby reducing morbidity and subsequent mortality from acute and chronic complications and improving quality of life.

The first screening program for SCD has been introduced in the USA since 1975 [32] and in the UK in 1993 [33].

In 1987, an NIH Consensus Conference stated that every child should be subjected at birth to screening for HbS to prevent the severe childhood complications of SCD, mainly infections and splenic sequestration, both potentially fatal [34]. Subsequently, a randomized study demonstrated the effectiveness of neonatal screening in dramatically reducing infant mortality from infection, allowing early initiation of prophylaxis with penicillin [35].

International Guidelines on the treatment of SCD recommend universal newborn screening on a national basis, best if integrated with existing neonatal screening programs and programs of *prix-en-charge* in specialized hematology reference centers [5, 36].

The recommendation is that newborn screening for identification of SCD is performed to all newborns. All patients must be identified promptly and taken in charge by dedicated and specialized services in order to begin penicillin prophylaxis within two months of age (Strength of Recommendation A).

Since the late 1980s numerous are the experiences of newborn screening programs, many organized by national health systems other confined to single-center experiences or supported by private funding.

2.1. Neonatal screening for SCD: major international experiences

United States—In the United States, the first neonatal screening program for SCD dates back to the 1970s (State of New York and Columbia), but after the publication of the NIH recommendations, all the states have organized a universal neonatal screening program for the S gene, associated with neonatal screening for other diseases. The analysis is performed at the birth from capillary blood taken by pricking the heel and using Guthrie paper. The analysis is done in most cases by Hygh performance liquid chromatography (HPLC).

The results of 20 years of the program (1989–2012) show an average incidence of the S gene in the general population of 1:64 (1.5%) and an average incidence of SCD of 1: 2000 (0.05%) [37]. The program in the United States was effective in significantly reducing the mortality of children with SCD [38].

Canada—In 1988 a targeted screening pilot program was started at the University of Montreal on babies with at least one African parent. The test, performed by HPLC, identified a proportion of 10% with trait and 0.8% of the affected. A significant number of non-enrolled patients was reported by the program, as many as 11 patients born in the reporting period: 5 of 72 of infants escaped enrollment in a care program, six infants were not identified as affected, and three false negatives and three inadequate samples were identified, stressing the importance of an absolute rigor in the organization of a screening program [39].

In 2006 a universal neonatal screening program for SCD, on a national basis, was initiated in Ontario and subsequently implemented in eight other Canadian provinces, comprising 10 provinces and three territories. The survey is performed on the cord blood or capillary blood on tissue paper by HPLC, using Iso-Electric-Focusing (IEF) or hemoglobin electrophoresis as a confirmatory test. A debate is ongoing on whether to inform parents of the carriers subject [36].

In *Brazil*, many states organized a neonatal screening program for the identification of patients with SCD. Since 2001 in the State of Janeiro Rio a universal neonatal screening program is active, funded by the National Health System, which includes the analysis by HPLC of the sample from the Guthrie test, performed on the baby after discharge in association with the first vaccine administration; the program provides for the subsequent taking charge of patients with SCD at the Reference Center.

The results of the first 10 years of experience (2001–2011) showed a SCD incidence of 1:1335 births and incidence of the trait by about 5% of births [40, 41]. The mortality was 3.7% significantly lower than the mortality of 25% of a cohort of Brazilian children not included in a screening program [42] but also significantly lower than that of a population of children undergoing neonatal screening, but not incorporated in a comprehensive program of follow-up. In fact, mortality in this population was found to be 5.6% [43]. The importance of integrating neonatal screening in an effective program of care of the patient at a specialized reference center has been more recently confirmed by another recent Brazilian study, which indicated in Minias Gerais State a mortality of 7.5% patients with SCD in the first 14 years of life, even though they were undergoing newborn screening, because of a non-effective care program [44].

In *Europe*, although there is strong evidence that hemoglobinopathies are an increasingly important public health problem [3], as a result of recent migration flows from the Mediterranean countries, Africa and Asia, there is very little data regarding the overall prevalence of SCD; the health policy of the governments, regarding the management of SCD, is uneven in the various nations. The European Network for Rare and Congenital Anemias (ENERCA) estimates that there are around 44,000 people in Europe suffering from hemoglobinopathises, 70% of which are SCD, and strongly recommends that the National Health Systems develop screening programs and specialized reference centers for the care of the patient and their family [6].

The United Kingdom (UK) was the first European country to organize, in 1993, a universal neonatal screening program for SCD. The initial pilot program, which began in England, was updated and since 2010 is extended to the whole of Britain. The program, supported by the National Health System (NHS), provides universal neonatal screening, performed with analysis of Guthrie test concurrently with other screenings. Samples are analyzed at 13 reference hematological laboratories by HPLC, each laboratory screening between 25,000 and 100,000 newborns a year. The organization provides for centralized analysis in reference laboratories, each with a minimum of 25,000 tests per year. The incidence of carriers in the UK is an average of 15/1000 (1.5%) and 1:1900 (0.05%) with significant variations by region and ethnicity [45].

A national program of universal newborn screening of Guthrie by HPLC [46] is active in the *Netherlands* since 2007. A debate on whether to notify the carrier state to avoid stigmatization is currently underway [10].

In *Belgium*, since 1994 in the city of Brussels and in 2004 in the city of Liege, all newborns are subjected to universal screening for SCD. The analysis of umbilical cord blood is performed by IEF and HPLC as a possible confirmatory test. The affected frequency is determined to be 1:1559 [47].

In *Spain*, since 2000 universal neonatal screening programs have been initiated in Extremadura, Basque Country, Madrid, Valencia and Catalonia with plans of extending it from 2016 to the whole country. The prevalence of the affected varies from 1:3900 in Catalonia to 1:5900 in the region of Madrid [8, 48, 49].

In *Germany*, pilot programs of universal newborn screening were organized since 2011, first in Berlin, then in Heidelberg and in the Southeast Region of Germany and then in Hamburg. The tests were offered to all newborns although the original population was not at risk of hemoglobinopathy. The goal was to provide information about the global prevalence in Germany of a disease that has high prevalence in immigrant populations, coming mainly from areas at risk. The test was carried out by PCR for S chain from Guthrie paper in Hamburg, and by HPLC in the other experiences; the incidence of the affected ranged from 1:2385 to 1:8348 [9].

The results of the pilot studies were considered adequate to justify a universal neonatal screening program on a national basis, extended to the entire Germany. The activation of the project is planned for 2016. The carrier status is not communicated for fear of stigma.

Since 1985, *France* has organized a universal neonatal screening program for SCD in Guadeloupe: in the following years, many pilots studies were initiated in France; since 2000 a national screening program targeted at infants at risk of hemoglobinopathy was extended to the entire country; the selection is based on ethnic belonging. Although the program is not universal, it appears to be effective in intercepting almost all affected infants, ensuring their ultimate takeover by the Reference Centres [50].

In *Italy*, some experiences of neonatal screening for SCD have been reported.

From 2010 to 2012 in Ferrara, 1992 newborns have been tested and 24 carriers identified (1.2%). Screening was universal, run on Guthrie by HPLC. The experience was suspended for lack of funding [51].

In 2013 in Novara a project of newborn screening targeted to babies with a parent coming from areas at risk of hemoglobinopathy was implemented. A total of 337 of 2447 were tested and 20 carriers identified (6%) [52].

In Modena, since 2011 an antenatal screening program targeted at at-risk women by ethnicity was developed. The pilot study showed the presence of hemoglobinopathy in 27% of the 330 women tested (coverage of 70% of the program). Successively, the screening of infants of carrier mothers, run on cordon and analyzed by HPLC, has identified 48 carriers and 9 HbSS [53]. The universal antenatal screening program, extended to all pregnant women and including infants at risk of maternal positivity, is currently ongoing and supported with funding from the Province of Ferrara.

Since 2010, a centralized program of targeted neonatal screening (at least one parent from outside the region) is active in Friuli Venezia Giulia, financed by the region. The figures, as yet unpublished, report 6018 infants tested from 2010 to 2015, a percentage of carriers between 1.74 and 4.7% depending on the provinces (F Zanolli, personal communication).

A pilot program of universal newborn screening has been running since May 2, 2016, in Padua and is currently being activated in Monza.

Africa bears the highest burden of SCD. In the past years, several pilot newborn screening programs have been implemented in Central Africa [21], Ghana [20, 22], Congo [24], Benin [25], Angola [26], Nigeria [23, 54, 55] and Uganda [56] and are underway in Tanzania [19]. Some of the most significant experiences are described in detail below.

The first program started in *Ghana* in 1995 [22], and after 10 years, a total of 202,244 infants were screened through public and private clinics in Kumasi, Tikrom and a nearby rural community. 3745 (1.9%) infants were identified as having possible SCD with IEF: 2047 (1.04%) SS, 1684 (0.83%) SC.

In *Central Africa*, between July 2004 and July 2006, 1825 newborn dried blood samples were collected onto filter papers in four maternity units from Burundi, Rwanda and the East of the Democratic Republic of Congo. The presence of hemoglobin C and S was tested in the eluted blood by an enzyme-linked immunosorbent assay (ELISA) test using a monoclonal antibody. All positive samples were confirmed by DNA analysis. Of the 1825 samples screened, 97 (5.32%) were positive. Of these, 60 (3.28%) samples were heterozygous for Hb S, and four (0.22%) for Hb C; two (0.11%) newborns were Hb SS homozygotes.

In *Uganda* [56], punch samples were obtained from dried blood spots routinely collected from HIV-exposed infants for the national Early Infant Diagnosis program. Between February 2014, and March 2015, 99,243 dried blood spots were analyzed through IEF, and results were available for 97,631. The overall number of children with sickle cell trait was 12,979 (13.3%) and with disease was 716 (0.7%), with extreme variability across regions.

Two pilot screenings from *Nigeria* are reported. Obaro et al. (54) screened HPLC children aged less than 5 years. Overall, 272 (2.76%) new cases from 9963 children who had not been previously tested were identified. The authors reported also the screening of 163 (1.6%) children whose parents indicated that their offspring had been previously tested. 31.2% of parents (51/163) did not know the result of their offspring's test.

Inusa et al. [55] from January 2010 to December 2011 screened children aged 0–60 months in 29 randomly selected local communities of three adjoining northern Nigerian states in a community-based study: Abuja, Kaduna and Katsina. For infants of 0–6 months, blood spots were used, and for infants of 7–60 months, EDTA blood samples were analyzed using HPLC. Thirty-one selected samples with high Hb A2 (3.5–7.4%) were further analyzed using molecular diagnosis to ascertain the presence of the Beta Thalassemia gene. Of the 10,001 infants and children screened, 269 (2.69%) had a SCD diagnosis, 90% of which were HbSS (n = 243), 5% HbSC (n = 13), 3% with high A2>6% (possible S with existence β thalassaemia (n = 9) and 1% HbSD (n = 2). A total of 74% of infants screened were HbAA (n = 7391). 2341 (23%) were carriers, 96% HbAS (n = 2236), 2% HbAC (n = 51), 1% HbAD (n = 25), and 1% HbABeta-thal (n = 22). HbSβo was confirmed by molecular analysis from the 31 selected samples.

3. Management of sickle cell disease in childhood

SCD is a chronic and complex multisystem disorder requiring comprehensive care that includes screening, prevention, health education, management of acute and chronic complications [5, 57]. Poor service organization and episodic health care cause higher rates of acute events and chronic complications, with subsequent increased burden on hospital structures and higher costs for health systems [58].

Neonatal screening program for SCD is not successful without a comprehensive care program at a specialized reference center for the treatment of the disease.

The organization of the Comprehensive Sickle Cell Centers proved crucial integration of screening programs, providing health education, preventive treatment (prophylaxis of infections, up-to-date vaccinations, stroke prevention), appropriate diagnostic therapeutic pathways for the treatment of acute and chronic complications, planning of blood transfusion and administration of HU, accompanying the transition to adult care for adolescents and young adults through structured transition programs. The care delivered by a specialized and multidisciplinary team in referral centers is effective in reducing mortality and improving the quality of life [38, 59]. Where these facilities were lacking, the effectiveness of neonatal screening program was reduced [60].

A recommended examinations schedule for yearly follow-up of children with SCD is shown in **Table 1** [61], while the services that a reference center should offer are displayed in **Table 2** [5].

	0 – 1 Year	2 years	3 - 5 years	6 - 9 years	10 – 15 years	16 -18 years
Physical examination	■	■	■	■	■	■
Transcutaneous O_2 saturation	■	■	■	■	■	■
Biological tests*	■	■	■	■	■	■
Adherence (treatments, appointments)	■	■	■	■	■	■
TCD		■	■	■	■	
Hepatic US			■	■	■	■
School success			■	■	■	■
Pulmonary function tests			■	■	■	■
Hip X-Ray				■	■	■
Electrocardiography				■	■	■
Ophtalmologic evaluation				**	■	■

* Complete blood count, liver profile, electrolytes, BUN, creatinine, γalbuminuria, ferritin if transfused, calcium metabolism including vitamin D and PTH, Parvovirus B19 serology until positive.

** Since the age of 6 y.o. if Hb SC disease

Table 1. Recommended examinations to be performed annually in children with SCD [60].

- Pediatrician or hematologist with hemoglobinopathies skills
- Dedicated outpatient clinic
- Network with the territory and the peripheral hospitals
- Diagnostic laboratory
- Newborn screening program
- Transcranial Doppler service
- Pediatric intensive care
- Transfusion service
- Pediatric specialist services (cardiology, urology, nephrology, pulmonology, endocrinology, orthopedics, surgery, anesthesia, ophthalmology, dentistry)
- Psychology service with availability of psychometric assessments
- Radiology and neuroradiology
- Bone marrow transplant unit
- Adult-specialist team for the transition program

Table 2. Characteristics of a specialized reference center [5] and services that it should be able to offer directly or in agreement with nearby centers.

A comprehensive approach to the care of children with SCD should include the following goals: to improve quality of life, by preventing and treating infections, adequate pain management and anemia control; to prevent organ damage, mainly stroke, renal and lung; to prevent SCD related mortality [61].

3.1. Management of sickle cell disease in childhood: open issues at a global level

In spite of the strong evidence to perform newborn screening and comprehensive care, these services are far from optimally delivered to patients with SCD not only in Europe and the USA, but mainly in areas of Africa and India where the majority of the children with SCD live. Many pilot programs were initiated in the last decade in many countries of Latin America, Middle East, Asia, and Africa; some were integrated with other screening programs. These data are encouraging but such programs need to be further enhanced.

Increased North-South, South-South and East-West collaboration could be an important way to increase service delivery to all affected children.

4. Cerebrovascular complications of sickle cell disease: stroke and silent infarcts

In the most severe forms of SCD, the homozygous SS and the double etherozygous Sβ°, the brain is frequently affected (**Figure 2**). Overt ischemic stroke occurs in 11% of untreated children as a result of stenosis or occlusion in the large arteries of the Circle of Willis [62, 63]. Cerebral silent infarcts (CSI), affecting 40% of children by the age of 14, are caused by small vessel disease [64, 65] although recent evidence suggests that also a combination of chronic hypoperfusion or hypoxic events, favored by an underlying artheropathy of the large vessels, can lead to CSI [66]. In the past 15 years, improvements have been made in the management of stroke and CSI [66, 67]. In fact, algorithms for screening, prevention and management of stroke and CSI based on neuroimaging techniques such as transcranial Doppler (TCD) and

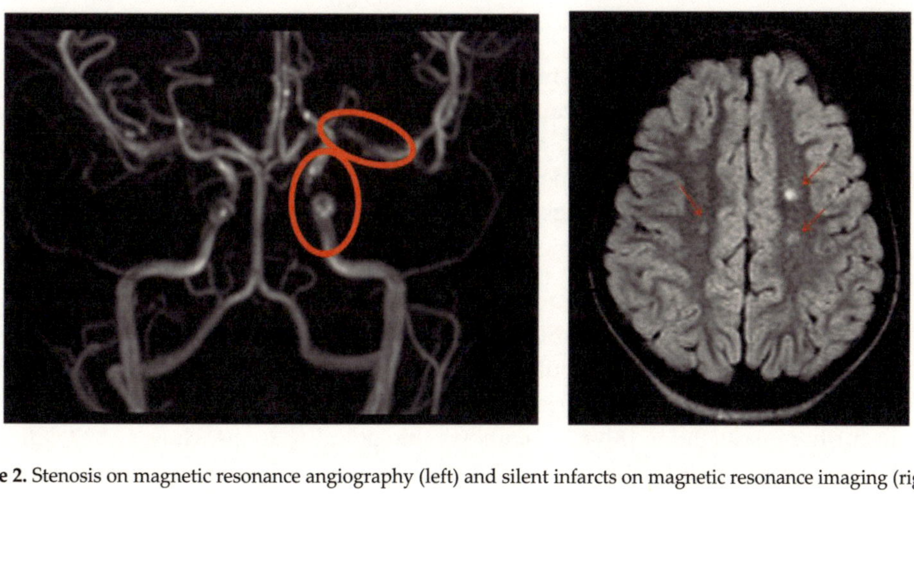

Figure 2. Stenosis on magnetic resonance angiography (left) and silent infarcts on magnetic resonance imaging (right).

magnetic resonance imaging/angiography (MRI/MRA) are routinely used in clinical practice [67–70].

TCD screening is recommended starting at age 2 years in children with HbSS and HbSβ°, and those identified at risk of stroke are offered chronic transfusion as stroke prevention [67]. Stroke can be virtually eliminated or dramatically reduced if a proper TCD screening program followed by chronic transfusion for at risk patients is established [59, 68]. Recently, a randomized study demonstrated that after one year of chronic transfusion, hydroxycarbamide (HU) can be safely offered to children with normal neuroimaging under strict surveillance [71]. While TCD allows identifying patients at risk of stroke and initiate appropriate treatment, it is not useful to screen for the other cerebrovascular complications of SCD such us CSI. Moreover, its usefulness in identifying risk of stroke in other genotypes of SCD such as HbSC and HbSβ+, in which stroke is less common, has yet to be evaluated.

Screening with MRI/MRA, although unable to indentify children at risk of developing CSI, is strongly recommended in many centers starting at age 5 years, when sedation is no longer necessary [66, 68, 72], to ensure diagnosis at young age and promptly start therapeutic or educational measures. In case of abnormal TCD, developmental delay or cognitive impairment or any other clinical reason, MRI is indicated even before 5 years of age. Both chronic transfusions and HU have been shown to stabilize CSI [66, 67, 73], but at present there is no general agreement on prevention strategies.

4.1. Stroke and silent infarcts: open issues at a global level

In spite of extensive research performed in the United States and Europe on the management of stroke and CSI in children with SCD in the past decades, the delivery of routine TCD screening to children with SCD has been quite low. Primary stroke prevention through TCD is recommended in all national and international guidelines, but less than 50% of children in the USA [74] and the United Kingdom benefit from this technique [75]. Data regarding the coverage of TCD screening are not available for other countries of Europe, South America or the Middle East at a national level, but only for single-center experiences [59, 66, 69, 72, 76], and this is a gap that should be filled.

TCD data are not yet available from many areas of the world like India, Northern and Sub-Saharian Africa. Nevertheless, personnel training on the correct protocol of TCD screening for SCD has been performed in Africa, and promising pilot studies are being conducted in Nigeria [77–79]. These studies demonstrate the feasibility of primary and secondary prevention programs in low-resource settings with huge numbers of patients. They also allow us to explore the efficacy of alternative protocols compared to those in use in the USA and Europe and to demonstrate the benefit of HU in reducing TCD velocities [80].

A challenge that a global approach to SCD can address is the reported variability of stroke and cerebrovascular complications in populations of different ethnic backgrounds. Stroke and CSI seem to occur with different frequencies across populations, although data are still poor and warrant further investigation [81–85]. Moreover, biological factors such as G6PD deficiency and alfa thalassemia co-inheritance as well as coagulation activation and single nucleotide

http://dx.doi.org/10.5772/64656

polymorphisms (SNPSs) do not seem to have the same role on the genesis of cerebrovascular complications in different populations [86–90].

In conclusion, more TCD and MRI/MRA data from SCD populations across the world could aid in designing wide population studies to explore genetic and biological modifying factors of cerebrovascular disease as currently performed in other pathologic conditions [91]. Coordinating cerebrovascular studies across countries and continents can be challenging [79, 92–95] but is now warranted to improve patients access to recommended screening tools and to better target treatment interventions according to biological disease-modifying factors, which may vary across ethnicities.

5. Future directions

The main objective would be to increase the access to the milestones of care:

- Expand universal newborn screening to all Countries with sufficient prevalence of disease
- Expand access to vaccinations, antibiotic prophylaxis and transcranial Doppler for stroke prevention, by increasing the number of skilled personnel and service availability
- Increase the use of disease-modifying treatments for the pediatric age, such as hydroxiurea, in formulations that are suitable for children (low dose tablets or syrups) in all countries

Strengthening collaboration at a global level and developing North-South, South-South and East-West partnerships could aid in reaching the above mentioned aims.

Acknowledgements

The research was performed with funding from the Fondazione Città della Speranza and Comitato Assistenza Sociosanitaria in Oncoematologia Pediatrica, C.A.S.O.P.

Author details

Laura Sainati, Maria Montanaro and Raffaella Colombatti*

*Address all correspondence to: rcolombatti@gmail.com

Department of Child and Maternal Health, Veneto Region Reference Center for the Diagnosis and Treatment of Sickle Cell Disease in Childhood, Clinic of Pediatric Hematology-Oncology, Azienda Ospedaliera-University of Padova, Padova, Italy

References

[1] Weatherall DJ, Clegg JB. Inherited haemoglobin disorders: an increasing global health problem. Bull World Health Organ 2001, 79:704–712.

[2] Piel FB, Patil AP, Howes RE, et al. Global epidemiology of sickle haemoglobin in neonates: a contemporary geostatistical model-based map and population estimates. Lancet 2013, 381(9861):142–51.

[3] Roberts I, de Montalambert M. Sickle cell disease as a paradigm of immigration haematology: new challenges for immigration hematologists in Europe. Haematologica 2007, 92:865–871.

[4] de Montalembert M, Girot R, Galactéros F. Sickle cell disease in France in 2006: results and challenges. Arch Pediatr 2006, 13:1191–1194.

[5] NHS Standard and Guidelines for Clinical Care. http://www.sct.screening.nhs.uk/standardsandguidelines

[6] Aguilar Martinez P, Angastiniotis M, Eleftheriou A, Gulbis B, Mañú Pereira Mdel M, Petrova-Benedict R, Corrons JL. Haemoglobinopathies in Europe: health & migration policy perspectives. Orphanet J Rare Dis 2014, 9:97.

[7] Colombatti R, Perrotta S, Samperi P, Casale M, Masera N, Palazzi G, Sainati L, Russo G; Italian Association of Pediatric Hematology-Oncology (AIEOP) Sickle Cell Disease Working Group. Organizing national responses for rare blood disorders: the Italian experience with sickle cell disease in childhood. Orphanet J Rare Dis 2013, 8:169.

[8] Mañú Pereira M, Corrons JL. Neonatal haemoglobinopathy screening in Spain. J Clin Pathol 2009, 62:22–25.

[9] Lobitz S, Frömmel C, Brose A, Klein J, Blankenstein O. Incidence of sickle cell disease in an unselected cohort of neonates born in Berlin, Germany. Eur J Hum Genet 2014, 22(8):1051–3.

[10] Jans SM, van El CG, Houwaart ES, Westerman MJ, Janssens RJ, Lagro-Janssen AL, Plass AM, Cornel MC. A case study of haemoglobinopathy screening in the Netherlands: witnessing the past, lessons for the future. Ethn Health 2012, 17(3):217–39.

[11] Serjeant GR, Ghosh K, Patel J. Sickle cell disease in India: a perspective. Indian J Med Res 2016, 143(1):21–4.

[12] Ansong D, Akoto AO, Ocloo D, Ohene-Frempong K. Sickle cell disease: management options and challenges in developing countries. Mediterr J Hematol Infect Dis 2013, 5(1):e2013062. doi: 10.4084/MJHID.2013.062. eCollection 2013

[13] Piel FB, Tatem AJ, Huang Z, Gupta S, Williams TN, Weatherall DJ. Global migration and the changing distribution of sickle haemoglobin: a quantitative study of temporal trends between 1960 and 2000. Lancet Glob Health 2014, 2(2):e80–9.

[14] Makani J, Ofori-Acquah SF, Nnodu O, Wonkam A, Ohene-Frempong K. Sickle cell disease: new opportunities and challenges in Africa. Scientific World J 2013, 2013:193252.

[15] Ndeezi G, Kiyaga C, Hernandez AG, Munube D, Howard TA, Ssewanyana I, Nsungwa J, Kiguli S, Ndugwa CM, Ware RE, Aceng JR. Burden of sickle cell trait and disease in the Uganda Sickle Surveillance Study (US3): a cross-sectional study. Lancet Glob Health 2016, 4(3):e195–200.

[16] Odame I, Kulkarni R, Ohene-Frempong K. Concerted global effort to combat sickle cell disease: the first global congress on sickle cell disease in Accra, Ghana. Am J Prev Med 2011, 41(6 Suppl. 4):S417–21.

[17] Rahimy MC, Gangbo A, Ahouignan G, Adjou R, Deguenon C, Goussanou S, Alihonou E. Effect of a comprehensive clinical care program on disease course in severely ill children with sickle cell anemia in a sub-Saharan African setting. Blood 2003, 102(3): 834–8.

[18] Aloni MN, Nkee L. Challenge of managing sickle cell disease in a pediatric population living in Kinshasa, democratic republic of congo: a sickle cell center experience. Hemoglobin 2014, 38(3):196–200.

[19] Makani J, Soka D, Rwezaula S, Krag M, Mghamba J, Ramaiya K, Cox SE, Grosse SD. Health policy for sickle cell disease in Africa: experience from Tanzania on interventions to reduce under-five mortality. Trop Med Int Health 2015, 20(2):184–7.

[20] Treadwell MJ, Anie KA, Grant AM, Ofori-Acquah SF, Ohene-Frempong K. Using formative research to develop a counselor training program for newborn screening in Ghana. J Genet Couns 2015, 24(2):267–77.

[21] Mutesa L, Boemer F, Ngendahayo L, Rulisa S, Rusingiza EK, Cwinya-Ay N, Mazina D, Kariyo PC, Bours V, Schoos R. Neonatal screening for sickle cell disease in Central Africa: a study of 1825 newborns with a new enzyme-linked immunosorbent assay test. J Med Screen 2007, 14(3):113–6.

[22] Ohene-Frempong K, Oduro J, Tetteh H, Nkrumah F. Screening Newborns for Sickle Cell Disease in Ghana. Pediatrics Jan 2008, 121 (Supplement 2) S120-S121

[23] Odunvbun ME, Okolo AA, Rahimy CM. Newborn screening for sickle cell disease in a Nigerian hospital. Public Health 2008, 122(10):1111–6.

[24] Tshilolo L, Aissi LM, Lukusa D, Kinsiama C, Wembonyama S, Gulbis B, Vertongen F. Neonatal screening for sickle cell anaemia in the Democratic Republic of the Congo: experience from a pioneer project on 31,204 newborns. J Clin Pathol 2009, 62(1):35–8.

[25] Rahimy MC, Gangbo A, Ahouignan G, Alihonou E. Newborn screening for sickle cell disease in the Republic of Benin. J Clin Pathol 2009, 62(1):46–8.

[26] McGann PT, Ferris MG, Ramamurthy U, Santos B, de Oliveira V, Bernardino L, Ware RE. A prospective newborn screening and treatment program for sickle cell anemia in Luanda, Angola. Am J Hematol 2013, 88(12):984–9.

[27] Ranque B, Menet A, Diop IB, Thiam MM, Diallo D, Diop S, Diagne I, Sanogo I, Kingue S, Chelo D, Wamba G, Diarra M, Anzouan JB, N'Guetta R, Diakite CO, Traore Y, Legueun G, Deme-Ly I, Belinga S, Boidy K, Kamara I, Tharaux PL, Jouven X. Early renal damage in patients with sickle cell disease in sub-Saharan Africa: a multinational, prospective, cross-sectional study. Lancet Haematol 2014, 1(2):e64–73.

[28] McGann PT, Tshilolo L, Santos B, Tomlinson GA, Stuber S, Latham T, Aygun B, Obaro SK, Olupot-Olupot P, Williams TN, Odame I, Ware RE; REACH Investigators. Hydroxyurea Therapy for children with sickle cell anemia in sub-Saharan Africa: rationale and design of the REACH trial. Pediatr Blood Cancer 2016, 63(1):98–104.

[29] Heeney MM, Hoppe CC, Abboud MR, Inusa B, Kanter J, Ogutu B, Brown PB, Heath LE, Jakubowski JA, Zhou C, Zamoryakhin D, Agbenyega T, Colombatti R, Hassab HM, Nduba VN, Oyieko JN, Robitaille N, Segbefia CI, Rees DC; DOVE Investigators. A multinational trial of prasugrel for sickle cell vaso-occlusive events. N Engl J Med 2016, 374(7):625–35.

[30] Christakis J, Vavatsi N, Hassapopoulou H, Papadopoulou M, Mandraveli K, Loukopoulos D, Morris JS, Serjeant BE, Serjeant GR. Comparison of homozygous sickle cell disease in northern Greece and Jamaica. Lancet 1990, 335(8690):637–40.

[31] Urio F, Lyimo M, Mtatiro SN, Cox SE, Mmbando BP, Makani J. High prevalence of individuals with low concentration of fetal hemoglobin in F-cells in sickle cell anemia in Tanzania. Am J Hematol 2016; 91(8):E324-4.

[32] Consensus Development Panel. NIH Newborn screening for sickle cell disease and other hemoglobinopathies. AM J Med Assoc 1987, 258:1205–9.

[33] Standing Medical Advisory Committee. Sickle cell, thalassemia and other haemoglobinopathies. London: HMSO, 1993.

[34] NIH Consensus Conference. Newborn screening for sickle cell disease and other heamoglobinopathies. JAMA 1987, 258:1205–9.

[35] Vichinsky E, et al. Newborn screening for sickle cell disease: effects on mortality. Pediatrics 1988, 81:749–55.

[36] Consensus Statement on the Care of Patients with Sickle Cell Disease in Canada. Accessed at: http://www.sicklecelldisease.ca/wp-content/uploads/2013/04/CANHAEM-Consensus-Statement-for-SCD-Guide2015_v10.pdf.

[37] Therell BL Jr, Lloyd-Puryear MA, Eckman JR, Mann MY. Newborn screening for SCD in the United States: a review of data spanning two decades. Semin Perinathol 2015, 39:238–51.

[38] Quinn CT, et al. Improved survival of children and adolescents with sickle cell disease. Blood 2010, 115(17):3447–52.

[39] Robitaille N. Newborn screening for SCD: a 1988–2003 Quebec experience. Paediatr Child Health 2006, 11(4):223–7.

[40] Therrell BL, Padilla CD, Loeber JG, Kneisser I, Saadallah A, Borrajo GJ, Adams J. Current status of newborn screening worldwide: 2015. Semin Perinatol 2015, 39(3):171–87.

[41] Lobo CL, Ballas SK, Domingos AC, Moura PG, do Nascimento EM, Cardoso GP, de Carvalho SM. Newborn screening program for hemoglobinopathies in Rio de Janeiro, Brazil. Pediatr Blood Cancer 2014, 61(1):34–9.

[42] Diniz D, Guedes C. Sickle cell anaemia: a Brazilian problem. A bioethical approach to the new genetics. Cad Saude Publica 2003, 19(6):1761–70.

[43] Fernandes AP, Januário JN, Cangussu CB, Macedo DL, Viana MB. Mortality of children with sickle cell disease: a population study. J Pediatr (Rio J) 2010, 86(4):279–84.

[44] Sabarense AP, Lima GO, Silva LM, Viana MB. Characterization of mortality in children with sickle cell disease diagnosed through the Newborn screening program. J Pediatr (Rio J) 2015, 91:242–7.

[45] Streetly A. Positive screening and carriers results for the England wide universal newborn sickle cell screening program by ethnicity and area for 2005–2007. J Clin Pathol 2010, 63 (7): 626–9

[46] Bouva MJ. Implement neonatal creening for haemoglobinopathies in the Netherlands. J Med Screen 2010, 17:58–65.

[47] Gulbis B, Cotton F, Ferster A, Ketelslegers O, Dresse MF, Rongé-Collard E, Minon JM, Lé PQ, Vertongen F. Neonatal haemoglobinopathy screening in Belgium. J Clin Pathol. 2009;62(1):49-52 Gulbis B. Neontal haemoglobinopathy screening in Belgium. J Clin Pathol 2009, (62):49–52.

[48] García Arias MB, Cantalejo López MA, Cela de Julián ME, Bravo Clouzet R, Galarón García P, Beléndez Bieler C. [Sickle cell disease: registry of the Spanish Society of Pediatric Hematology].An Pediatr (Barc). 2006;64(1):78-84

[49] Cela de Julián E, Dulín Iñiguez E, Guerrero Soler M, Arranz Leirado M, Galarón García P, Beléndez Bieler C, Bellón Cano JM, García Arias M, Cantalejo López A. [Evaluation of systematic neonatal screening for sickle cell diseases in Madrid three years after its introduction]. An Pediatr (Barc). 2007;66(4):382-6

[50] Badens C. Neonatal screening for sickle cell disease in France. J Clin Pathol 2009, 62(1): 31–33.

[51] Ballardini E, et al. Universal neonatal screening for sickle cell disease and other haemoglobinopathies in Ferrara, Italy. Tranfus Blood 2013, 11(2):245–9.

[52] Rolla R. Neonatal screening forsickle cell disease and other hemoglobinophaties in the changing Europe. Clin Lab 2014, 60(12):2089–93.

[53] Venturelli D. Sickle cell disease in the areas of immigration of high-risk populations: a low cost and reproducible method of screening in northern Italy. Tranfusion Blood 2014, 12:346–51.

[54] Obaro SK, Daniel Y, Lawson JO, Hsu WW, Dada J, Essen U, Ibrahim K, Akindele A, Brooks K, Olanipekun G, Ajose T, Stewart CE, Inusa BP. Sickle-cell disease in Nigerian children: parental knowledge and laboratory results. Public Health Genomics 2016, 19(2):102–7.

[55] Inusa BP, Daniel Y, Lawson JO, Dada J, Matthews CE, Momi S, Obaro SK. Sickle cell disease screening in Northern Nigeria: the co-existence of B-thalassemia inheritance. Pediat Therapeut 2015, 5:3.

[56] Ndeezi G, Kiyaga C, Hernandez AG, Munube D, Howard TA, Ssewanyana I, Nsungwa J, Kiguli S, Ndugwa CM, Ware RE, Aceng JR. Burden of sickle cell trait and disease in the Uganda Sickle Surveillance Study (US3): a cross-sectional study. Lancet Glob Health 2016, 4(3):e195–200.

[57] Section on Hematology/Oncology Committee on Genetics; American Academy of Pediatrics. Health supervision for children with sickle cell disease. Pediatrics 2002, 109(3):526–35.

[58] Kauf TL, et al. The cost of health care for children and adults with sickle cell disease. Am J Hematol 2009, 84(6):323–7.

[59] Telfer P, et al. Clinical outcomes in children with sickle cell disease living in England: a neonatal cohort in East London. Haematologica 2007, 92(7):905–12.

[60] McGann P. Improving survival for children with SCD: newborn screening is only the first step. Paediatric Inte Child Heath 2015, 35(4):285–6.

[61] de Montalembert M, Ferster A, Colombatti R, Rees DC, Gulbis B; European Network for Rare and Congenital Anaemias. ENERCA clinical recommendations for disease management and prevention of complications of sickle cell disease in children. Am J Hematol 2011, 86(1):72–5.

[62] Ohene-Frempong K, Weiner SJ, Sleeper LA, et al. Cerebrovascular accidents in sickle cell disease: rates and risk factors. Blood 1998, 91(1):288–94.

[63] Bernaudin F, Verlhac S, Fréard F, et al. Multicenter prospective study of children with sickle cell disease: radiographic and psychometric correlation. J Child Neurol 2000, 15:333–43.

[64] Debaun MR, Amstrong FD, McKinstry RC, et al. Silent cerebral infarcts: a review on a prevalent and progressive cause of neurologic injury in sickle cell anemia. Blood 2012, 119:4587–4596.

[65] Connes P, Verlhac S, Bernaudin F. Advances in understanding the pathogenesis of cerebrovascular vasculopathy in Sickle Cell Anemia. Br J Haematol 2000, 161:484–94.

[66] Bernaudin F, Verlhac S, Arnaud C, et al. Chronic and acute anemia and extracranial internal carotid stenosis are risk factors for silent cerebral infarcts in sickle cell anemia. Blood 2015, 125(10):1653–61.

[67] Adams RJ, McKie VC, Hsu L, et al. Prevention of a first stroke by transfusions in children with sickle cell anemia and abnormal results on transcranial Doppler ultrasonography. N Engl J Med 1998, 339:5–11.

[68] Brousse V, Kossorotoff M, de Montalembert M. How I manage cerebral vasculopathy in children with sickle cell disease. Br J Haematol 2015, 170(5):615–25.

[69] Bernaudin F, Verlhac S, Arnaud C, et al. Impact of early transcranial Doppler screening and intensive therapy on cerebral vasculopathy outcome in a newborn sickle cell anemia cohort. Blood 2011, 117(4):1130–40; quiz 1436.

[70] DeBaun MR, Kirkham FJ. Central nervous system complications and management in sickle cell disease. Blood. 2016;127(7):829-38.

[71] Ware RE, Davis BR, Schultz WH, Brown RC, Aygun B, Sarnaik S, et al. Hydroxycarbamide versus chronic transfusion for maintenance of transcranial doppler flow velocities in children with sickle cell anaemia-TCD with transfusions changing to hydroxyurea (TWiTCH): a multicentre, open-label, phase 3, non-inferiority trial. Lancet 2016, 387(10019):661–70.

[72] Colombatti R, Montanaro M, Guasti F, Rampazzo P, Meneghetti G, Giordan M, Basso G, Sainati L. Comprehensive care for sickle cell disease immigrant patients: a reproducible model achieving high adherence to minimum standards of care. Pediatr Blood Cancer 2012, 59(7):1275–9.

[73] DeBaun MR, Gordon M, McKinstry RC, Noetzel MJ, White DA, Sarnaik SA, et al. Controlled trial of transfusions for silent cerebral infarcts in sickle cell anemia. N Engl J Med 2014, 371(8):699–710.

[74] Reeves SL, Madden B, Freed GL, Dombkowski KJ.Transcranial Doppler Screening Among Children and Adolescents With Sickle Cell Anemia. JAMA Pediatr. 2016;170(6): 550-6.

[75] Deane CR, Goss D, O'Driscoll S, et al. Transcranial Doppler scanning and the assessment of stroke risk in children with HbSC disease. Arch Dis Child 2008, 93:138–41.

[76] Bavarsad Shahripour R, Mortazavi MM, Barlinn K, Keikhaei B, et al. Can STOP trial velocity criteria be applied to Iranian children with sickle cell Disease? J Stroke 2014, 16(2):97–101.

[77] Lagunju I, Sodeinde O, Telfer P. Prevalence of transcranial Doppler abnormalities in Nigerian children with sickle cell disease. Am J Hematol 2012, 87(5):544–7.

[78] Soyebi K, Adeyemo T, Ojewunmi O, James F, Adefalujo K, Akinyanju O. Capacity building and stroke risk assessment in Nigerian children with sickle cell anaemia. Pediatr Blood Cancer 2014, 61(12):2263–6.

[79] Galadanci NA, Abdullahi SU, Tabari MA, Abubakar S, Belonwu R, Salihu A, et al. Primary stroke prevention in Nigerian children with sickle cell disease (SPIN): challenges of conducting a feasibility trial. Pediatr Blood Cancer 2015, 62(3):395–401.

[80] Lagunju I, Brown BJ, Sodeinde O. Hydroxyurea lowers transcranial Doppler flow velocities in children with sickle cell anaemia in a Nigerian cohort. Pediatr Blood Cancer 2015, 62(9):1587–91.

[81] Njamnshi AK, Mbong EN, Wonkam A, Ongolo-Zogo P, Djientcheu VD, Sunjoh FL, Wiysonge CS, Sztajzel R, Mbanya D, Blackett KN, Dongmo L, Muna WF. The epidemiology of stroke in sickle cell patients in Yaounde, Cameroon. J Neurol Sci 2006, 250(1–2):79–84.

[82] Njamnshi AK, Wonkam A, Djientcheu Vde P, Ongolo-Zogo P, Obama MT, Muna WF, Sztajzel R. Stroke may appear to be rare in Saudi-Arabian and Nigerian children with sickle cell disease, but not in Cameroonian sickle cell patients. Br J Haematol 2006, 133(2):210; author reply 211.

[83] Asbeutah A, Gupta R, Al-Saeid O, Ashebu S, Al-Sharida S, Mullah-Ali A, Mustafa NY, Adekile A. Transcranial Doppler and brain MRI in children with sickle cell disease and high hemoglobin F levels. Pediatr Blood Cancer 2014, 61(1):25–8.

[84] Inati A, Jradi O, Tarabay H, Moallem H, Rachkidi Y, El Accaoui R, Isma'eel H, Wehbe R, Mfarrej BG, Dabbous I, Taher A. Sickle cell disease: the Lebanese experience. Int J Lab Hematol 2007, 29(6):399–408.

[85] Italia K, Kangne H, Shanmukaiah C, Nadkarni AH, Ghosh K, Colah RB. Variable phenotypes of sickle cell disease in India with the Arab-Indian haplotype. Br J Haematol 2015, 168(1):156–9.

[86] Belisário AR, Rodrigues Sales R, Evelin Toledo N, Velloso-Rodrigues C, Maria Silva C, Borato Viana M. Glucose-6-phosphate dehydrogenase deficiency in Brazilian children with sickle cell anemia is not associated with clinical ischemic stroke or high-risk transcranial Doppler. Pediatr Blood Cancer 2016, 63(6):1046–9.

[87] Joly P, Garnier N, Kebaili K, Renoux C, Dony A, Cheikh N, et al. G6PD deficiency and absence of α-thalassemia increase the risk for cerebral vasculopathy in children with sickle cell anemia. Eur J Haematol 2016, 96(4):404–8.

[88] Belisário AR, Sales RR, Toledo NE, Velloso-Rodrigues C, Silva CM, Viana MB. Association between ENPP1 K173Q and stroke in a newborn cohort of 395 Brazilian children with sickle cell anemia. Blood 2015, 126(10):1259–60.

[89] Flanagan JM, Sheehan V, Linder H, Howard TA, Wang YD, Hoppe CC, Aygun B, Adams RJ, Neale GA, Ware RE. Genetic mapping and exome sequencing identify 2 mutations

associated with stroke protection in pediatric patients with sickle cell anemia. Blood 2013, 121(16):3237–45.

[90] Mourad H, Fadel W, El Batch M, Rowisha M. Heamostatic and genetic predisposing factors for stroke in children with sickle cell anemia. Egypt J Immunol 2008, 15(1):25–37.

[91] Liu H, Xia P, Liu M, et al. PON gene polymorphisms and ischaemic stroke: a systematic review and meta-analysis. International J Stroke 2013, 8(2):111–23.

[92] Padayachee ST, Thomas N, Arnold AJ, Inusa B. Problems with implementing a standardised transcranial Doppler screening programme: impact of instrumentation variation on STOP classification. Pediatr Radiol 2012, 42(4):470–4.

[93] Inusa B, Sainati L, Colombatti L, McMahon C, Hemmaway C, Padayachee S. The impact of a standardised transcranial Doppler training programme in screening children with sickle cell disease: a European Multicenter Perspective. Blood 2013, 122 (21):983.

[94] Colombatti R, Meneghetti G, Ermani M, Pierobon M, Sainati L. Primary stroke prevention for sickle cell disease in north-east Italy: the role of ethnic issues in establishing a Transcranial Doppler screening program. Ital J Pediatr 2009, 35:15.

[95] Nimgaonkar V, Krishnamurti L, Prabhakar H, Menon N. Comprehensive integrated care for patients with sickle cell disease in a remote aboriginal tribal population in southern India. Pediatr Blood Cancer 2014, 61(4):702–5.

Section 2

Diagnostic Strategies for Sickle Cell Disease

Chapter 3

New Perspectives in Prenatal Diagnosis of Sickle Cell Anemia

Ebru Dündar Yenilmez and Abdullah Tuli

Additional information is available at the end of the chapter

http://dx.doi.org/10.5772/64646

Abstract

Hemoglobin disorders such as thalassemias and sickle cell anemias can be avoided by detecting carriers, ensuring genetic counseling and prenatal diagnosis. Nowadays Chorionic villus sampling (CVS amniocentesis, and cordocentesis are still the most widely used invasive sampling methods for prenatal diagnosis of the fetus. These traditional methods are associated with a risk of fetal loss. The revelation of cell-free fetal DNA (cffDNA) in maternal plasma and serum provides the opportunity of noninvasive prenatal diagnosis (NIPD). Different encouraging clinical applications have arose such as noninvasive identification of fetal sexing, fetal Rhesus D, and the determination of the paternal alleles in maternal plasma. The determination of the presence or absence of paternally inherited alleles in maternal plasma of sickle cell disease (SCD) and β-thalassemia would allow the diagnosis of autosomal dominant diseases or the exclusion of autosomal recessive diseases of the fetuses, respectively. prenatal diagnosis of genetic diseases. Analysis of cffDNA in maternal plasma for NIPD has the advantage of being safer versus the invasive methods. Different technologies were used since the discovery of cffDNA for NIPD—especially high-resolution melting (HRM) analysis is one of those methods. Genotyping can be done with HRM without using labeled probes and more complex regions can be analyzed with unlabeled hybridization probes. High-resolution melting is a rapid and useful method to detect paternal alleles for the NIPD of SCD and thalassemias when the fetus has a risk for double heterozygote.

Keywords: noninvasive prenatal diagnosis, sickle cell disease, cell-free fetal DNA, high-resolution melting, paternal mutation, maternal plasma

1. Introduction

Hemoglobinopathies caused by mutations in the α- or β-like globin gene clusters are the most common inherited disorders in humans, with around 7% of the world population being carriers of a globin gene mutation [1].

Hemoglobinopathies are caused by variants that affect the direct synthesis of the globin chains of hemoglobin, and may result in different synthesis (thalassemia syndromes, etc.) or structural changes (sickling of the red blood cells, hemolytic anemia). Thalassemia variants and various abnormal hemoglobins interact to produce a wide variety of disorders. Sickle cell disease was first described in 1910, and in the following years, similar cases were described, supporting the idea that this was a new disease and providing enough evidence for a preliminary clinical and pathological description [2]. Linus Pauling was the first to hypothesize in 1945 that the disease might originate from an abnormality in the hemoglobin molecule [3]. The sickle mutation was characterized several years later by Ingram et al. as a glutamine to valine substitution at the sixth residue of the β-globin polypeptide [4].

Sickle cell disease causes a very destructive condition and is an autosomal recessive-inherited hemoglobinopathy. The disease affects millions of people which results in serious complications due to vaso-occlusive phenomenon and hemolysis [5].

Prevention of the disease through carrier identification, genetic counseling, and prenatal diagnosis (PD) remains the only realistic approach to diminish the impact of the disease and allows better use of available resources for the existing patient populations [6–8]. In addition, for monogenic diseases the parental mutation(s) have to be characterized before analysis of the fetal sample [9].

Polymerase chain reaction (PCR) is commonly in use as a traditional molecular method for prenatal diagnosis of hemoglobinopathies. The PCR-based technologies differ in genotyping hemoglobin variants. Amplification refractory mutation system (ARMS), denaturing gradient gel electrophoresis (DGGE), restriction endonuclease PCR (RE-PCR), sequencing analysis (Sanger), microarrays, pyrosequencing, real-time PCR, and high-resolution melting analysis (HRM) can be counted among these PCR-based detecting methods [10].

2. Prenatal diagnosis in sickle cell disease

The prenatal diagnosis (PD) for the disease gives the opportunity for expectant couples to have an accurate, rapid result about the genotype of their fetus. This process offers an option for the parents to terminate the pregnancy at an early period in case of positive result and to prepare them psychologically and medically for the arrival of the new child when abortion is not an option. This practice is usually carried out using either chorionic villus sampling (CVS) or amniocentesis. Both procedures are invasive with CVS being done between the 10th and 12th week of pregnancy while amniocentesis is usually carried out later (between the 14th and 20th week) [5, 11].

http://dx.doi.org/10.5772/64646

Four main categories have been identified for severe disease states, for which genetic counseling, and possibly prenatal diagnosis, is indicated. The category for some SCD is shown in **Table 1** [10, 12].

Genotype interaction	Disorder expected	Appropriate to offer PND
Homozygous		
Hb S	Sickle cell disease	Yes
Compound heterozygous		
Hb S/β^{o}- or severe β^{+}-thalassemia	Sickle cell disease	Yes
Hb S/mild β^{+}-thalassemia	Mild sickle cell disease	Occasionally*
Hb S/Hb C	Sickle cell disease (variable severity)	Yes
Hb S/Hb D-Punjab	Sickle cell disease	Yes
Hb S/Hbs I-Toulouse, Shelby, Hope, North Shore	Hemolytic anemia	No
Hb S/Hb E	Mild to severe sickle cell disease	Occasionally*

Note: The decision to have prenatal diagnosis belongs to the couple, once they have had comprehensive counseling.
*Couples with genotypes that may lead to offspring with unpredictable phenotypes occasionally select to have prenatal diagnosis or PGD.

Table 1. Sickle cell disorders—interactions and indications for prenatal diagnosis and preimplantation genetic diagnosis (PND) [10].

These conventional methods for sampling fetal genetic material are invasive and associated with a risk for fetal miscarriage [13] (**Table 2**).

Sample	Fetal risk	Analysis	Current status
Fetal blood	1–2%	Hb separation	Disused
Amniotic cells	>0.5%	DNA	Clinically available
Trophoblastic cells	>0.5%	DNA	Clinically available
Fetal Cell/DNA in maternal circulation	0%	DNA	Investigational

Table 2. The sampling methods used in prenatal diagnosis for hemoglobinopathies at past and present [6].

2.1. Invasive methods

The main testing procedures include amniocentesis and CVS, together with ultrasonography, ultrasound, serum markers, and genetic screening. Amniocentesis and CVS continue to be the gold standards for prenatal diagnosis of genetic disorders. Though these procedures are minimally invasive and cause some risk to the mother and fetus, they are routinely and safely conducted. Each of these procedures must be applied during a specific time period to achieve accurate results, and the test sensitivity of these tests is limited. Chorionic villus sampling is not applicable before 9 weeks of gestation. On the other hand, for amniocentesis the correct time interval is proposed to 15 and 20 weeks of gestation. Both these procedures were associated with a risk of fetal miscarriage of $<1.0\%$. Fetal sexing cannot be determined in the early first trimester using ultrasonography. Thus, the noninvasive applications that clarify fetal sexing, fetal Rhesus D, single gene disorders, and chromosome abnormalities at the early stage of first trimester were a fascinating development [14].

2.2. Noninvasive methods

The well-known presence of fetal cells and free fetal nucleic acids (including DNA and RNA) in the maternal circulation has accelerated the research area toward developing new methods for noninvasive prenatal diagnosis (NIPD), applicable to the exclusion of both single gene and chromosome disorders [15]. This is in contrast to cell-free fetal DNA (cffDNA) where only paternally inherited alleles that differ from those carried by the mother can be distinguished with most current methods [12, 15].

2.2.1. Circulating fetal cells in maternal plasma

Fetal cells represent the ideal source of fetal genetic material for NIPD, since they offer the potential of achieving a "full" genetic analysis. Among fetal cell categories found in the circulation are trophoblasts, fetal leukocytes, and fetal nucleated erythroblasts (nucleated red blood cells (NRBCs)). Fetal nucleated cells that are present in the maternal circulation have been explored as a source of fetal genetic materials for NIPD [16, 17]. Typically, fetal cells exist at a concentration of several cells per milliliter of maternal blood. The rarity of circulating fetal cells has prevented their robust detection, thus hampering the general use of this approach. Due to their limitations, an alternative form of fetal genetic materials for diagnostic test development would be needed [18].

2.2.2. Cell-free fetal DNA in maternal plasma

The discovery of cell-free fetal DNA (cffDNA) in the maternal blood circulation has offered new possibilities for NIPD [19]. Many fascinating clinical experiments such as noninvasive detection of fetal sexing and fetal Rhesus D status have been developed which is the bases for the detection of paternal alleles in maternal plasma [20, 21]. Detecting the presence or absence of paternally inherited alleles in maternal plasma in inherited diseases such as β-thalassemia and SCD would allow the diagnosis or the exclusion of those diseases in the fetus, respectively [22–24].

3. Genotyping applications with high-resolution melting

High-resolution melting (HRM) is a novel, closed-tube, post-PCR technique allowing genomic researchers to easily analyze genetic variations in PCR amplicons. This method was introduced in 2002 as a simplest approach for genotyping and mutation scanning. After PCR amplification,

http://dx.doi.org/10.5772/64646

melting curves are generated by monitoring the fluorescence of a saturating dye that does not inhibit PCR [25].

This technique enables researchers to rapidly and efficiently discover genetic variations (e.g., single nucleotide polymorphisms (SNPs), mutations, methylations). In HRM experiments, the target sequence is amplified by PCR in the presence of a saturating fluorescent dye (e.g., LightCycler® 480 ResoLight Dye). Dyes that stain double-stranded DNA are commonly used to identify products by their melting temperature (T_m). Alternatively, hybridization probes allow genotyping by melting of product/probe duplexes [26].

High-resolution DNA melting analysis with saturation dyes for either mutation detection of PCR products or genotyping with unlabeled probes, PCR product scanning, and probe genotyping in the same reaction has been reported [27]. Modern HRM is facilitated by novel saturation dyes and high-resolution instruments. Asymmetric cyanine dyes such as SYBR Green I and LCGreen are dyes of choice in fluorescence melting analysis [26].

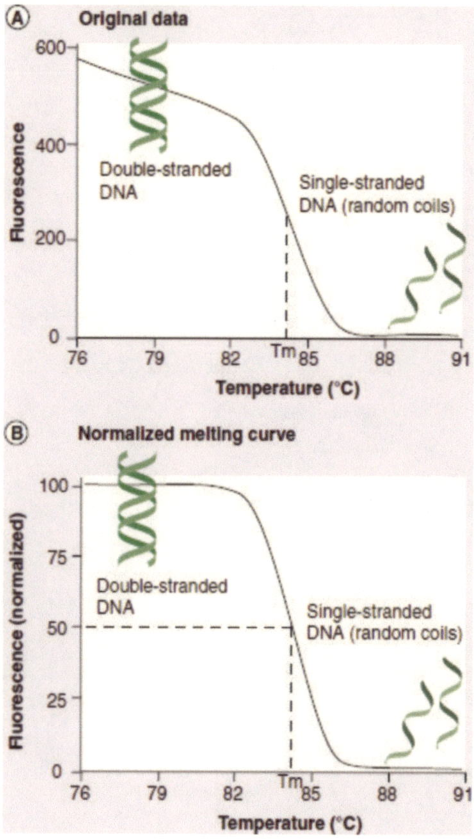

Figure 1. (A) The linear decrease of fluorescence at low temperature and a rapid decrease at melting temperature (T_m). (B) The normalized data (between 0 and 100%) shown after the background subtraction and the curve is seen horizontal outside of the transition period [26].

High-resolution melting analysis requires only the usual unlabeled primers and a generic double-stranded DNA dye added before PCR for amplicon genotyping, and is a promising method for mutation screening.

The HRM analysis of the related sequence (amplicon) has a unique DNA melting temperature in the presence of saturating DNA-binding dyes. The melting behavior depends on the base content (primarily the GC bases) and the length of the sequence when the temperature of the solution is increased. The graph of the fluorescence signal against the temperature plotted as the intensity decreases and the double-stranded DNA becomes single stranded as the dye is released (**Figure 1**). To estimate the T_m at which 50% of the DNA is in the double-stranded state, the derivative of the curve can be considered. The difference or the derivative plot and the melting curve may be used for analysis of the sequence (**Figure 2**) [28].

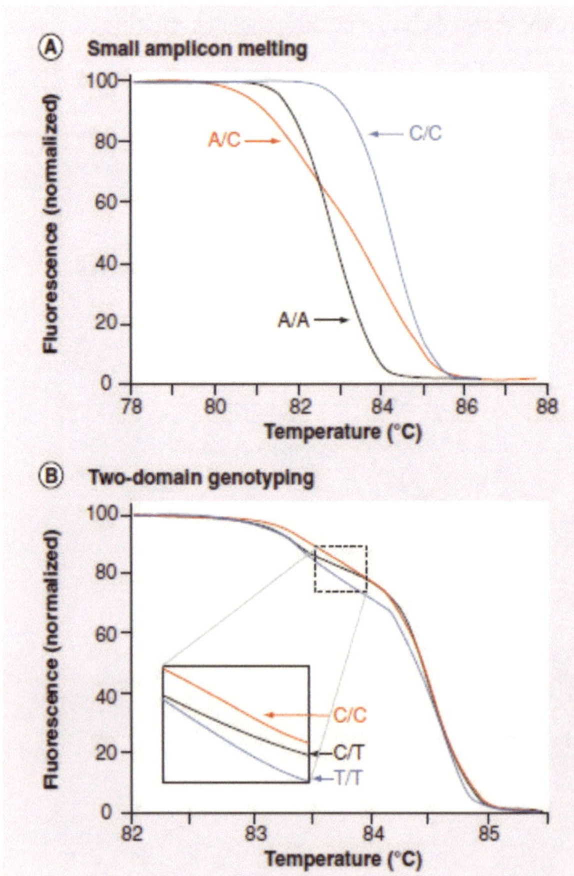

Figure 2. (A) Melting of a small amplicon (B) A large amplicon melting that melts in two-domains.

High-resolution method has been successfully applied in many studies for NIPD [29, 30]. Specific primers that are used in the assay can detect the mutations when compared to hybridization or restriction enzyme-based methods [31, 32]. Recently, it has also been used in the detection of α- and β-thalassemia variants [32, 33].

4. Materials

4.1. Equipment

The method described in this chapter was performed with a LightCycler LC 480 instrument and version 1.5 (Roche Diagnostics, Basel, Switzerland). The other important equipment includes the following:

- LightCycler 480 Multiwell Plate 96 (Roche Diagnostics 4729692001), in which the real-time PCR reactions are run in LightCycler instrument.
- LightCycler 480 Sealing Foil—50 foils (Roche Diagnostics 04729757001)—is used to cover the multiwell plates.
- MagNa pure compact instrument (Roche Diagnostics, Basel, Switzerland), for the extraction of couples genomic DNA, plasma cffDNA, and chorion villus DNA of fetus.
- A bench centrifuge, to separate the maternal plasma and to centrifuge the multiwell plates before real-time PCR.

4.2. Reagents

The reagents used are as follows:

- MagNA Pure LC DNA Extraction Kit—Large Volume (Roche).
- Hemoglobin S/C ToolSet™ for LightCycler™ (Roche Diagnostics) (β-globin, sickle cells, Hb S, Hb C) (see **Table 2**).
- LightCycler master hybridization probes (Roche).
- LightCycler HRM master mix ×2 (Roche).
- Primers for HRM analysis of beta-globin gene mutations (see **Table 4**).

4.3. Storage of the PCR reagents

Storage of the PCR reagents is as follows:

- The PCR primers to be used on the LightCycler are diluted from 100-μM stock solutions. The diluted primers are divided into aliquots and stored at −20°C. The stock solutions are diluted to 10 μM for preparing primer working solutions. These working solutions can be stored at 4°C for up to 3 months.
- LightCycler master hybridization probes and HRM master mix are stored in aliquots of small volume (e.g., 20 μL) at −20°C (when thawed, an aliquot does not refreeze; it can be used up to 1 month at 4°C.

5. Methods

5.1. Cell-free fetal DNA extraction

Maternal blood (10 mL) and peripheral blood (5 mL) samples from parents of each fetus were collected in ethylenediaminetetraacetic acid (EDTA) tubes. Two steps were used during centrifugation (1600 *g* for 10 min and 16,000 *g* for 10 min) for separating the plasma from maternal blood within 1 h. The plasma samples were stored at −20°C for the next step [33]. The plasma samples were taken before chorionic villus sampling. Magna Pure Large Volume Isolation Kit (Roche Diagnostics, Basel, Switzerland) according to the total nucleic acid plasma extraction protocol of the MagNa Pure Compact instrument is used for DNA extraction. Extracted DNA was eluted in elution buffer (50 μL) and stored at −80°C. Whole blood (500 μL) of each parent's DNA was extracted by the same method.

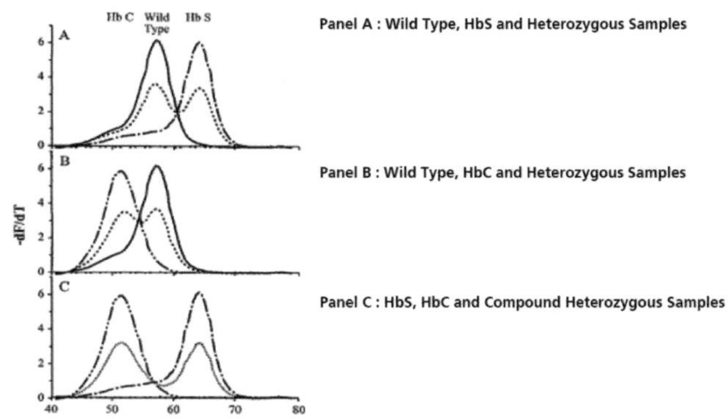

Figure 3. Melting curve analysis of Hb S/Hb C locus in β-globin gene.

5.2. Real-time PCR and melting curve analysis

5.2.1. Genotyping Hb S mutation using Hb S/C Toolset

Genotyping Hb S mutation using Hb S/C Toolset includes the following:

1. The Hb S/C genotyping in cffDNA was detected by real-time PCR and HRM analyses in the same run in a LightCycler 480 (Roche Applied Science) instrument.

2. The hemoglobin S/C kit (Ratiogen) for the LightCycler™ (Neftenbach, Switzerland) was used to examine the human β-globin gene for the presence of Hb S/C variant using LightCycler PCR with melting curve analysis (**Figures 3** and **4**).

3. The primer pair and fluorescent detection/anchor probes were optimized to specifically amplify a 214-bp segment of exon 1 of the human β-globin gene. In a final volume of 20 μL, the reaction mixture included 9.6μL of Hb S/C Solvent, 2.8μL of HbS/C Oligo Tool, 25mM 1.6 μL MgCl2, and 2 μL Master Hybridization probe (10×) (**Table 3**).

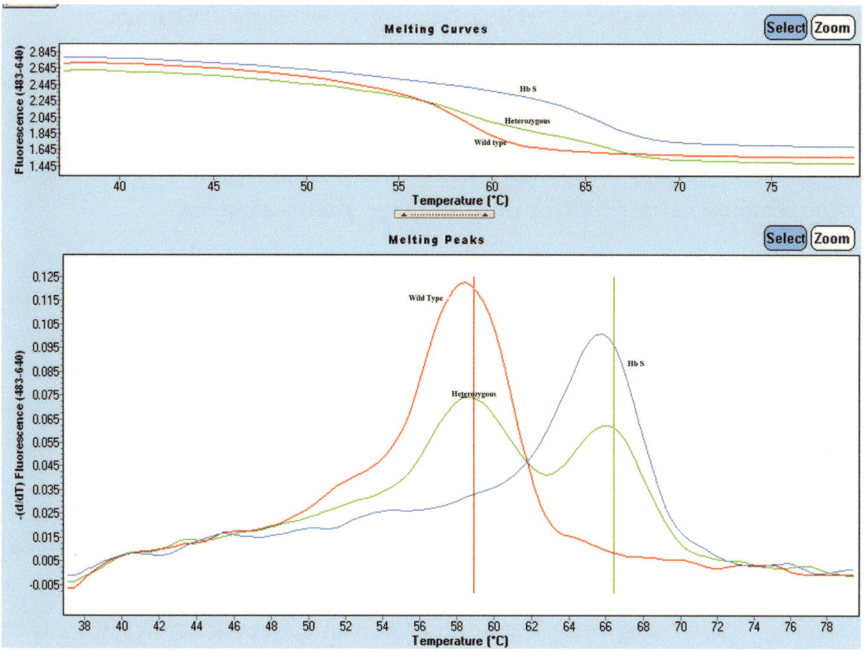

Figure 4. Genotyping of Hb S. Melting curve analysis of Hb S genotypes of the Hb S locus in the beta-globin gene. (T_m values: wild type 56°C; Hb S: 63°C; Hb C: 50°C (not shown). Note: The values for the respective melting temperatures may vary for ±2.5°C).

Reagent	Volume (μL)
OligoTool Hb S/C	2.8
Solvent Hb S/C	9.6
$MgCl_2$, 25 mM	1.6 (final 3mM)
Master hybridization probes 10×	2
Total reaction mix	16
DNA or control Hb S heterozygous	4
Total	20

Table 3. Reaction mix preparation.

5.2.1.1. PCR protocol

- The PCR protocol consisted of an initial denaturation step at 95°C for 1 min, followed by 35 cycles of 1 s at 95°C, 30 s at 63°C, and 1 s at 72°C.
- After the amplification step, the LightCycler is programmed for the melting step; 95°C for 60 s, 35°C for 20 s, and melting at 80°C with continuous fluorescence reading at 25 acquisitions per 1°C.
- Control samples (negative and positive) were suggested to use for each run.

5.2.2. *High-resolution melting design and gene scanning for Hb S/beta thalassemia*

- Four overlapping DNA fragments were synthesized to cover the regions of interest in the β-globin gene. The oligonucleotide primers are shown in **Table 4**.
- Perform PCR amplifications in a total volume of 20 μL, use high-resolution melting master ×2 (Roche Diagnostics) and 5 μL of DNA from the plasma samples.
- For the β-globin gene mutation assay, we use 300-nM primers and 2.5 mM $MgCl_2$. Control samples with known β-globin gene mutations and the wild type should be included in each assay.

Location	Amplicon	Primer sequences	
	length (bp)	Forward primer (5′–3′)	Reverse primer (5′–3′)
P1 (promoter-exon 1)	351	F1-CAATTTGTACTGATGGTATGG	R1-CTTCATCCACGTTCACCTTGC
P2 (5′ UTR-Exon 2)	425	F2-CACTAGCAACCTCAAACAGAC	R2-CACTCAGTGTGGCAAAGGTG
P3 (Exon 2-IVS 2)	318	F3-TTTGAGTCCTTTGGGGATCTG	R3-CCACACTGATGCAATCATTCG
P4 (IVS 2-3′ UTR)	354	F4-GTTAAGGCAATAGCAATATTTCT	R4-TGGACAGCAAGAAAGCGAGC

Table 4. Primers for HRM analysis of beta-globin gene mutations.

5.2.2.1. *PCR protocol*

1. The PCR program requires SYBR Green I (533 nm) and it consists of an initial denaturation-activation step at 95°C for 10 min followed by 45 cycles of 3 s at 95°C, 5 s at 58°C, and 20 s at 72°C.
2. The melting step at 95°C for 60 s, 35°C for 20 s, and the melting at 80°C with continuous fluorescence reading at 25 acquisitions per 1°C.
3. Gene Scanning software was used to perform the melting curve analysis in three steps: normalization, shifting of the temperature axis of the normalized melting curves, and analysis of the difference plot of the difference between the melting curve shapes derived by subtracting the wild type and mutant DNA curves.
4. The difference plots cluster the samples into groups. High-resolution melting results were confirmed by sequencing in samples that had not been identified using conventional PCR.

5.2.3. *High-resolution melting analysis*

- The HRM technique was standardized by analyzing genomic DNA from Hb S and β-thalassemia heterozygous parents with known mutations. A melting curve program is used to detect the Hb S mutation in the samples. The melting temperature (T_m) was 63°C for the S allele and 56°C for the A allele.

- The related primer sets P1-P4 (**Table 4**) were used to analyze the β-thalassemia mutations by HRM analysis. Heterozygous and homozygous samples were included in each PCR run as a positive control to check the mutation.
- The contamination was monitored using a DNA-free blank. In all steps in the assay, for each mutation, the wild-type samples were separated from the heterozygous or homozygous samples by the melting curves, as expected (**Figure 4**).
- The majority of mutations seen in our Mediterranean population can be detected using P1, P2, and P3 set primers. Paternal alleles have been detected in cffDNA using primer set P1 in exon 1 and promoter region (ex. -30 (T>A), -101 (C>T), CAP+1 (A>C)_ of beta-globin gene. The mutations of 5′ UTR-exon 2 region (ex. HbS (A>T), IVSI-1 (G>A), IVSI-5 (G>A), IVSI-6 (T>C), IVSI-110 (G>A), Cd8 (-AA), Cd9/10 (+T), Cd15 (G>A), Cd39 (C>T)) were detected with primer set P2. The most detected mutations in exon 2-IVS 2 region were IVSII-1 (G>A), IVSII-745 (C>G), and IVSII-848 (C>A) using primer set P3 [33].

6. Conclusion

The invention of cffDNA in maternal plasma provided new opportunities for NIPD during pregnancy [19]. Many fascinating clinical studies such as fetal sexing and fetal Rhesus D genotyping have been developed according to the detection of the paternal alleles, which differ from the mother in maternal plasma [34]. The parents with different carrier status have a chance of 50% for having a sick (thalassemia or SCD) fetus, if the paternal allele is detected in maternal plasma. If the mutation of the father is not detected in maternal plasma, there is no need to perform invasive prenatal processes. High-resolution melting analysis can be applicable to find paternal mutations in cffDNA that differs from the mother. The double-heterozygote-affected fetuses can be diagnosed using HRM analysis. The results should be confirmed by invasive methods. The maternal background could affect the results in cffDNA when the gestational age is under <7 weeks. The low levels of cffDNA may be the reason at this point.

Determination of the paternal alleles in cffDNA avoids the risk for a double heterozygous fetus. High-resolution melting method is easy to practice when compared to other complicated methods. This method is useful for NIPD of hemoglobinopathies and does not require any modification of PCR protocols. The couples that carry the same mutation, genotype determination of the cffDNA in maternal plasma is difficult but not impossible. Specific SNPs might be used instead of mutations for the best accuracy of the HRM method. In conclusion to compare with invasive methods, HRM has the lowest risk for PCR contamination because of being a closed-tube method. Small amounts of fetal DNA in maternal plasma can be detected and analyzed for mutations of single-gene disorders such as hemoglobinopathies in the early stage of pregnancy. The HRM method is applicable for other genetic disorders to detect the known mutations in cffDNA from maternal plasma.

Author details

Ebru Dündar Yenilmez* and Abdullah Tuli

*Address all correspondence to: edundar@cu.edu.tr

Faculty of Medicine, Department of Medical Biochemistry, Çukurova University, Adana, Turkey

References

[1] Sebastiani P, Ramoni MF, Nolan V, Baldwin CT, Steinberg MH. Genetic dissection and prognostic modeling of overt stroke in sickle cell anemia. Nature Genetics. 2005;37(4): 435–40.

[2] Frenette PS, Atweh GF. Sickle cell disease: old discoveries, new concepts, and future promise. The Journal of Clinical Investigation. 2007;117(4):850–8.

[3] Scriver JB, Waugh T. Studies on a case of sickle-cell anaemia. Canadian Medical Association Journal. 1930;23(3):375.

[4] Ingram V. Abnormal human haemoglobins. III. The chemical difference between normal and sickle cell haemoglobins. Biochimica et Biophysica Acta. 1959;36(2):402–11.

[5] Kaur M, Dangi CBS, Singh M. An overview on sickle cell disease profile. Asian Journal of Pharmaceutical and Clinical Research. 2013;6(suppl 1):25–37.

[6] Angastiniotis M, Modell B. Global epidemiology of hemoglobin disorders. Annals of the New York Academy of Sciences. 1998;850(1):251–69.

[7] Group WW. Community control of hereditary anaemias. Bulletin of the World Health Organization. 1983;61:63–80.

[8] Cao A, Pirastu M, Rosatelli C. The prenatal diagnosis of thalassaemia. British Journal of Haematology. 1986;63(2):215–20.

[9] Traeger-Synodinos J, Vrettou C, Kanavakis E. Rapid detection of fetal Mendelian disorders: thalassemia and sickle cell syndromes. Prenatal Diagnosis. 2008:133–45.

[10] Traeger-Synodinos J, Harteveld CL, Old JM, Petrou M, Galanello R, Giordano P, et al. EMQN Best Practice Guidelines for molecular and haematology methods for carrier identification and prenatal diagnosis of the haemoglobinopathies. European Journal of Human Genetics. 2015;23(4):426–37.

[11] Wapner RJ, editor. Invasive prenatal diagnostic techniques. Seminars in Perinatology; 2005: Philadelphia Elsevier Publishing Company.

[12] Traeger-Synodinos J, Vrettou C, Kanavakis E. Prenatal, noninvasive and preimplantation genetic diagnosis of inherited disorders: hemoglobinopathies. Expert Review of Molecular Diagnostics. 2011;11(3):299–312.

[13] Chiu RW, Lo YM. Clinical applications of maternal plasma fetal DNA analysis: translating the fruits of 15 years of research. Clinical Chemistry and Laboratory Medicine: CCLM/FESCC. 2013;51(1):197–204.

[14] Gahan PB. Circulating nucleic acids in plasma and serum: applications in diagnostic techniques for noninvasive prenatal diagnosis. International Journal of Women's Health. 2013;5:177.

[15] Hahn S, Jackson LG, Kolla V, Mahyuddin AP, Choolani M. Noninvasive prenatal diagnosis of fetal aneuploidies and Mendelian disorders: new innovative strategies. Expert Review of Molecular Diagnostics. 2009;9(6):613–21.

[16] Bianchi DW, Flint AF, Pizzimenti MF, Knoll J, Latt SA. Isolation of fetal DNA from nucleated erythrocytes in maternal blood. Proceedings of the National Academy of Sciences. 1990;87(9):3279–83.

[17] Cheung M-C, Goldberg JD, Kan YW. Prenatal diagnosis of sickle cell anaemia and thalassaemia by analysis of fetal cells in maternal blood. Nature Genetics. 1996;14(3): 264–8.

[18] Bianchi DW, Simpson J, Jackson L, Elias S, Holzgreve W, Evans M, et al. Fetal gender and aneuploidy detection using fetal cells in maternal blood: analysis of NIFTY I data. Prenatal Diagnosis. 2002;22(7):609–15.

[19] Lo YMD, Corbetta N, Chamberlain PF, Rai V, Sargent IL, Redman CWG, et al. Presence of fetal DNA in maternal plasma and serum. The Lancet. 1997;350(9076):485–7.

[20] Bustamante-Aragones A, Pérez-Cerdá C, Pérez B, Rodriguez de Alba M, Ugarte M, Ramos C. Prenatal diagnosis in maternal plasma of a fetal mutation causing propionic acidemia. Molecular Genetics and Metabolism. 2008;95(1–2):101–3.

[21] Finning KM, Chitty LS. Non-invasive fetal sex determination: Impact on clinical practice. Seminars in Fetal and Neonatal Medicine. 2008;13(2):69–75.

[22] Chiu RWK, Lau TK, Leung TN, Chow KCK, Chui DHK, Lo YMD. Prenatal exclusion of β thalassaemia major by examination of maternal plasma. The Lancet. 2002;360(9338):998–1000.

[23] Saito H, Sekizawa A, Morimoto T, Suzuki M, Yanaihara T. Prenatal DNA diagnosis of a single-gene disorder from maternal plasma. The Lancet. 2000;356(9236):1170.

[24] Ding C, Chiu RW, Lau TK, Leung TN, Chan LC, Chan AY, et al. MS analysis of single-nucleotide differences in circulating nucleic acids: application to noninvasive prenatal diagnosis. Proceedings of the National Academy of Sciences of the United States of America. 2004;101(29):10762–7.

[25] Reed H KJ, Wittwer CT. High resolution DNA melting analysis for simple and efficient molecular diagnostics. Pharmacogenomics. 2007;8(6):597–608.

[26] Wittwer CT, Kusakawa N. Real-time PCR. In: Persing DH, Tenover FC, Versalovic J, Tang JW, Unger ER, Relman DA, White TJ, eds. Molecular microbiology: diagnostic principles and practice. Washington: ASM Press; 2004. p 71–84.

[27] Zhou L, Wang L, Palais R, Pryor R, Wittwer CT. High-resolution DNA melting analysis for simultaneous mutation scanning and genotyping in solution. Clinical Chemistry. 2005;51(10):1770–7.

[28] Maria Erali KVV, Carl T. Wittwer. High resolution melting applications for clinical laboratory medicine. Experimental and Molecular Pathology. 2008;85:50–8.

[29] Phylipsen M, Yamsri S, Treffers EE, Jansen DT, Kanhai WA, Boon EM, et al. Non-invasive prenatal diagnosis of beta-thalassemia and sickle-cell disease using pyrophosphorolysis-activated polymerization and melting curve analysis. Prenatal Diagnosis. 2012;32(6):578–87.

[30] Macher HC, Martinez-Broca MA, Rubio-Calvo A, Leon-Garcia C, Conde-Sanchez M, Costa A, et al. Non-invasive prenatal diagnosis of multiple endocrine neoplasia type 2A using COLD-PCR combined with HRM genotyping analysis from maternal serum. PLoS One. 2012;7(12):e51024.

[31] Prathomtanapong P, Pornprasert S, Phusua A, Suanta S, Saetung R, Sanguansermsri T. Detection and identification of β-thalassemia 3.5 kb deletion by SYBR Green1 and high resolution melting analysis. European Journal of Haematology. 2009;82(2):159–60.

[32] Shih H-C, Er T-K, Chang T-J, Chang Y-S, Liu T-C, Chang J-G. Rapid identification of HBB gene mutations by high-resolution melting analysis. Clinical Biochemistry. 2009;42(16):1667–76.

[33] Yenilmez ED, Tuli A, Evruke IC. Noninvasive prenatal diagnosis experience in the Çukurova Region of Southern Turkey: detecting paternal mutations of sickle cell anemia and beta-thalassemia in cell-free fetal DNA using high-resolution melting analysis. Prenatal Diagnosis. 2013;33(11):1054–62.

[34] Lazaros L, Hatzi E, Bouba I, Makrydimas G, Dalkalitsis N, Stefos T, et al. Non-invasive first-trimester detection of paternal beta-globin gene mutations and polymorphisms as predictors of thalassemia risk at chorionic villous sampling. European Journal of Obstetrics, Gynecology, and Reproductive Biology. 2008;140(1):17–20.

Chapter 4

Point-of-Care Testing in Sickle Cell Disease

Julie Kanter

Additional information is available at the end of the chapter

http://dx.doi.org/10.5772/64862

Abstract

Sickle cell disease is one of the most common inherited blood disorders. Universal screening and central laboratory diagnostics have improved early identification of affected individuals and helped to reduce childhood mortality in high-resource countries. Additional methods of centralized diagnostics have also been developed in some low resource areas in partnership with private companies, local governments and academic US-based institutions. However, these techniques require expansive infrastructure and government partnership for success. Thus, many individuals living in low-resource settings are often not diagnosed until late childhood when they present with clinical symptoms. In addition, confirmation of disease in affected individuals in the urgent care setting remains limited in both high- and low-resource areas due to the use of batched testing methods. All of the current diagnostic methods rely on advanced laboratory systems and are often prohibitively expensive and time-consuming. To address this need and improve the capacity for timely diagnosis, novel methods for point-of-care testing for sickle cell disease are currently in process.

Keywords: point of care, sickle cell, diagnosis

1. Introduction

Approximately 5% of the world's population carries traits for hemoglobin disorder (majority sickle cell disease, thalassemia). The global incidence of sickle cell disease (SCD) is 300,000 births/year of which 90% are estimated to occur in sub-Saharan African and India, many of whom reside in low-resource areas. In many of these areas, 50–80% of children die before five years of age [1]. In contrast, a small margin of affected individuals are born in the USA, England, France and other high-resource countries where 98% of children are living >18 years of age. In these high-resource countries, early diagnosis remains a key reason for the improved longevity [2, 3].

Newborn screening provides an early diagnosis of SCD which has demonstrated efficacy in reducing infant mortality through initiation of penicillin prophylaxis and delivery of care/ education prior to the onset of clinical complications [4, 5]. However, current newborn screening programs are dependent on central laboratories with capabilities to perform cost-efficient, high-throughput screening [6]. In addition to high-cost laboratory equipment, these programs require complex work-flow including skilled individuals, sample transport and advanced systems of medical care. Additionally, most newborn screening samples are collected at outlying hospitals and are shipped to centralized laboratories where tests are batched and run on a scheduled basis and results are then sent to primary care providers or public health officials to communicate with affected families. Screening is two-tiered starting with testing in the hospital and complementary, confirmatory testing performed at follow-up to confirm the diagnosis (and validate the sample was sent on the correct patient). Thus, all individuals are tested while in the hospital during the newborn period, and the results are often not available for communication until several weeks after discharge. While systems of care exist in many developed countries for communicating these results, these options are not available in other, less resourced areas. Even in some high-resource areas, it can also be difficult to find the newborn and bring them back to the provider for confirmatory testing.

While newborn screening is limited in low-resource areas, many high-resource countries are unable to diagnose and confirm sickle cell disease at the point of care (POC). Similar to tests used during newborn screening, diagnostic tests for SCD are expensive and time consuming. As a result, the testing is often batched and run on specific days with limited availability for diagnosis at the point of care or when the patient presents. While this limitation does not affect most patients who have been previously identified within a health system, the inability to confirm the diagnosis at the point of care can lead to delays in treatment in outside hospitals (where the individual is not usually treated) or inappropriate treatment for an affected individual. Due to the painful nature of this disease, many patients face undue stigmatization for having sickle cell disease. Without "proof" of disease, patients may not be able to receive the care they need in a timely manner. Conversely, there are also anecdotal reports of individuals without SCD who falsely claim to be affected by the condition to receive opioid therapy in the emergency room setting. For those patients not established within a hospital system, a point-of-care test may enhance the ability of acute care physicians to provide appropriate therapy.

Research has clearly demonstrated that the health burden of hemoglobin disorders can be reduced through screening and early diagnosis, prevention and management [5, 7, 8]. While these cost-effective lifesaving strategies/therapies are already known, many are not universally available [9]. Thus, options for enhancing access to early diagnosis include the development of centralized laboratories in low-resource areas and novel point-of-care testing method which remain in development.

2. Traditional diagnostic testing in SCD

The diagnosis of a hemoglobin disorder is usually performed by confirmatory testing in hospital, private or academic laboratories. The majority of current labs in high-resource areas utilize methods of protein chemistry methods such as isoelectric focusing (IEF) or high-performance liquid chromatography (HPLC) and (Sebia) capillary electrophoresis (CE) [10]. Some additional laboratories utilize hemoglobin electrophoresis with either cellulose acetate or citrate agar. Specifically, acid citrate agar is used for conformation of hemoglobin SC disease. See **Table 1** for a list of testing methods.

Isoelectric focusing utilizes agarose gels to separate hemoglobin (Hb) fractions and variants based on their isoelectric points [11]. Hb A and Hb F are clearly resolved by this method. Hb C can also be distinguished from Hb E and Hb O, and Hb S can be distinguished from Hb.

High-performance liquid chromatography separates hemoglobin in sample by passing them through a column filled with a solid adsorbent material. Specifically, HPLC uses the principles of cation exchange for the separation and determination of the relative percentage of normal and abnormal hemoglobin. Each component in the sample interacts slightly differently with the adsorbent material, causing different flow rates for the different components and leading to the separation of the components as they flow out the column. This is the method used to identify and quantify relative fractions of Hb F, Hb A2, Hb S, Hb C, Hb Barts and other Hb variants. HPLC is also used to quantify Hb A2 and Hb F for carrier screening [12, 13].

Hemoglobin electrophoresis at alkaline or acidic pH can be used as a primary or confirmatory method of identification. Electrophoresis separates molecules based on size and charge. Different hemoglobin has a different charge, and according to those charges and the amount, hemoglobin moves at different speeds in the gel whether in alkaline gel or acid gel. This method separates hemoglobin based on the relative mobility of the variant hemoglobin into characteristic bands [10, 14].

Novel diagnostic testing in hemoglobinopathies. A variety of novel methods of hemoglobinopathy testing are now available at select laboratories in high-resource areas. These newer techniques expand the analysis and complexity of hemoglobinopathy testing and identification. Techniques include molecular methods of identification, such as the linear array assay, a multiplexed reverse dot blot genotyping method, used to simultaneously test for a panel of common beta-globin variants (Hb S, C, E, D and O), as well as majority (>95%) of common beta-thalassemia mutations[1]. Another newer method uses multiplex gap PCR assays to detect common alpha thalassemia deletion mutations, alpha globin gene duplications and other globin gene deletions, such as Hb Lepore and HPFH. Finally, DNA sequence analysis of alpha, beta or gamma globin genes can also be performed to definitively identify unknown point mutations or sequence variation. At present, however, these more advanced techniques remain sequestered in advanced laboratories and are not universally available.

---

[1] (http://www.rbclab.com/Pages/200/220/116%20LA/220%20116.html)

Type of test	Method	Results	PRO	CON
Traditional testing methods				
Isoelectric focusing	Agarose gels to separate hemoglobin based on isoelectric points	Hb A, Hb F, Hb C, Hb S, Hb E and Hb OArab	Reliable, able to distinguish most types of sickle cell disease including compound heterozygotes	Expensive, requires skilled technicians, often batched and run every few days
High-performance liquid chromotography	Separates hemoglobin by principles of cation exchange	Identify and quantify Hb F, Hb A, Hb A2, Hb S, Hb C, Hb Barts and others	Reliable, able to distinguish most types of sickle cell disease, including compound heterozygotes	Expensive, requires skilled technicians, often batched and run
Hemoglobin electrophoresis	Separates Hb based on size and charge	Identify and quantify HbF, Hb A, Hb A2, Hb S, Hb C, Hb Barts and others	Reliable, able to distinguish most types of sickle cell disease including compound heterozygotes	Expensive, requires skilled technicians, often batched and run
Novel diagnostic testing methods				
AMPS	Density based test to separate Hb in different density fluids	Identifies Hb S and Hb A	Inexpensive, done at the point of care	Interpretation is more difficult, Less reliable results, difficult to distinguish HbSC disease
Paper-based Sickle test	Microfluidic assessment	Identifies Hb S and A and C and company has a separate test that can identify Hb F	Inexpensive, done at the point of care, reliable diagnosis of HbSS disease, easily performed by non-skilled personnel	Requires a scanner for final results, can be difficult to distinguish HbAS (trait) from HbSC, test could be altered in different humidities
Sickle SCAN	Lateral flow assay	Distinguishes Hb A, Hb S, Hb C	Reliably identifies HbA, HbS, and HbC, easily performed by non-skilled personnel, easily interpreted, rapid test at the point of care	More expensive than the other point of care tests above. Does not identify hemoglobin F. Limit of detection of Hb A is 2%
HemeChip	Micro-elecrophoresis assay	Distinguishes Hb F, S, C, A, and D	Reliable, able to distinguish most types of sickle cell disease including compound heterozygotes	Requires a skilled interpretation, web-based image processing application for automated results

Table 1. Hemoglobinopathy testing methods.

http://dx.doi.org/10.5772/64862

3. Centralized laboratory efforts in low-resource settings

In regions of the world where sickle cell trait and SCD are very prevalent, partnership between private and public organizations and researchers and local hospitals has resulted in impressive newborn screening/diagnostics for SCD. Examples of such efforts include Angola, Uganda and Jamaica.

3.1. Angola

Angola's newborn screening program for SCD was born out of the government mandated public health initiative for perinatal HIV screening and a partnership with Chevron. Chevron is one of the leading producers of petroleum in Angola. Thus, Chevron provides support for many Angola-based health initiatives. This initiative was undertaken in partnership with a US academic hospital to assess whether a centralized newborn screening program for SCD was feasible in a low-resource setting. Additional emphasis in this initiative was placed on local training and capacity building for the region. The laboratory was set up in the only pediatric hospital in Angola, and the program was designed to send all collected samples to this location for analysis [15].

For the pilot program in Angola, researchers selected two large maternity hospitals in Luanda as initial sites of blood collection from newborn infants. To enhance local capacity building, obstetrical nurses were trained in the techniques of blood collection and then retrained monthly, and then retrained approximately once a month. All samples were drawn using a heel stick procedure to fill bloodspots on a custom-designed Whatman screening card. Individual cards were distinguished by unique barcodes linked to a database containing necessary demographic information. Additionally, a detachable portion of the card was provided to the mother. Bloodspots were dried and placed in a plastic bag for storage until specimen pickup, as all testing was performed at the central laboratory.

Isoelectric focusing (IEF, RESOLVE® neonatal hemoglobin system, PerkinElmer, Inc.) was used to perform testing of the dried bloodspot samples within one to two days of arrival in the NBS laboratory. Samples were batched for testing (as done in the USA). Once resulted, the samples were scored first by the laboratory technician and the laboratory supervisor subsequently scored each gel independently to ensure accuracy of results. All IEF results with an FAS, FS or other abnormal hemoglobin patterns, or in the rare instance of an indeterminate result, were selected for repeat analysis by capillary electrophoresis (CE).

Attempts were made to contact all families of all newborns with HbSC or HbSS results between 6 and 8 weeks of age. Attempted contact was made by telephone. If the family could be reached, infants had repeat samples drawn for confirmatory testing and enrollment in the local sickle cell clinic. However, due to the low-resource area and limited telephone access, 46% of families of infants (with +tests) could not be contacted highlighting the difficulties of centralized laboratory testing in low-resource areas [15, 16].

3.2. Uganda

Similar to Angola, the Ugandan Ministry of Health already had an active program for prevention of mother-to-child transmission of HIV based on identifying and treated infected mother and exposed newborns. It identifies and treats infected mothers and their exposed infants. For this program, dried blood spots are collected from exposed infants at health-care facilities across the country, carried by motorcycle to laboratory hubs at the subdistrict level, and shipped by courier to the Central Public Health Laboratories in the capital. A sickle cell laboratory was initiated within the same central public health laboratories to test for normal and abnormal hemoglobin. Also like Angola, the initiation of the sickle cell NBS program was initiated through a partnership between a US academic center and the local hospital and ministry of health [17–19].

The laboratory methods for sickle cell disease in Uganda were the same as those discussed in Angola. Again, local staff at the Central Public Health Laboratories received on-site training by a technical, US-based team on the study protocol, isoelectric focusing procedures and interpretation of results. Additional sessions and re-teaching sessions were also provided as well as ongoing laboratory support. The system for reporting positive results in Uganda was more advanced than that of Angola. Here, the hemoglobin results were communicated to the collection sites with the existing HIV notification system [20].

3.3. Jamaica

Jamaica initiated newborn screening in 1973 with the development of the well-described Jamaican Sickle Cell Cohort Study. In this initial effort, 100,000 consecutive live births were screened at the main Government Maternity Hospital (Victoria Jubilee Hospital, Kingston). Obstetric and labor nurses were trained to collect cord blood specimens, and self-adhesive labels were provided in every labor ward. These labels were duplicated and consecutively numbered so that identical labels were applied to the blood tube and a data card for each patient. The blood tubes were stored at room temperature, collected each morning. These were utilized to form hemolysates which were then used for hemoglobin electrophoresis [21, 22].

Following this initial work, Jamaica initiated a second centralized screening program in 1995 including both the main Government Maternity Hospital in Kingston (Victoria Jubilee Hospital) as well as both the University Hospital of the West Indies, Kingston (added in 1997) and the Spanish Town Hospital (added in 1998) to include 43% of births in Jamaica. Cord blood samples were collected at birth on a Guthrie card instead of in tubes as done in the initial study. All hemoglobin electrophoresis testing was performed by the newborn screening program at the Sickle Cell Unit (SCU), Tropical Medicine Research Institute, Jamaica. Patient demographics were collected with the Guthrie card and recorded in the newborn screening database. After testing was completed, infants with positive screening results suggestive of a hemoglobinopathy or with an inappropriate specimen or unclear results were notified by letter to come in for confirmatory testing. For those babies who fail to come in, a research nurse found them to encourage parents to bring their infant to the SCU for further testing.

From 1995 to 2006, 150,803 infants had undergone cord blood screening and approximately 889 infants had phenotype results suggestive of possible SCD in the initial testing [3].

While the efforts described above are successful, they rely on a significant amount of government or partnership support to establish the infrastructure needed for testing patients, confirming the diagnosis and re-identifying/contacting the affected families. Additionally, a large enough patient population is needed within specific areas to justify the cost of this type of infrastructure. Thus, it remains a priority to validate a POC testing device for the diagnosis of SCD.

4. Point-of-care testing for SCD

4.1. Methodology

To be an effective diagnostic test at the point of care (POC), all testing methods/devices must contain some similar properties. By definition, POC testing requires that testing must occur at or near the site of patient care. The goal of POC is to improve medical and economic outcomes by promoting rapid response and faster therapeutic turnaround time which requires rapid testing in close proximity to the patient. POC tests should also be simple. "Simple" means that the device/test uses unprocessed samples, is easy to read and interpret, does not require medical personnel for testing and includes instructions for confirmatory testing when needed. The test must demonstrate "insignificant risk of erroneous result" through risk analysis which can be overcome for hemoglobinopathy testing through the obligation to perform confirmatory testing. Finally, one of the advantages of diagnostic POC testing is the opportunity for immediate feedback for the patient [23, 24]. A POC gives the tester (or clinician) the capability to interact at the time of testing, taking advantage of the counseling and educational opportunity.

These devices must have high specificity to detect HbS (including in the presence of hemoglobin F), the capacity to distinguish sickle cell trait (HbAS) from samples with SCD. These point-of-care testing methods for SCD and sickle cell trait must be scalable, portable and easy to use. Results must be available within the same visit/time period for the affected patient (no follow-up required to receive tests results). For low-resource areas, devices need to be low cost, compact, and light weight to enhance portability. Finally, testing must be easy to perform with a simple design and rapid interpretation that does not require complex evaluation (i.e., does not require a medical professional) [25, 26].

4.1.1. POC tests in development

There are several testing methods and devices currently in development to achieve the aims above. These tests rely in different ways on the pathophysiologic properties of the sickle hemoglobin that differentiate it from other hemoglobin. While this list likely not exhaustive, it includes the current published tests in development. The testing methods are in various stages of evaluation and validation, and many companies and individuals are seeking device agency approvals. Current testing methodologies are listed in **Table 1** and include in the following.

4.2. Density-based test

One of the main properties of cells containing hemoglobin S is that these cells sickle upon deoxygenation. The degree of sickling is relative to the quantitative amount of S hemoglobin within the red cell. As cells sickle, this increases their density which allows red blood cells (RBCs) containing hemoglobin to be separated by cell density. Red blood cells in SCD have a specific distribution of cell densities which can be distinguished using Aqueous Multiphase Systems (AMPS). This system includes a combination of polymers and/or surfactants in water than form distinct, immiscible phases which allows the separation of cells based on density. For this testing device, whole blood must be centrifuged and separated into components prior to the red cells being placed in the AMPS solution. To allow for centrifugation in low-resource areas, investigators have identified battery operated mini-centrifuges capable of successfully separating the red cell fragment and allowing for testing. Devices are stable and densities can be tuned to distinguish very small differences ($\Delta\rho$ ~0.0005 g/cm^3). However, potential negatives include difficult in interpretation in the field and inability to successfully distinguish hemoglobin SC disease (**Figure 1**) [27, 28].

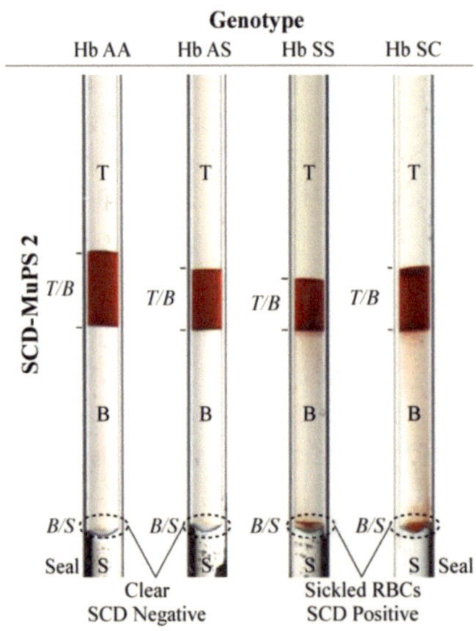

Figure 1. AMPS-based sickle cell disease POC test [27].

4.3. Microfluidic-paper-based test

Paper-based testing utilizes similar methodology to conventional hemoglobin solubility assays (e.g. SickleDex™, SA and ASI test), which have been used routinely by blood banks and clinical laboratories to verify the presence of HbS in blood samples for many years [10]. When deoxygenated, sickle hemoglobin forms polymers, which are more soluble in solution. Specific solubility buffers contain:

1. Saponin irreversibly lyses red blood cells (RBCs) by creating holes in the lipid bilayer that releases hemoglobin into the buffer.

2. Sodium hydrosulfite converts the released hemoglobin into deoxy-Hb that is either soluble (HbA, HbE, HbF or HbC) or insoluble (HbS) in the phosphate buffer.

When these solutions of hemolyzed samples are placed on paper, the delay in transit time caused by the sickle polymers results in a characteristic blood stain pattern which distinguishes normal, sickle cell trait and SCD samples. In other words, paper-based assay identifies the presence of HbS by measuring the separation of HbS from non-HbS by differential wicking/ transit of insoluble Hb S vs. soluble Hb in a paper matrix. Blood stain patterns are produced on the chromatography paper based on solubility. However, instead of measuring turbidity (as in Sickledex test), the paper blood stain reflects the amount of polymerized HbS trapped within the paper fibers while the soluble (non-polymerized) hemoglobin continues to spread on the paper. Because hemoglobin is naturally colored, the assay read out uses the red color count in the region of the polymerized hemoglobin and soluble hemoglobin [29].

Testing results (the blood stain) can then be scanned using portable scanners (on a cell phone) to quantify the density of the blood stain and differentiate SCD vs SC trait vs. sickle SC disease. However, this test remains dependent on a low percent of fetal hemoglobin which makes it less ideal in newborn screening. A newer version of the test in development may resolve this complication but results are pending at this time. This device successfully reduces the required blood sample volume, lowering the per-test cost and significantly simplifying the interpretation of results. Sickle cell anemia can be distinguished easily but scanning is required for further hemoglobin differentiating. Scanned results are easy to interpret which makes the test highly adaptable in the non-medical population (**Figure 2**) [30].

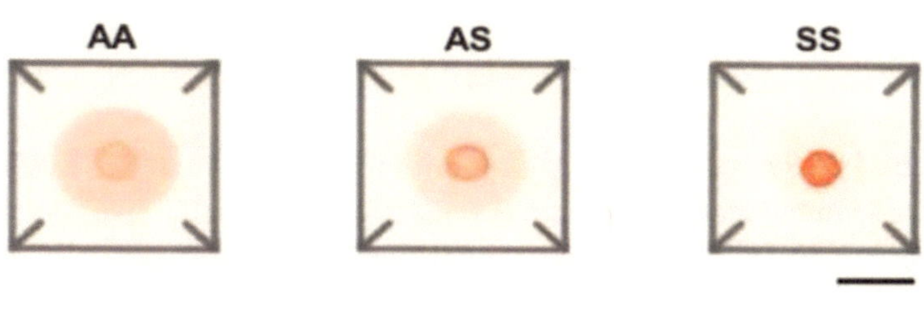

Figure 2. Characteristic blood stain patterns produced by paper-based SCD assay.

4.4. Lateral flow assays

Lateral flow assays are simple devices intended to detect the presence (or absence) of a target analyte. For this type of test, the analyte is hemoglobin. Antibodies are utilized to bind to the human alpha globin chain and are conjugated to colored nanoparticles. These antibodies are conjugated to yellow-colored nanoparticles bind the antigen (Hb) as they migrate toward the test lines. Conjugated antibodies with bound Hb (antigen) bind to capture antibodies (polyclonal antibodies for specific hemoglobin S, C, A) on each of three test lines (producing positive result). Nanoparticles without antigens bind to the control line (proof of validity of the testing device) (**Figure 3**) [32].

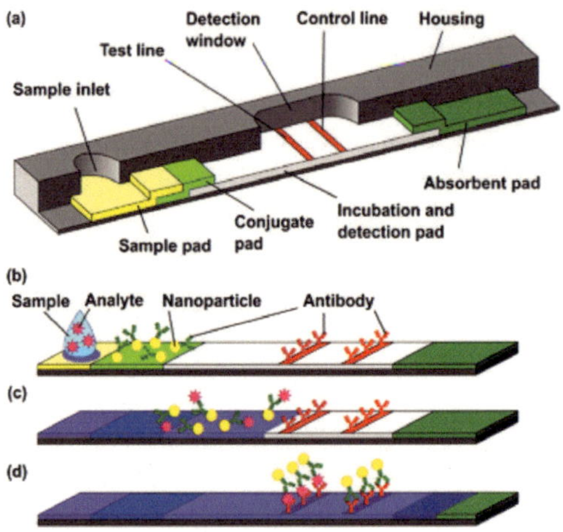

Figure 3. (a–d) Lateral testing method [31].

Current tests in development utilize polyclonal antibodies that can bind to hemoglobin S, C, A and F. The result is a single test line for each specific hemoglobin (identifying the presence of that particular hemoglobin). Importantly, this type of test is electricity/battery free, can be performed with capillary whole blood that does not require centrifugation and produces rapid results. Because lateral flow tests can demonstrate the result of more than one hemoglobin at a time, these devices can also detect heterozygotes (patients carrying two or more distinctive hemoglobin or patients who have been transfused with a differing hemoglobin).

4.5. HemeChip (micro-electrophoresis assay)

The newest published device for point-of-care testing in SCD is a small version of a hemoglobin electrophoresis. Minimal amount of blood (from a capillary stick) is required and placed on a piece of cellulose paper in alkaline buffer. The paper is then inserted into a device (**Figure 4**) that houses a micro-engineered plastic chip for cellulose acetate electrophoresis and uses a battery powered electric field to separate hemoglobin based on charge as described in standard hemoglobin electrophoresis. The result requires image quantitation using an intensity-based application on a mobile phone image. Results validated against standard EP and HPLC with correlation >0.96 for all hemoglobin tested including the ability to distinguish Hb F, S, C, A, D. This test utilizes the principles of electrophoresis to detect and distinguish hemoglobin based on the traveling distance from the sample application point and displays quantitative % hemoglobin fractions. A web-based image processing application for automated and objective quantification of HemeChip results at the POC using cloud computing resources [33].

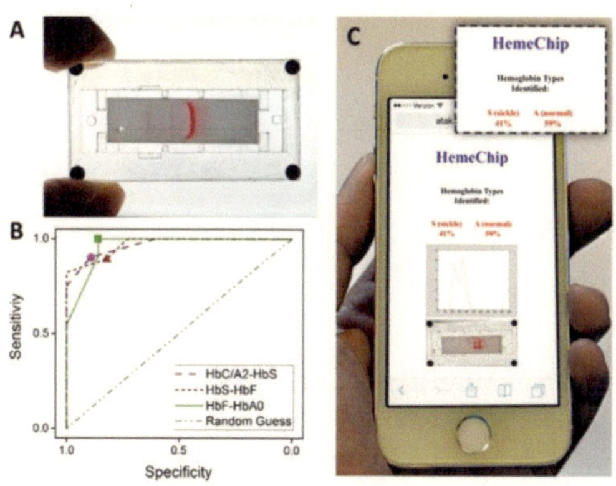

Figure 4. (a–c) Hemechip [33].

5. Discussion

Multiple point-of-care tests are currently in development for the identification of sickle cell disease at the point of care. It is important for confirmatory hematology testing, a multiplex device should be available for clinicians to make proper clinical assessments. As discussed, the device and method must distinguish target hemoglobin from interfering substances in blood that cause false-positive or negative results. It is clear that the pathophysiology of SCD, specifically the point mutations in the genome leading to the hemoglobin expression and the polymer formation that occurs upon cellular dehydration have been well utilized in the design of these testing devices. The optimal testing method will be the device that can produce at the lowest cost, easily utilized in a low-resource setting, with easy-to-interpret results and low false-negative results.

Based on the testing method described above, the lateral flow test is currently the most easily utilized in the field without requiring specialists for interpretation. This test has the capacity to clearly distinguish the majority of hemoglobin within a rapid period of time. However, it is unclear whether lateral flow tests will be cost prohibitive for widespread use. Alternatively, the Hemechip provides an excellent method for sickle cell disease confirmation also easily utilized in point-of-care settings although the interpretation requires additional skill as well as the use of mobile phone and internet access.

6. Conclusions

There are significant therapeutic and diagnostic health disparities that exist between SCD and other, inherited and acquired health conditions. Recent literature demonstrates that point-of-care diagnostics for sickle cell disease are feasible and accurate. Thus, it is hopeful that novel point-of-care diagnostics will change the screening paradigm for some areas in which central lab testing is not available.

Author details

Julie Kanter

Address all correspondence to: kanter@musc.edu

Medical University of South Carolina, Charleston, SC, USA

References

[1] Piel FB, Hay SI, Gupta S, Weatherall DJ, Williams TN. Global burden of sickle cell anaemia in children under five, 2010–2050: modelling based on demographics, excess mortality, and interventions. PLoS Med. 2013;10(7):e1001484.

[2] Grosse SD, Odame I, Atrash HK, Amendah DD, Piel FB, Williams TN. Sickle cell disease in Africa: a neglected cause of early childhood mortality. Am J Prev Med. 2011;41(6 Suppl. 4):S398–405.

[3] King L, Knight-Madden J, Reid M. Newborn screening for sickle cell disease in Jamaica: a review – past, present and future. West Indian Med J. 2014;63(2):147–150.

[4] Woods GM, Jorgensen JH, Waclawiw MA, et al. Influence of penicillin prophylaxis on antimicrobial resistance in nasopharyngeal S. pneumoniae among children with sickle cell anemia. The ancillary nasopharyngeal culture study of prophylactic penicillin study II. J Pediatr Hematol Oncol. 1997;19(4):327–333.

[5] Platt OS, Brambilla DJ, Rosse WF, et al. Mortality in sickle cell disease. Life expectancy and risk factors for early death. N Engl J Med. 1994;330(23):1639–1644.

[6] Newborn Screening. A blueprint for the future executive summary: newborn screening task force report. Pediatrics. 2000;106(2 Pt 2):386–388.

[7] Blinder MA, Vekeman F, Sasane M, Trahey A, Paley C, Duh MS. Age-related treatment patterns in sickle cell disease patients and the associated sickle cell complications and healthcare costs. Pediatr Blood Cancer. 2013;60(5):828–835.

[8] Gaston M. Screening for sickle cell disease. South Med J. 1974;67(3):257–258.

[9] Piel FB, Patil AP, Howes RE, et al. Global epidemiology of sickle haemoglobin in neonates: a contemporary geostatistical model-based map and population estimates. Lancet. 2013;381(9861):142–151.

[10] Clarke GM, Higgins TN. Laboratory investigation of hemoglobinopathies and thalassemias: review and update. Clin Chem. 2000;46(8 Pt 2):1284–1290.

[11] Jenkins MA, Ratnaike S. Capillary isoelectric focusing of haemoglobin variants in the clinical laboratory. Clin Chim Acta. 1999;289(1–2):121–132.

[12] Kutlar F, Kutlar A, Huisman TH. Separation of normal and abnormal hemoglobin chains by reversed-phase high-performance liquid chromatography. J Chromatogr. 1986;357(1):147–153.

[13] Kutlar A, Kutlar F, Wilson JB, Headlee MG, Huisman TH. Quantitation of hemoglobin components by high-performance cation-exchange liquid chromatography: its use in diagnosis and in the assessment of cellular distribution of hemoglobin variants. Am J Hematol. 1984;17(1):39–53.

[14] ITANO HA. Interpretation of electrophoretic, solubility and denaturation data in the study of hemoglobin differences. Fed Proc. 1957;16(3):748–756.

[15] McGann PT, Ferris MG, Ramamurthy U, et al. A prospective newborn screening and treatment program for sickle cell anemia in Luanda, Angola. Am J Hematol. 2013;88(12):984–989.

[16] McGann PT, Grosse SD, Santos B, et al. A cost-effectiveness analysis of a pilot neonatal screening program for sickle cell anemia in the Republic of Angola. J Pediatr. 2015;167(6):1314–1319.

[17] Serjeant GR, Ndugwa CM. Sickle cell disease in Uganda: a time for action. East Afr Med J. 2003;80(7):384–387.

[18] Okwi AL, Ocaido M, Byarugaba W, Ndugwa CM, Parkes A. Sickling and solubility tests and the peripheral blood film method for screening for sickle cell disease [corrected]. S Afr Med J. 2009;99(12):887–891.

[19] Ndugwa C, Higgs D, Fisher C, et al. Homozygous sickle cell disease in Uganda and Jamaica a comparison of Bantu and Benin haplotypes. West Indian Med J. 2012;61(7): 684–691.

[20] Rukundo H, Tumwesigye N, Wakwe VC. Screening for HIV I through the regional blood transfusion service in southwest Uganda: the Mbarara experience. Health Transit Rev. 1997;7(Suppl.):101–104.

[21] Serjeant GR. Jamaica, the Caribbean and sickle cell disease. West Indian Med J. 2012;61(4):331–337.

[22] Knight-Madden J, Serjeant GR. Invasive pneumococcal disease in homozygous sickle cell disease: Jamaican experience 1973–1997. J Pediatr. 2001;138(1):65–70.

[23] Collinson PO. The need for a point of care testing: an evidence-based appraisal. Scand J Clin Lab Invest Suppl. 1999;230:67–73.

[24] Kost GJ. Guidelines for point-of-care testing. Improving patient outcomes. Am J Clin Pathol. 1995;104(4 Suppl. 1):S111–S127.

[25] Alper SL. Harnessing red cell membrane pathophysiology towards point-of-care diagnosis for sickle cell disease. J Physiol. 2013;591(6):1403–1404.

[26] Kost GJ. Optimizing point-of-care testing in clinical systems management. Clin Lab Manage Rev. 1998;12(5):353–363.

[27] Kumar AA, Patton MR, Hennek JW, et al. Density-based separation in multiphase systems provides a simple method to identify sickle cell disease. Proc Natl Acad Sci USA. 2014;111(41):14864–14869.

[28] Kumar AA, Chunda-Liyoka C, Hennek JW, et al. Evaluation of a density-based rapid diagnostic test for sickle cell disease in a clinical setting in Zambia. PLoS One. 2014;9(12):e114540.

[29] Yang X, Kanter J, Piety NZ, Benton MS, Vignes SM, Shevkoplyas SS. A simple, rapid, low-cost diagnostic test for sickle cell disease. Lab Chip. 2013;13(8):1464–1467.

[30] Piety NZ, Yang X, Kanter J, Vignes SM, George A, Shevkoplyas SS. Validation of a low-cost paper-based screening test for sickle cell anemia. PLoS One. 2016;11(1):e0144901.

[31] Mark D, Haeberle S, Roth G, von Stetten F, Zengerle R. Microfluidic lab-on-a-chip platforms: requirements, characteristics and applications. Chem Soc Rev. 2010;39(3): 1153–1182.

[32] Kanter J, Telen MJ, Hoppe C, Roberts CL, Kim JS, Yang X. Validation of a novel point of care testing device for sickle cell disease. BMC Med. 2015;13:225.

[33] Ung R, Alapan Y, Hasan M et al. Point-of-Care Screening for Sickle Cell Disease By a Mobile Micro-Electrophoresis Platform. Blood 2015 126:3379.

Section 3

Mechanism of Pain in Sickle Cell Disease

Chapter 5

Mechanisms of Pain in Sickle Cell Disease

Anupam Aich, Alvin J Beitz and Kalpna Gupta

Additional information is available at the end of the chapter

http://dx.doi.org/10.5772/64647

Abstract

Pain is one of the most common features of sickle cell disease (SCD) lacking effective therapy. Pain in SCD is relatively more complicated than other conditions associated with pain requiring understanding of the pathobiology of pain specific to SCD. The characterization of pain to define the diverse modalities of nociception in SCD is currently under progress via human studies accompanied by transgenic mouse models of SCD. Sickle pathobiology characterized by oxidative stress, inflammation and vascular dysfunction contributes to both peripheral and central nociceptive sensitization via mast cell activation in the periphery, and reactive oxygen species and glial activation and endoplasmic reticulum stress in the spinal cord among other effectors. These effects are mediated via several cellular receptors, which can be targeted to produce positive therapeutic outcomes. In this chapter, we will discuss the present understanding of molecular mechanisms of SCD pain and outline the mechanism-based translational potential of novel actionable targets to treat SCD pain.

Keywords: pain, sickle cell disease, neurogenic inflammation, substance P, mast cell

1. Introduction

Pain is a hallmark feature of sickle cell disease (SCD), which can start in infancy, leading to hospitalization, reduced survival and poor quality of life. Pain in SCD is unique because of unpredictable and recurrent episodes of acute pain due to vaso-occlusive crises (VOC), in addition to chronic pain experienced by a majority of adult patients on a daily basis [1]. Treatment choices remain limited to opioids, which impose liabilities of their own including constipation, mast cell activation, fear of addiction and respiratory depression [2]. Moreover, significantly larger doses of opioids are required to treat pain in SCD as compared to other acute and chronic pain conditions [1]. Pain can be lifelong in SCD and may therefore influence cognitive function and lead to depression and anxiety, which can in turn promote the perception of pain [1].

Treatment of chronic pain remains unsatisfactory overall, perhaps due to the diverse pathobiology in different diseases. Therefore, it is critical to understand the mechanisms specific to the genesis of sickle pain to develop targeted therapies. Vascular dysfunction, inflammation, ischemia/reperfusion injury and oxidative stress in the wake of VOC can each evoke activation of the nociceptive nerve fibers leading to acute pain. On the other hand, constant endothelial activation, inflammation and reactive oxygen species (ROS) generation may underlie the nerve injury leading to chronic inflammatory and/or neuropathic pain. Endothelial activation, inflammation and oxidative stress have been extensively characterized in the periphery [1] but not in the central nervous system in SCD. Both peripheral and central mechanisms may underlie the nociceptor activation leading to pain. In this chapter, we describe the sickle pathobiology that may contribute to pain and define possible treatable targets.

1.1. Presentation of pain in SCD

Current research in characterizing pain in SCD patients indicates that both acute and chronic pain are prevalent among the adult patients, while infants and children mostly suffer from acute pain [3–5]. The shift from acute to chronic pain may therefore occur during the transition from childhood to adolescence. Young children with a median age of 3.8 years (range 0.3–7.6 years) exhibited less frequent pain, occurring on 1.6% of a total of 141,197 days [3]. Yet, only 14% of these episodes required hospitalization, and infants between the age of 0 and 12 months had the most pain (80%) associated with dactylitis [3]. In another study on 100 young subjects, about 40% of children and adolescents in the age range of 8–18 years reported chronic pain with another 40% exhibiting episodic pain, and the remainder had no pain [4]. Though the pain intensity and quality of life were comparable among the young patients with chronic and episodic pain, the patients with chronic pain suffered from greater functional disability, depression and hospital admissions compared to the episodic pain group [4]. The adult patients recruited in the Pain in Sickle Cell Epidemiology Study (PiSCES) reported chronic SCD pain on 54.5% of 31,017 days at home [5]. Opioids have remained the major strategy to treat acute sickle pain, while chronic pain is managed with the combination of non-steroidal anti-inflammatory drugs (NSAIDs), opioids, anti-depressants and anticonvulsant medications [6]. However, to date no satisfactory therapy exists.

2. Characteristics of pain in SCD

Based on transgenic mouse models of SCD and presentation of pain in patients, four major characteristics of pain have been described (**Table 1**). These characteristics include increased sensitivity to (i) mechanical, (ii) heat and (iii) cold stimuli and (iv) decreased grip force ([3, 7–12, 14–17, 22–27], Lei et al., 2016, under review). Characterization of SCD pain in patients has been quite challenging due to the episodic and sudden nature of the acute pain, often requiring hospitalization. The characterization of chronic pain is challenging owing to the complex and

Characteristics of pain	Pain phenotyping method	
	Subjects with SCD	Transgenic mice expressing sickle hemoglobin
Mechanical hyperalgesia	QST—tactile sensation using a cotton ball, hand-held soft brush and non-penetrating pin-pick on the left/right forearm [7] and reported via visual analog scale QST—using von Frey filaments at the thenar eminence of non-dominant hands and lateral dorsum of randomly selected foot [8]	Paw withdrawal responses to von Frey monofilaments in NY1DD & S+S^{antilles} mice [9], in BERK mice [9–13] and in Townes mice [Lei et al., communicated]
Heat hyperalgesia	QST—using Thermal Sensory Analyzer (Medoc: Israel) which employs cold temperature to the skin via a peltier-based thermode [7, 8]	Paw withdrawal latency and frequency in response to static heat stimuli in BERK mice [9, 11–13] and in Townes mice [14], Lei et al., 2016, under review]
Cold hyperalgesia	QST—using Thermal Sensory Analyzer (Medoc: Israel) which employs cold temperature to the skin via a peltier-based thermode [7, 8, 15] Case-crossover study and retrospective statistical analysis of occurrence of pain/VOCs in relation to weather conditions [16–20]	Paw withdrawal latency and frequency in response to static cold stimuli in S+S^{antilles} mice [9], in BERK mice [9, 10, 12, 13] and in Townes mice [[14], Lei et al., 2016, under review] Temperature preference assay for BERK mice [21]
Deep-tissue/ musculoskeletal hyperalgesia	Questionnaire-based assessment using the Nordic musculoskeletal symptoms questionnaire and the SF-36 Health Survey [22]	Tensile force of peak forelimb exertion measured using grip force meter—in NY1DD & S+S^{antilles} mice [9], in BERK mice [9–12] and in Townes mice [Lei et al., 2016, under review]
Observer-based Quantification	Not documented	Observer-based quantification of facial expression measured by action units and body parameters from changes in the back curvature [23]

Table 1. Characteristics of pain in SCD.

intractable nature of SCD pain, which may have a combination of inflammatory, nociceptive and/or neuropathic origin. Clinical studies have used the patient-reported questionnaire-based assessment and quantitative sensory testing (QST) approaches to evaluating the nature and characteristics of pain in patients [7, 15, 28–30]. In a recent QST of 48 children with SCD, 13 individuals exhibited increased mechanical allodynia and also decreased sensitivity to heat or cold detection (hypoesthesia) [7]. A similar study of 27 SCD patients aged 10.3–18.3 years with race-matched control patients corroborated the heat-cold sensation features but demonstrated an increased cold-pain feature in SCD patients [15]. In contrast, Brandow et al. [8].

found a decreased threshold for cold and heat detection in a cohort of 55 SCD patients (≥7 years old) compared to 57 race-matched healthy controls [8]. In contrast, no significant differences were observed in these patients in response to mechanical stimuli [8]. Cold hypersensitivity under cold weather conditions has been found to be associated with pain and VOC in pediatric [18]. and adult patients [19, 20]. Musculoskeletal/deep-tissue pain has been found to be present at multiple sites including the arms, chest and lower back in a questionnaire-based study of 27 adult patients with mean age of 31.77 years [22].

In parallel, transgenic mouse models expressing human sickle hemoglobin, which mimic the SCD pathobiology and pain, have been highly instructive in developing the understanding of sickle pain [9]. Transgenic sickle mouse models have been able to recapitulate the features of SCD with variable severity depending upon the extent of expression of human sickle hemoglobin (HbS) and the presence/or absence of mouse hemoglobin α and β [31]. NY1DD sickle mice developed by Fabry et al. contain a single copy of the human α and β^s transgene with deletion of mouse major β genes, but express mouse α chains and express about 26% HbS leading to a mild phenotype [32]. S+S^{antilles} mice carry an additional mutation and express about 42% of human β^s showing a stronger phenotype than NY1DD mice [33]. These mice with milder pathology do not show significant characteristics of chronic or acute pain [9], which can be induced by hypoxia/reoxygenation. On the other hand, homozygous Townes [34] and Berkeley (BERK) [35] transgenic mice express exclusively human α and β hemoglobins without mouse α or β chains and express >99% human HbS. Consequently, these mice demonstrate a severe SCD phenotype including excessive hemolysis, inflammation, organ damage and shorter life span [26, 31, 34–37]. BERK and Townes models show constitutive chronic hyperalgesia early in life ([12], Lei et al., 2016, under review). Moreover, hypoxia/reoxygenation treatment evokes a further increase in hyperalgesia simulating acute pain during VOC, compared to their specific background strains expressing normal human hemoglobin A ([12], Lei et al., 2016, under review). Therefore, BERK and Townes homozygous sickle mice exhibit human sickle pathology as well as pain similar to patients with SCD. Hence, both of these models are well suited to understand how sickle pathobiology leads to the genesis and progression of pain in SCD recalcitrant to therapy.

3. Sickle pathobiology underlying pain

Sickling of RBCs under low oxygen due to a point mutation in the beta hemoglobin chain of hemoglobin is the primary pathogenic condition in SCD [13]. Sickle RBCs have impaired oxygen-carrying ability and cause jamming of micro-capillaries via adhesion to endothelial walls in the event known as VOC [21]. Resultant SCD pathobiology is characterized by inflammation, oxidative stress, ischemia reperfusion injury and organ damage [21], all of which can independently and/or cumulatively lead to activation of the nociceptive system (**Figure 1**). For example, the increased levels of inflammatory cytokines, such as TNFα and IL-6 [38] in the periphery and the central nervous system (CNS) can activate nociceptors and spinal nociceptive neurons, which may in turn be an outcome of activated macrophages or mast cells in the periphery and glial cells in the CNS driving a vicious cycle of inflammation

http://dx.doi.org/10.5772/64647

and pain (**Figure 1**). Decreased oxygenation and reduced blood supply due to vascular occlusion during VOC may impair oxygenation and nutrient supply to the nerve fibers, thus causing nerve damage and activation of nociceptors. Hematologic, inflammatory and vascular dysfunctions have been well characterized in the periphery, but not in the CNS in subjects with SCD and in sickle mice [21, 39]. Our laboratory demonstrated oxidative stress, increased inflammatory cytokines and neuropeptides in the spinal cord of sickle mice as compared to control mice [12, 40]. Thus, sickling of RBCs affects the periphery and the CNS, which may lead to a complex pathobiology of pain in SCD leading to inflammatory, nociceptive and neuropathic pain. SCD is also characterized by phenotypic heterogeneity and unpredictable episodes of VOC, which may vary in frequency, recurrence and intensity among patients [21]. Therefore, SCD pain displays a marked heterogeneity in the context of neurobiology.

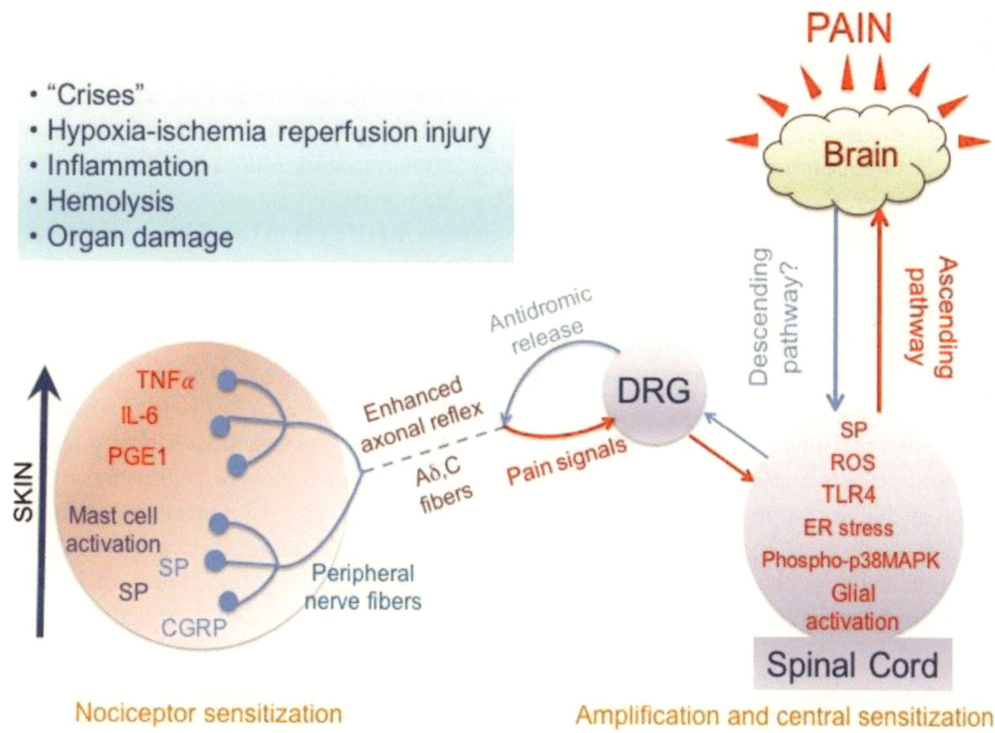

Figure 1. Sickle pathobiology evoked peripheral and central mechanisms of pain: Sickle pathobiology comprising vaso-occlusive crises, hypoxia/reoxygenation injury, hemolysis, inflammation and organ damage can sensitize nerve fibers in the periphery. Activated mast cells release neuropeptide substance P (SP) and other mediators in the skin further sensitizing peripheral nociceptors. Pain signals are transmitted from periphery through dorsal root ganglion (DRG) and spinal cord to the brain. Increased reactive oxygen species (ROS) and endoplasmic reticulum (ER) stress, inflammatory milieu, glial activation accompanied by increased toll-like receptor 4 (TLR4) phosphorylation of p38MAPK with correlative nociceptor sensitization in the spinal cord of sickle mice suggest persistent central sensitization. Sustained and enhanced central sensitization contributes to antidromic release of neuropeptides and nociceptive mediators in the periphery, which in turn accentuates peripheral nociception without noxious stimuli. Thus, a vicious feed-forward cycle of peripheral and central sensitization continues and chronic pain persists in sickle pathobiology.

4. Peripheral and central mechanisms of pain in SCD

Transgenic mouse models described above have been highly instructive in examining the mechanisms specific to sickle pain. Pain can be both chronic as well as acute following VOC and the underlying mechanisms may or may not vary between the two. BERK sickle mice show significantly higher chronic hyperalgesia as compared to age- and gender-matched Townes sickle mice (Lei et al., 2016, under review). Most of the mechanisms have been examined in BERK sickle mice for both chronic hyperalgesia constitutively existent in these mice and acute pain following hypoxia/reoxygenation to simulate VOC [9]. Structural analysis of the skin of homozygous BERK mice (expressing human sickle hemoglobin) compared to control mice (expressing normal human hemoglobin) showed alterations in nerve fibers and blood vessels [12]. Vascular and nerve plexi as well as normal branching is diminished in BERK sickle mice skin, showing nerve sprouting indicative of inflammatory and neuropathic pain [12]. These structural changes are accompanied by increased expression of neuropeptides substance P (SP) and calcitonin-gene-related peptides (CGRP) in the skin [12]. Concomitantly, skin in BERK sickle mice is significantly thinner with a comparatively thinner epidermis, similar to that observed in other murine models of pain such as diabetes [41]. These structural and neuro-chemical alterations in association with well-known inflammatory milieu may likely activate nociceptors on the peripheral nerve terminals as demonstrated by activation of transient receptor potential cation channel subfamily V member 1 (TRPV1) in the skin of BERK sickle mice [11]. This peripheral nociceptor activation leads to the activation of glial cells and neuronal activating transcription factor 3 (ATF3) in the dorsal root ganglion (DRG) [10], which may lead to the transmission of increased action potentials to the second-order neurons of the spinal cord. Indeed, second-order neurons in the dorsal horn of the spinal cord show constitutive nociceptor sensitization in electrophysiological recordings in the BERK sickle mice [42]. Nociceptive neurons in the dorsal horn of sickle mice show increased excitability and an increased rate of spontaneous activity [42]. These electrophysiological responses are accompanied by higher response to mechanical stimuli and prolonged after-discharges following the mechanical stimulus, suggestive of central sensitization [42]. This sustained and continuous activation of spinal neurons may lead to increased release of neuropeptides and nociceptive mediators, which may be released into the periphery antidromically, in turn activating the peripheral nerve terminals without noxious insult. This vicious feed-forward cycle of peripheral and central sensitization may underlie chronic pain recalcitrant to therapy. Also, increased phosphorylation of mitogen-activated protein kinases related to neuronal hyper-excitability is supportive of central sensitization in sickle mice [42]. Concurrently, Darbari et al. evaluated brain connectivity in 25 adolescent and young patients using functional magnetic resonance imaging (fMRI), and these patients were divided into low and high pain groups based on their hospitalization frequency [25]. In the fMRI analysis, the high pain group exhibited excessive pronociceptive connectivity while the low pain group displayed greater association with brain regions implicated in anti-nociception [25]. In this study, although all the patients were on hydroxyurea, the expression of fetal hemoglobin (HbF) was higher in the low pain group and was in positive correlation with anti-nociceptive connectivity [25]. These results suggest involvement of central mechanisms in sickle pain. Moreover, central sensitization in sickle patients was recently evaluated using QST, questionnaires and daily pain diaries [29]. Those patients with higher scores for central sensitization exhibited worse manifestations of SCD. Therefore, understanding the molecular mechanisms that drive peripheral nociceptor and central nociceptive neuronal activation is cardinal to developing effective therapies.

We found that mast cells, a tissue-resident granulocyte, are activated in the skin of sickle mice and contribute to neurogenic inflammation, inflammation and pain [43]. Mast cells from sickle mouse skin show significantly higher transcripts for toll-like receptor 4 (TLR4) as compared to mast cells from control mice [43]. Moreover, heme, the product of excessive hemolysis, a significant feature of SCD, can activate mast cells in the periphery. Additionally, spinal TLR4 expression and cell-free heme are significantly higher in sickle mice compared to control mice (Lei et al., under preparation). It has been shown that excess heme can induce spinal microglial activation via TLR4 in vitro [44], and thus, this may be a mechanism contributing to central sensitization in sickle patients. In this regard, spinal microglial activation is suggested to be a contributor to central sensitization leading to pain [45]. Spinal microglial and astroglial activation is correlative to increased ROS production and SP in the spinal cord of sickle mice [40]. Spinal microglial activation and ROS production via TLR4 can also be an accessory to the central sensitization process [44]. Most of these studies were performed in male mice. Recently, Sorge et al. have demonstrated that nerve injury-induced pain in male mice (not in female mice) are mediated via TLR4 (possibly via microglial activation) [46], but via T-lymphocytes instead of microglial cells in female mice [47]. Though the PiSCES report (from extensive multi-center human study on sickle pain) found no significant difference in pain sensation and intensity according to gender differences [48], it is yet to be demonstrated/verified whether sickle pain is mediated via gender-specific pathways.

Peripheral injury due to acute VOC evokes acute pain, but it is likely that the chronic inflammatory state, oxidative stress, vascular dysfunction and nerve injury lead to sustained sensitization of both peripheral and central nociceptive neurons. SCD pain can also be of neuropathic origin, which has been demonstrated in patient-reported [49, 50] and QST-based studies [30]. Circulating glial fibrillary acidic protein (GFAP) and SP expression are significantly higher in subjects with SCD as compared to normal healthy subjects [51, 52]. In a group of 2–18-year-old SCD patients, serum SP levels were found to be elevated, which increased further during VOC [52]. SP possibly acts on neurokinin 2 (NK2) receptors to sensitize TRPV1 leading to an enhancement of afferent excitability and an increase in peripheral nociception [11]. SP can further contribute to plasma extravasation due to its vasodilatory effect leading to neurogenic inflammation, in addition to activating mast cells [43, 53]. The painful dactylitis in children with SCD [3] may be due to neurogenic inflammation in response to increased release of SP from the peripheral nerve terminals. Increased GFAP has been associated with stroke in children with SCD and supports increased glial cell activity observed in the DRG and dorsal horn of the spinal cord of sickle mice [12, 40, 51]. Zappia et al. found that cold hyperalgesia in sickle mice increases with age [54], and these data are in accord with the finding that sickle patients experience increased thermal hypersensitivity as they age [8]. Additionally, the expression of endothelin 1 and tachykinin receptor 1 were increased by 2.7- and 1.6-fold, respectively, in the DRG of sickle mice, compared to control mice [54]. Endothelin 1 may contribute to cold hyperalgesia via endothelin receptors [55], and SP can contribute to hyperalgesia via tachykinin 1 [56] located in the peripheral nervous system. These findings suggest that diverse SCD pathobiology underlies the genesis and progression of recalcitrant pain in SCD. Therefore, multimodal targeting may be required in a case-specific manner to achieve satisfactory analgesic outcomes.

5. Treatable targets for ameliorating sickle pain

5.1. Opioid receptors (ORs)

The current mainstay of treatment for acute and chronic pain in SCD is opioids. To assess opioid effects on chronic SCD pain in adult patients, 15,778 home pain days of 219 patients were monitored [57]. On 78% of the pain days, the patients used opioids—38% of the total patients used long-acting opioids and 47% used short-acting opioids. The striking outcome of this study was that the opioid usage significantly correlates with the severity of pain intensity and other manifestations of SCD—suggestive of negative impact of the opioids on the pathophysiology of chronic SCD [57].

Although the analgesic action of morphine is vital for pain remission, the effects of morphine can be multifactorial leading to opioid-induced hyperalgesia [58] and possible exacerbation of other complications of SCD [2]. Morphine exacerbates renal pathology in sickle mice [59], and its interaction with TLR4 may promote neuroinflammation [60]. Morphine-induced angiogenesis and co-activation of receptor tyrosine kinases may influence organ pathology including retinopathy, nephropathy, stroke and pulmonary arterial hypertension [2].

Among four different opioid receptors, mu opioid receptor (MOR) facilitates analgesic action of opioids [2]. Repeated activation of MORs can lead to tolerance to opioids. Morphine transactivates platelet-derived growth factor receptor—beta (PDGFR-β) [61]—and inhibition of PDGFR-β by imatinib (a tyrosine kinase inhibitor) attenuates morphine tolerance [62]. Reversal of tolerance to morphine by Imatinib can also be a consequence of reduced activation of mast cells as discussed below. Therefore, strategies to ameliorate the side effects and reduce tolerance are required to optimize pain control with opioids.

Nociceptin opioid receptor (NOP/OR) is another member of opioid receptor family which contributes to nociceptive signaling [63]. The endogenous ligand of NOP/OR is nociceptin/orphanin FQ (N/OFQ), and it is known to attenuate secretion of neuropeptides (SP and CGRP) from peripheral nerve endings [64] and from mast cells [65]. Our recent findings demonstrate that a small molecule agonist of NOP/OR, AT200, is able to decrease hyperalgesia in sickle mice by reducing inflammation and mast cell activation [66]. Continuous treatment of sickle mice with AT200 did not produce any tolerance, suggestive of a feasible opioid drug devoid of tolerance. This approach of targeting other ORs with potential to attenuate underlying sickle pathobiology needs to be investigated further.

http://dx.doi.org/10.5772/64647

5.2. Mast cells

Mast cells are tissue resident granulocytes, well known for their role in pruritis and anaphylaxis [67]. We (Gupta et al.) found that mast cell activation contributes to pain in sickle mice [43]. Constitutive mast cell activation leads to inflammation characterized by the release of inflammatory cytokines in the skin and neurogenic inflammation in sickle mice. Cromolyn sodium, a mast cell stabilizer, and imatinib, an inhibitor of mast cell c-kit, attenuated these mast cell associated effects in mice [43]. Neurogenic inflammation characterized by excessive plasma leakage from the vasculature in response to SP released from the nerve terminals is reminiscent of painful dactylitis in children with SCD. Activated mast cells release tryptase, which activates protease-activator receptor 2 (PAR2) on peripheral nerve endings stimulating the release of SP [43]. In turn, SP then stimulates vascular leakage and vasodilation as well as further activation of mast cells, leading to a vicious cycle of inflammation, neurogenic inflammation and hyperalgesia [43]. Pharmacological and genetic inhibition of mast cells contributes to reduction in sickle pain in mice [43].

Morphine is an activator of mast cell degranulation [67]. Sickle mice pre-treated with cromolyn or imatinib show increased analgesic response to a sub-optimal dose of morphine [43]. It is therefore likely that morphine acts on the CNS to induce analgesia but promotes hyperalgesia by simultaneously activating mast cells, resulting in reduced analgesic efficacy. Therefore, co-treatment strategies with mast cell stabilizers or imatinib may improve analgesic outcomes and reduce tolerance (as discussed above) and may even minimize the side effects of opioids.

Products released from activated mast cells include SP, cytokines and growth factors, such as PDGF and VEGF, which can directly act on the vasculature in the vicinity [67]. We have recently observed that mast cell-derived mediators cause increased permeability in monolayers of mouse brain microvascular endothelial cells by stimulating endoplasmic reticulum (ER) stress [Luk et al., communicated]. Additionally, ER stress has been shown to mediate pain in diabetic neuropathic rats [68]. Thus, inhibiting mast cells in combination with ER stress inhibitors may have an impact on endothelial dysfunction and pain—two critical characteristic features of SCD. Therefore, common targets influencing vascular, inflammatory and nociceptive mechanisms may provide comparatively more effective treatable targets that reduce pain, inflammation and vascular complications without inadvertent effects on SCD.

5.3. Cannabinoid receptors (CBRs)

Cannabinoid receptors (CBRs) CB1R and CB2R are 7-transmembrane G-protein coupled receptors, expressed in the CNS, as well as on vascular and inflammatory cells [69]. Like opioids, cannabinoids that bind to CBRs have been used for centuries for medical and recreational purposes. Cannabinoids have remained controversial due to their misuse for recreational and euphoric effects [69]. Moreover, the schedule 1 status and stringent regulatory requirements have been a major deterrent in the development of these drugs for analgesia. The presence of CB1R and CB2R in the neuro-immune system makes them an attractive target for treating sickle pain. Several specific CB2R agonists have been developed to prevent the adverse effects of cannabinoids on CB1R, which is known to promote the euphoric and CNS-related effects. We found that CP55,940, a non-selective CBR agonist, which binds to both CB1R and

CB2R, ameliorates chronic and hypoxia/reoxygenation evoked hyperalgesia in sickle mice [9, 12]. However, subsequent studies targeting the contribution of individual CBRs in sickle mice show that CB1R agonists reduce mechanical, thermal and deep tissue hyperalgesia, while CB2R agonists reduce deep tissue hyperalgesia only in both chronic and acute hypoxia-/reoxygenation-evoked hyperalgesia [24]. Importantly, CB1R agonists ameliorated neurogenic inflammation, while CB2R agonists reduced mast cell activation in sickle mice, suggesting that both CB1Rs and CB2Rs are potentially critical to treat sickle pain and its underlying pathobiology.

Recently, multiple sclerosis patients experiencing spasticity and neuropathic pain exhibited significantly improved response to Sativex, a cannabis-derived oromucosal spray [70, 71]. Efficacy of Sativex for treating cancer pain is currently being tested [72], and use of cannabinoids also potentiates and improves the analgesic action of opioids in chronic pain conditions [73]. Additionally, cannabinoids attenuate ischemia/reperfusion injury [74], which is a hallmark feature of VOC in SCD.

Collectively, these results suggest that targeting CBRs may provide analgesia via not only anti-nociceptive mechanisms but also due to its potential to ameliorate the complex pathobiology of SCD—consequently improving the overall efficacy of the treatment. A questionnaire-based study found that 52% of the sickle patients, who self-administered marijuana, used it to relieve, reduce or prevent acute or chronic pain [75]. Therefore, CBRs offer an effective target to ameliorate pain in SCD.

5.4. Toll-like receptor 4 (TLR4)

TLR4 is the first discovered cell surface receptor of this family, which is essential for pathogen detection in innate immunity via lipopolysaccharide (LPS) recognition [76]. TLR4 has been shown to be associated with several modalities of pain including inflammatory pain [46, 77], neuropathic pain [46, 78–80], post-operative cognitive dysfunction [81], cancer pain [82], etc. Recent studies in the SCD field suggest that TLR4 activation may be a significant contributor to the multifactorial effects in SCD ranging from vaso-occlusion and inflammation to pain [83]. Heme is a product of excessive hemolysis in SCD, and heme acts as an activator for TLR4 [84]. In transgenic sickle mice, heme-activated TLR4 signaling contributes to acute lung injury (a major feature of SCD) [85] and heme-induced endothelial TLR4 activation contributes to VOC [86].

We (Gupta et al.) found that in transgenic sickle mice TLR4 expression is elevated in the spinal cord compared to control mice [12]. Spinal microglial cells are known to be involved in nociceptive signaling [46]. These cells isolated from sickle and control mice, when stimulated with hemin, exhibited activation dependent on TLR4, and this activation was mediated via ROS production and ER stress [44]. Additionally, we have observed increased expression of TLR4 in cultures of skin mast cells from sickle mice vs control mice [43]. Subsequently, genetic [87] and pharmacological [88] inhibition of TLR4 in sickle mice led to amelioration of hyperalgesia and neurogenic inflammation in transgenic sickle mice. Morphine tolerance exhibited by the SCD patients may also be a result of morphine's potential for TLR4 activation [2, 89, 90]. However, it is suggested that TLR4 may be involved in pain processing only in males [46], whereas knocking out TLR4 affected cisplatin-induced mechanical allodynia in both male and female mice [91]. No adverse off-target effects of targeting of TLR4 in other disease conditions have been observed so far [92, 93]. Therefore, the contribution of TLR4 in sickle pain needs to be evaluated.

5.5. Other targets

A calcium-modulating serine/threonine protein kinase present in the CNS, Ca^{2+}/calmodulin protein kinase IIα (CaMKIIα), has been of recent interest as a modulator of neuropathic pain and is an important contributor to initiation and maintenance of opioid-induced hyperalgesia [94]. Recently, in a limited clinical trial, 18 SCD patients were treated with single dosage of trifluoperazine (a CaMKIIα inhibitor) going up to 10 mg, and eight subjects reported almost 50% reduction in their chronic pain. This study established 10 mg as the toxicity limit, and the improvement in patients' health without any adverse effect warrants a randomized clinical trial to evaluate efficacy of this treatment strategy in SCD patients [95].

Dexmedetomidine, a specific α_2-adrenoreceptor agonist, provides anti-nociception independent of opioid receptor action and via inhibition of sensory neurons [96]. This molecule also provides protection from ischemia/reperfusion injury [96]. These properties of dexmedomidine led to a study of its efficacy in sickle mice, and Calhoun et al. found that transgenic sickle mice receiving dexmedomidine had improved analgesia [97]. This may provide an adjuvant to existing analgesic treatment strategies used for reducing pain in SCD patients.

5.6. Integrative approaches

We observed that curcumin, an active ingredient of turmeric and Coenzyme Q10 independently ameliorated chronic hyperalgesia in sickle mice when used over a period of 4 weeks [40]. These treatments also reduced oxidative stress, microglial activation and SP in the spinal cords of sickle mice. In a clinical study on sickle patients, treatment with Coenzyme Q10 reduced the incidence of VOC [98]. In rheumatoid- and osteo-arthritis, curcumin or Theracurcumin with higher bioavailability was effective in reducing pain, inflammation and oxidative stress and symptoms of osteoarthritis in separate studies, including a randomized, double-blind, placebo-controlled trial [99, 100]. Curcumin lowered the oxidative stress and iron overload in the spleen and liver of rats with chronic iron overload [101]. Importantly, in thalassemia patients, curcumin reduced oxidative stress [102]. Thalassemia often co-exists with SCD [103], and increased iron in the tissues due to hemolysis is a characteristic feature of SCD [104]. Therefore, these dietary supplements may provide an advantage in treating sickle pathobiology and pain without the inadvertent side effects of pharmacologics discussed above.

Acupuncture has been evolving as a promising approach to relieve chronic pain. Along with several case reports [105–107], a retrospective study of 47 adult SCD patients demonstrated significant improvement in analgesia using acupuncture treatment [108]. Therefore, we developed a novel electroacupuncture (EA) method to treat awake/conscious mice to elucidate central and peripheral mechanisms contributing to acupuncture-induced analgesia without the influence of anesthesia. We found that EA in awake sickle BERK mice significantly reduces mechanical, deep tissue and cold hyperalgesia [Wang et al., in preparation]. Response to EA was variable, but majority of sickle mice showed a high analgesic response, exhibiting reduced systemic inflammation, in addition to reduced peripheral inflammation and neuroinflammation. Integrative approaches such as acupuncture for pain control could be potentially beneficial in treating pain in SCD.

5.7. Co-treatment strategies

Mechanism-driven understanding of SCD pain pathology from basic research provides us with a variety of treatable targets as mentioned above. The promise of these different modulators of SCD pain is quite exciting; but to become viable treatment options for the SCD patients, they require systematic and rigorous clinical trials for evaluating their efficacy and any side effects that they may pose.

6. Translational potential of treatable targets-based pharmacologics

From the discussion above, it is clear that targeting sickle pain may require multiple pharmacologics due to the complex nature of SCD pathobiology and associated nociceptive mechanisms. In this regard, we can first evaluate FDA approved drugs for sickle pain based on preclinical data. Imatinib is approved by the FDA for managing chronic myeloid leukemia systemic mastocytosis [109]. Thus, mast cell inhibition via imatinib can reduce morphine-induced mast cell activation and may also enhance the efficacy of sub-optimal doses of morphine. A small study in a cohort of 17 patients using a nasal spray form of the mast cell stabilizer, cromolyn, in combination with hydroxyurea indicated that these patients experienced reduced pain when compared to placebo or to the use of cromolyn or hydroxyurea alone [110]. Thus, FDA-approved mast cell stabilizers available for reducing airway inflammation can be potentially effective as adjuvants for sickle pain.

SP acts via NK-1 receptors and NK-1 receptor antagonists have been effective in different pain pathologies in animal models, but have failed to show efficacy in clinical trials [111]. Aprepitant, an FDA-approved NK-1 receptor antagonist for chemotherapy-induced nausea and vomiting, has been assessed for the effects on electrical hyperalgesia models of human volunteers, but did not show any efficacy [112]. However, in a separate study acute doses of aprepitant were shown to significantly increase the magnitude of *mu* agonist signs and symptoms in response to oxycodone [113]. Considering the role of SP in sickle pain and neurogenic inflammation, NK-1 receptor antagonists require further examination in preclinical models of SCD as co-drugs.

Additionally, TLR4 inhibitors such as TAK-242 and eritoran showed promising responses in animal studies for severe sepsis, but failed to show any efficacy in reducing 28-day mortality in phase III clinical trials [114, 115]. Though these molecules are still being evaluated for other pathologic conditions such as obesity in type 2 diabetic subjects [116], no clinical trials have been undertaken using these compounds to ameliorate chronic pain conditions. Interestingly, a nonspecific phosphodiesterase (PDE4) inhibitor, ibudilast, has been shown to inhibit TLR4 and microglial activation in animal models [117] and is currently in separate clinical trials for migraine pain, multiple sclerosis and opioid abuse [118–120].

Stemming from our animal research, we are currently conducting a trial to evaluate the effect of vaporized cannabis on pain in human subjects with SCD [121]. Vaporized cannabis offers an advantage over systemically administered cannabis, because it is not metabolized by the liver and may therefore not influence organ pathology in SCD.

Apart from the targets discussed in this section, other targets such as calcium signaling and oxidative stress can be managed using pharmacologics such as trifluoperazine and curcumin/CoQ10, respectively. Curcumin and/or CoQ10 showed reduction in pain in sickle mice and CoQ10 showed reduced "crises" in a small cohort of sickle patients [40, 98]. Other integrative approaches including arginine therapy and acupuncture show reduced pain/crises in patients with SCD [108, 122]. Thus, in addition to pharmacologics, integrative approaches offer the potential to reduce sickle pain. Finally, gene therapy vectors are a new tool for the development of molecularly selective pain therapies, which have been shown to provide reliable analgesia in preclinical models [123]. The use of gene therapy may lead to a new class of analgesic treatments based on the molecular selectivity of analgesic genes.

7. Future directions

Sickle cell disease comprises highly complex pathobiology and the associated pain involves a complicated pathophysiology that we are only beginning to appreciate. Therefore, treatment strategies solely targeting the nervous system do not promise pain remission in an effective manner. Rather, as discussed in this chapter, as our understanding of the mechanistic biological targets that potentiate pain and neurogenic inflammation in SCD increases, we must incorporate multiple approaches towards alleviation of this morbid pain syndrome. The tortuous nature of SCD pain involving both central and peripheral nervous systems requires co-treatment strategies, which will ameliorate simultaneously RBC pathology leading to vaso-occlusion, mast cell activation leading to neurogenic inflammation and pain, microglial activation via increased oxidative stress, heme-induced TLR4-mediated neuronal and vascular complications, hemolysis-driven high iron/calcium-mediated pathologies, etc. Translational and clinical studies are required to evaluate the physiological relevance of these targets in order to develop effective analgesics devoid of inadvertent adverse effects. The issue of transition from acute to chronic pain is an unanswered question in SCD and other pathologies, which remains to be understood.

Acknowledgements

We thank Yann Lamarre, PhD, for the artistic illustration of **Figure 1**. Authors are also thankful to the Institute for Engineering in Medicine, University of Minnesota and NIH grants, RO1 103773 and UO1 HL117664 to K.G for funding support. The content is solely the responsibility of the authors and does not necessarily represent the official views of the National Institutes of Health.

Author details

Anupam Aich[1], Alvin J Beitz[2] and Kalpna Gupta[1*]

*Address all correspondence to: gupta014@umn.edu

1 Vascular Biology Center, Division of Hematology, Oncology and Transplantation, Department of Medicine, University of Minnesota, Minneapolis, MN, USA

2 Department of Veterinary and Biomedical Sciences, University of Minnesota, Minneapolis, MN, USA

References

[1] Ballas SK, Gupta K, Adams-Graves P. Sickle cell pain: a critical reappraisal. Blood. 2012;12018:3647–56.

[2] Gupta M, Msambichaka L, Ballas SK, Gupta K. Morphine for the treatment of pain in sickle cell disease. Sci World J. 2015;2015:10.

[3] Dampier C, Ely B, Brodecki D, Coleman C, Aertker L, Sendecki JA, et al. Pain characteristics and age-related pain trajectories in infants and young children with sickle cell disease. Pediatr Blood Cancer. 2014;612:291–6.

[4] Sil S, Cohen LL, Dampier C. Psychosocial and functional outcomes in youth with chronic sickle cell pain. Clin J Pain. 2015;16:16.

[5] Smith WR, Penberthy LT, Bovbjerg VE, McClish DK, Roberts JD, Dahman B, et al. Daily assessment of pain in adults with sickle cell disease. Ann Intern Med. 2008;1482:94–101.

[6] Lutz B, Meiler SE, Bekker A, Tao Y-X. Updated mechanisms of sickle cell disease-associated chronic pain. Transl Periop Pain Med. 2015;22:8–17.

[7] Jacob E, Chan VW, Hodge C, Zeltzer L, Zurakowski D, Sethna NF. Sensory and thermal quantitative testing in children with sickle cell disease. J Pediatr Hematol Oncol. 2015;373:185–9.

[8] Brandow AM, Stucky CL, Hillery CA, Hoffmann RG, Panepinto JA. Patients with sickle cell disease have increased sensitivity to cold and heat. Am J Hema. 2013;881:37–43.

[9] Cain DM, Vang D, Simone DA, Hebbel RP, Gupta K. Mouse models for studying pain in sickle disease: effects of strain, age, and acuteness. Br J Haematol. 2012;1564:535–44.

[10] Garrison SR, Kramer AA, Gerges NZ, Hillery CA, Stucky CL. Sickle cell mice exhibit mechanical allodynia and enhanced responsiveness in light touch cutaneous mechanoreceptors. Mol Pain. 2012;862:1744–8069.

[11] Hillery CA, Kerstein PC, Vilceanu D, Barabas ME, Retherford D, Brandow AM, et al. Transient receptor potential vanilloid 1 mediates pain in mice with severe sickle cell disease. Blood. 2011;11812:3376–83.

[12] Kohli DR, Li Y, Khasabov SG, Gupta P, Kehl LJ, Ericson ME, et al. Pain-related behaviors and neurochemical alterations in mice expressing sickle hemoglobin: modulation by cannabinoids. Blood. 2010;1163:456–65.

[13] Vekilov PG. Sickle-cell haemoglobin polymerization: is it the primary pathogenic event of sickle-cell anaemia? Br J Haematol. 2007;1392:173–84.

[14] Kenyon N, Wang L, Spornick N, Khaibullina A, Almeida LE, Cheng Y, et al. Sickle cell disease in mice is associated with sensitization of sensory nerve fibers. Exp Bio Med. 2015;2401:87–98.

[15] O'Leary JD, Crawford MW, Odame I, Shorten GD, McGrath PA. Thermal pain and sensory processing in children with sickle cell disease. Clin J Pain. 2014;303: 244–50.

[16] Ibrahim AS. Relationship between meteorological changes and occurrence of painful sickle cell crises in Kuwait. Trans Royal Soc Trop Med Hyg. 1980;742:159–61.

[17] Redwood AM, Williams EM, Desal P, Serjeant GR. Climate and painful crisis of sickle-cell disease in Jamaica. British Medical Journal. 1976;16001:66–8.

[18] Rogovik AL, Persaud J, Friedman JN, Kirby MA, Goldman RD. Pediatric vasoocclusive crisis and weather conditions. J Emerg Med. 2011;415:559–65.

[19] Smith WR, Bauserman RL, Ballas SK, McCarthy WF, Steinberg MH, Swerdlow PS, et al. Climatic and geographic temporal patterns of pain in the Multicenter Study of Hydroxyurea. Pain. 2009;1461–2:91–8.

[20] Nolan VG, Zhang Y, Lash T, Sebastiani P, Steinberg MH. Association between wind speed and the occurrence of sickle cell acute painful episodes: results of a case-crossover study. Br J Haematol. 2008;1433:433–8.

[21] Rees DC, Williams TN, Gladwin MT. Sickle-cell disease. Lancet. 2010;376(9757):2018–31.

[22] Ohara DG, Ruas G, Castro SS, Martins PR, Walsh IA. Musculoskeletal pain, profile and quality of life of individuals with sickle cell disease. Rev Bras Fisioter. 2012;165:431–8.

[23] Mittal A, Gupta M, Lamarre Y, Jahagirdar B, Gupta K. Quantification of pain in sickle mice using facial expressions and body measurements. Blood Cells Mol Dis. 2016;57:58–66.

[24] Vincent L, Vang D, Nguyen J, Benson B, Lei J, Gupta K. Cannabinoid receptor-specific mechanisms to ameliorate pain in sickle cell anemia via inhibition of mast cell activation and neurogenic inflammation. Haematologica. 2015;24:136523.

[25] Darbari DS, Hampson JP, Ichesco E, Kadom N, Vezina G, Evangelou I, et al. Frequency of hospitalizations for pain and association with altered brain network connectivity in sickle cell disease. J Pain. 2015;1611:1077–86.

[26] Manci EA, Hillery CA, Bodian CA, Zhang ZG, Lutty GA, Coller BS. Pathology of Berkeley sickle cell mice: similarities and differences with human sickle cell disease. Blood. 2006;1074:1651–8.

[27] Dampier C, Ely E, Brodecki D, O'Neal P. Home management of pain in sickle cell disease: a daily diary study in children and adolescents. J Pediatr Hematol Oncol. 2002;248:643–7.

[28] Brandow AM, Farley RA, Panepinto JA. Early insights into the neurobiology of pain in sickle cell disease: a systematic review of the literature. Pediatr Blood Cancer. 2015;629:1501–11.

[29] Campbell CM, Moscou-Jackson G, Carroll CP, Kiley K, Haywood C, Jr., Lanzkron S, et al. An evaluation of central sensitization in patients with sickle cell disease. J Pain. 2016;1516:00517–4.

[30] Ezenwa MO, Molokie RE, Wang ZJ, Yao Y, Suarez ML, Pullum C, et al. Safety and utility of quantitative sensory testing among adults with sickle cell disease: indicators of neuropathic pain? Pain Pract. 2015;1210:12279.

[31] Nguyen J, Abdulla F, Chen C, Nguyen P, Nguyen M, Tittle B, et al. Phenotypic characterization the townes sickle mice. Blood. 2014;124(21):4916.

[32] Fabry ME, Costantini F, Pachnis A, Suzuka SM, Bank N, Aynedjian HS, et al. High expression of human beta S- and alpha-globins in transgenic mice: erythrocyte abnormalities, organ damage, and the effect of hypoxia. Proc Natl Acad Sci USA. 1992;8924:12155–9.

[33] Fabry M, Sengupta A, Suzuka S, Costantini F, Rubin E, Hofrichter J, et al. A second generation transgenic mouse model expressing both hemoglobin S (HbS) and HbS-Antilles results in increased phenotypic severity. Blood. 1995;866:2419–28.

[34] Ryan TM, Ciavatta DJ, Townes TM. Knockout-transgenic mouse model of sickle cell disease. Science. 1997;278(5339):873–6.

[35] Paszty C, Brion CM, Manci E, Witkowska HE, Stevens ME, Mohandas N, et al. Transgenic knockout mice with exclusively human sickle hemoglobin and sickle cell disease. Science. 1997;278(5339):876–8.

[36] Hanna J, Wernig M, Markoulaki S, Sun CW, Meissner A, Cassady JP, et al. Treatment of sickle cell anemia mouse model with iPS cells generated from autologous skin. Science. 2007;318(5858):1920–3.

[37] Wu LC, Sun CW, Ryan TM, Pawlik KM, Ren J, Townes TM. Correction of sickle cell disease by homologous recombination in embryonic stem cells. Blood. 2006;1084:1183–8.

[38] Sarray S, Saleh LR, Lisa Saldanha F, Al-Habboubi HH, Mahdi N, Almawi WY. Serum IL-6, IL-10, and TNFalpha levels in pediatric sickle cell disease patients during vaso-occlusive crisis and steady state condition. Cytokine. 2015;721:43–7.

[39] Frenette PS, Atweh GF. Sickle cell disease: old discoveries, new concepts, and future promise. J Clin Invest. 2007;1174:850–8.

[40] Valverde Y, Benson B, Gupta M, Gupta K. Spinal glial activation and oxidative stress are alleviated by treatment with curcumin or coenzyme Q in sickle mice. Haematologica. 2016;1012:e44–e7.

[41] Beiswenger KK, Calcutt NA, Mizisin AP. Epidermal nerve fiber quantification in the assessment of diabetic neuropathy. Acta Histoch. 2008;1105:351–62.

[42] Cataldo G, Rajput S, Gupta K, Simone DA. Sensitization of nociceptive spinal neurons contributes to pain in a transgenic model of sickle cell disease. Pain. 2015;1564:722–30.

[43] Vincent L, Vang D, Nguyen J, Gupta M, Luk K, Ericson ME, et al. Mast cell activation contributes to sickle cell pathobiology and pain in mice. Blood. 2013;12211:1853–62.

[44] Paul J, Lei J, Jha R, Nguyen J, Simone DA, Gupta K. Heme induced spinal microglial cell activation by TLR4 and endoplasmic reticulum stress in sickle mice. Blood. 2014;124(21):452.

[45] Grace PM, Hutchinson MR, Maier SF, Watkins LR. Pathological pain and the neuroimmune interface. Nat Rev Immunol. 2014;144:217–31.

[46] Sorge RE, LaCroix-Fralish ML, Tuttle AH, Sotocinal SG, Austin J-S, Ritchie J, et al. Spinal cord Toll-like receptor 4 mediates inflammatory and neuropathic hypersensitivity in male but not female mice. J Neurosci. 2011;3143:15450–4.

[47] Sorge RE, Mapplebeck JCS, Rosen S, Beggs S, Taves S, Alexander JK, et al. Different immune cells mediate mechanical pain hypersensitivity in male and female mice. Nat Neurosci. 2015;188:1081–3.

[48] McClish DK, Levenson JL, Penberthy LT, Roseff SD, Bovbjerg VE, Roberts JD, et al. Gender differences in pain and healthcare utilization for adult sickle cell patients: the PiSCES project. JWH. 2006;152:146–54.

[49] Wilkie DJ, Molokie R, Boyd-Seal D, Suarez ML, Kim YO, Zong S, et al. Patient-reported outcomes: descriptors of nociceptive and neuropathic pain and barriers to effective pain

management in adult outpatients with sickle cell disease. J Natl Med Assoc. 2010;1021:18–27.

[50] Brandow AM, Farley RA, Panepinto JA. Neuropathic pain in patients with sickle cell disease. Pediatr Blood Cancer. 2014;613:512–7.

[51] Savage WJ, Everett AD, Casella JF. Plasma glial fibrillary acidic protein levels in a child with sickle cell disease and stroke. Acta Haemato. 2011;1253:103–6.

[52] Michaels LA, Ohene-Frempong K, Zhao H, Douglas SD. Serum levels of substance P are elevated in patients with sickle cell disease and increase further during vaso-occlusive crisis. Blood. 1998;929:3148–51.

[53] Li WW, Guo TZ, Liang DY, Sun Y, Kingery WS, Clark JD. Substance P signaling controls mast cell activation, degranulation, and nociceptive sensitization in a rat fracture model of complex regional pain syndrome. Anesthesiology. 2012;1164:882–95.

[54] Zappia KJ, Garrison SR, Hillery CA, Stucky CL. Cold hypersensitivity increases with age in mice with sickle cell disease. Pain. 2014;15512:2476–85.

[55] Werner MF, Trevisani M, Campi B, Andre E, Geppetti P, Rae GA. Contribution of peripheral endothelin ETA and ETB receptors in neuropathic pain induced by spinal nerve ligation in rats. Eur J Pain. 2010;149:911–7.

[56] Teodoro FC, Tronco Júnior MF, Zampronio AR, Martini AC, Rae GA, Chichorro JG. Peripheral substance P and neurokinin-1 receptors have a role in inflammatory and neuropathic orofacial pain models. Neuropeptides. 2013;473:199–206.

[57] Smith M, Wally R, McClish P, Donna K, Dahman P, Bassam A, Levenson M, James L, Aisiku M, Imoigele P, Citero M, Vanessa de A, et al. Daily home opioid use in adults with sickle cell disease: the PiSCES project. J Opioid Manag. 2015;113:11.

[58] Chu LF, Angst MS, Clark D. Opioid-induced hyperalgesia in humans: molecular mechanisms and clinical considerations. Clin J Pain. 2008;246:479–96.

[59] Weber ML, Vang D, Velho PE, Gupta P, Crosson JT, Hebbel RP, et al. Morphine promotes renal pathology in sickle mice. Int J Nephrol Renovasc Dis. 2012;5:109–18.

[60] Wang X, Loram LC, Ramos K, de Jesus AJ, Thomas J, Cheng K, et al. Morphine activates neuroinflammation in a manner parallel to endotoxin. Proc Natl Acad Sci USA. 2012;10916:6325–30.

[61] Chen C, Farooqui M, Gupta K. Morphine stimulates vascular endothelial growth factor-like signaling in mouse retinal endothelial cells. Curr Neurovasc Res. 2006;33:171–80.

[62] Wang Y, Barker K, Shi S, Diaz M, Mo B, Gutstein HB. Blockade of PDGFR-[beta] activation eliminates morphine analgesic tolerance. Nat Med. 2012;183:385–7. DOI: 10.1038/nm.2633

[63] Zaveri NT. The nociceptin/orphanin FQ receptor (NOP) as a target for drug abuse medications. Curr Top Med Chem. 2011;119:1151–6.

[64] Helyes Z, Nemeth J, Pinter E, Szolcsanyi J. Inhibition by nociceptin of neurogenic inflammation and the release of SP and CGRP from sensory nerve terminals. Br J Pharmacol. 1997;1214:613–5.

[65] Nemeth J, Helyes Z, Oroszi G, Than M, Pinter E, Szolcsanyi J. Inhibition of nociceptin on sensory neuropeptide release and mast cell-mediated plasma extravasation in rats. Eur J Pharmacol. 1998;3471:101–4.

[66] Vang D, Paul JA, Nguyen J, Tran H, Vincent L, Yasuda D, et al. Small-molecule nociceptin receptor agonist ameliorates mast cell activation and pain in sickle mice. Haematologica. 2015;10012:1517–25.

[67] Aich A, Afrin L, Gupta K. Mast cell-mediated mechanisms of nociception. Intl J Mol Sci. 2015;1612:26151.

[68] Inceoglu B, Bettaieb A, Trindade da Silva CA, Lee KSS, Haj FG, Hammock BD. Endoplasmic reticulum stress in the peripheral nervous system is a significant driver of neuropathic pain. Proc Natl Acad Sci USA. 2015;112(29):9082–7.

[69] Gupta M, Thompson S, Gupta K, Abrams DI. Cannabis in the treatment of pain in sickle cell disease. JSCDH. 2016. In press.

[70] Collin C, Ehler E, Waberzinek G, Alsindi Z, Davies P, Powell K, et al. A double-blind, randomized, placebo-controlled, parallel-group study of Sativex, in subjects with symptoms of spasticity due to multiple sclerosis. Neurol Res. 2010;325:451–9.

[71] Barnes MP. Sativex: clinical efficacy and tolerability in the treatment of symptoms of multiple sclerosis and neuropathic pain. Expert Opin Pharmacother. 2006;75:607–15.

[72] Brower V. New pain drugs in pipeline, but challenges to usage remain. J Nat Can Inst. 2012;1047:503–5.

[73] Abrams DI, Couey P, Shade SB, Kelly ME, Benowitz NL. Cannabinoid-opioid interaction in chronic pain. Clin Pharmacol Ther. 2011;906:844–51.

[74] Zhang M, Adler MW, Abood ME, Ganea D, Jallo J, Tuma RF. CB2 receptor activation attenuates microcirculatory dysfunction during cerebral ischemic/reperfusion injury. Microvasc Res. 2009;781:86–94.

[75] Howard J, Anie KA, Holdcroft A, Korn S, Davies SC. Cannabis use in sickle cell disease: a questionnaire study. Br J Haematol. 2005;1311:123–8.

[76] Takeda K, Akira S. Toll-like receptors in innate immunity. Intl Immun. 2005;171:1–14.

[77] Qian B, Li F, Zhao L-X, Dong Y-L, Gao Y-J, Zhang Z-J. Ligustilide ameliorates inflammatory pain and inhibits TLR4 upregulation in spinal astrocytes following complete Freund's adjuvant peripheral injection. Cell Mol Neurob. 2015;361:143–9.

[78] Bettoni I, Comelli F, Rossini C, Granucci F, Giagnoni G, Peri F, et al. Glial TLR4 receptor as new target to treat neuropathic pain: efficacy of a new receptor antagonist in a model of peripheral nerve injury in mice. Glia. 2008;5612:1312–9.

[79] Jurga AM, Rojewska E, Piotrowska A, Makuch W, Pilat D, Przewlocka B, et al. Blockade of toll-like receptors (TLR2, TLR4) attenuates pain and potentiates buprenorphine analgesia in a rat neuropathic pain model. Neural Plasticity. 2016;2016:12.

[80] Wu F-x, Bian J-j, Miao X-r, Huang S-d, Xu X-w, Gong D-j, et al. Intrathecal siRNA against toll-like receptor 4 reduces nociception in a rat model of neuropathic pain. Intl J Med Sci. 2010;75:251–9.

[81] Lu S-M, Yu C-J, Liu Y-H, Dong H-Q, Zhang X, Zhang S-S, et al. S100A8 contributes to postoperative cognitive dysfunction in mice undergoing tibial fracture surgery by activating the TLR4/MyD88 pathway. Brain Behav Immun. 2015;44:221–34.

[82] Lan LS, Ping YJ, Na WL, Miao J, Cheng QQ, Ni MZ, et al. Down-regulation of Toll-like receptor 4 gene expression by short interfering RNA attenuates bone cancer pain in a rat model. Mol Pain. 2010;61:1–13.

[83] Gupta K. HMGB1 takes a "Toll" in sickle cell disease. Blood. 2014;124(26):3837–8.

[84] Figueiredo RT, Fernandez PL, Mourao-Sa DS, Porto BN, Dutra FF, Alves LS, et al. Characterization of heme as activator of Toll-like receptor 4. J Biol Chem. 2007;282(28):20221–9.

[85] Ghosh S, Adisa OA, Chappa P, Tan F, Jackson KA, Archer DR, et al. Extracellular hemin crisis triggers acute chest syndrome in sickle mice. J Clin Invest. 2013;123(11):4809–20.

[86] Belcher JD, Chen C, Nguyen J, Milbauer L, Abdulla F, Alayash AI, et al. Heme triggers TLR4 signaling leading to endothelial cell activation and vaso-occlusion in murine sickle cell disease. Blood. 2014;123(3):377–90.

[87] Vang D, Pena RDS, Robiner SA, Gupta K. Toll-like receptor 4 knockout attenuates neurogenic inflammation and hyperalgesia in sickle mice. Blood. 2013;122(21):732.

[88] Lei J, Wang Y, Paul J, Thompson S, Jha R, Gupta K, editors. Pharmacological inhibition of TLR4 reduces mast cell activation, neuroinflammation and hyperalgesia in sickle mice. ASH 57th Annual Meeting & Exposition, Orlando, Florida; 2015.

[89] Grace PM, Strand KA, Galer EL, Zhang Y, Berkelhammer D, Greene LI, et al. Therapeutic morphine prolongs neuropathic pain in rats: a role for TLR4 and inflammasome signaling in the lumbar spinal cord. Brain Behav Imm. 2014;40(Suppl.):e9–e10.

[90] Hutchinson MR, Shavit Y, Grace PM, Rice KC, Maier SF, Watkins LR. Exploring the neuroimmunopharmacology of opioids: an integrative review of mechanisms of central immune signaling and their implications for opioid analgesia. Pharmacol Rev. 2011;633:772–810.

[91] Woller SA, Corr M, Yaksh TL. Differences in cisplatin-induced mechanical allodynia in male and female mice. Eur J Pain. 2015;1910:1476–85.

[92] Hutchinson MR, Loram LC, Zhang Y, Shridhar M, Rezvani N, Berkelhammer D, et al. Evidence that tricyclic small molecules may possess toll-like receptor and MD-2 activity. Neuroscience. 2010;1682:551–63.

[93] Savva A, Roger T. Targeting toll-like receptors: promising therapeutic strategies for the management of sepsis-associated pathology and infectious diseases. Front Immun. 2013;4:4 387–N/A.

[94] Chen Y, Yang C, Wang ZJ. Ca2+/calmodulin-dependent protein kinase IIα is required for the initiation and maintenance of opioid-induced hyperalgesia. J Neurosci. 2010;301:38–46.

[95] Molokie RE, Wilkie DJ, Wittert H, Suarez ML, Yao Y, Zhao Z, et al. Mechanism-driven phase I translational study of trifluoperazine in adults with sickle cell disease. Eur J Pharmacol. 2014;723:419–24.

[96] Yoshitomi O, Cho S, Hara T, Shibata I, Maekawa T, Ureshino H, et al. Direct protective effects of dexmedetomidine against myocardial ischemia-reperfusion injury in anesthetized pigs. Shock. 2012;381:92–7.

[97] Calhoun G, Wang L, Almeida LEF, Kenyon N, Afsar N, Nouraie M, et al. Dexmedetomidine ameliorates nocifensive behavior in humanized sickle cell mice. Eur J Pharmacol. 2015;754:125–33.

[98] Thakur AS, Littaru GP, Moesgaard S, Dan Sindberg C, Khan Y, Singh CM. Hematological parameters and RBC TBARS level of Q 10 supplemented tribal sickle cell patients: a hospital based study. Indian J Clin Biochem. 2013;282:185–8.

[99] Gupta SC, Patchva S, Aggarwal BB. Therapeutic roles of curcumin: lessons learned from clinical trials. Aaps J. 2013;151:195–218.

[100] Nakagawa Y, Mukai S, Yamada S, Matsuoka M, Tarumi E, Hashimoto T, et al. Short-term effects of highly-bioavailable curcumin for treating knee osteoarthritis: a randomized, double-blind, placebo-controlled prospective study. J Orthop Sci. 2014;196:933–9.

[101] Badria FA, Ibrahim AS, Badria AF, Elmarakby AA. Curcumin attenuates iron accumulation and oxidative stress in the liver and spleen of chronic iron-overloaded rats. PLoS One. 2015;107:e0134156–N/A.

[102] Kalpravidh RW, Siritanaratkul N, Insain P, Charoensakdi R, Panichkul N, Hatairaktham S, et al. Improvement in oxidative stress and antioxidant parameters in beta-thalassemia/Hb E patients treated with curcuminoids. Clin Biochem. 2010;434–5:424–9.

[103] King A, Shenoy S. Evidence-based focused review of the status of hematopoietic stem cell transplantation as treatment of sickle cell disease and thalassemia. Blood. 2014;12320:3089–94.

[104] Raghupathy R, Manwani D, Little JA. Iron overload in sickle cell disease. Adv Hema. 2010;2010:272940–N/A.

[105] Marques CVP. Laser acupuncture to manage pain in child with sickle cell disease. Case report. Relato de caso. Revista Dor. 2014;15:70–3.

[106] Tsai S-L, McDaniel D, Taromina K, Lee MT. Acupuncture for sickle cell pain management in a pediatric emergency department, hematology clinic, and inpatient unit. Med Acccup. 2015;276:510–4.

[107] Bhushan D, Conner K, Ellen JM, Sibinga EMS. Adjuvant acupuncture for youth with sickle cell pain: a proof of concept study. Med Acccup. 2015;276:461–6.

[108] Lu K, Cheng MC, Ge X, Berger A, Xu D, Kato GJ, et al. A retrospective review of acupuncture use for the treatment of pain in sickle cell disease patients: descriptive analysis from a single institution. Clin J Pain. 2014;309:825–30.

[109] Iqbal N, Iqbal N. Imatinib: A breakthrough of targeted therapy in cancer. Chemother Res Pract. 2014;2014:9.

[110] Karimi M, Zekavat OR, Sharifzadeh S, Mousavizadeh K. Clinical response of patients with sickle cell anemia to cromolyn sodium nasal spray. Am J Hematol. 2006;8111:809–16.

[111] Garcia-Recio S, Gascón P. Biological and pharmacological aspects of the NK1-receptor. BioMed Res Inter. 2015;2015:14.

[112] Chizh BA, Gohring M, Troster A, Quartey GK, Schmelz M, Koppert W. Effects of oral pregabalin and aprepitant on pain and central sensitization in the electrical hyperalgesia model in human volunteers. Br J Anaesth. 2007;982:246–54.

[113] Walsh SL, Heilig M, Nuzzo PA, Henderson P, Lofwall MR. Effects of the NK1 antagonist, aprepitant, on response to oral and intranasal oxycodone in prescription opioid abusers. Addict Biol. 2013;182:332–43.

[114] Opal SM, Laterre PF, Francois B, LaRosa SP, Angus DC, Mira JP, et al. Effect of eritoran, an antagonist of MD2-TLR4, on mortality in patients with severe sepsis: the ACCESS randomized trial. JAMA. 2013;30911:1154–62.

[115] Rice TW, Wheeler AP, Bernard GR, Vincent JL, Angus DC, Aikawa N, et al. A randomized, double-blind, placebo-controlled trial of TAK-242 for the treatment of severe sepsis. Crit Care Med. 2010;388:1685–94.

[116] Musi N. The effect of TLR4 inhibtion in obese and type 2 diabetic subjects (Eritoran 2). Available from: https://clinicaltrials.gov/ct2/show/NCT02267317 [cited 2016 April 19].

[117] Zhaleh M, Panahi M, Ghafurian Broujerdnia M, Ghorbani R, Ahmadi Angali K, Saki G. Role of phosphodiesterase inhibitor Ibudilast in morphine-induced hippocampal injury. J Inj Violence Res. 2014;62:72–8.

[118] Rolan P, Gazerani P. Ibudilast in the treatment of patients with chronic migraine (IBU-003). Available from: https://clinicaltrials.gov/ct2/show/NCT01389193?term=ibudilast&rank=2 [cited 2016 April 19].

[119] Fox RJ. Safety, tolerability and activity study of ibudilast in subjects with progressive multiple sclerosis. Available from: https://clinicaltrials.gov/ct2/show/NCT01982942?term=ibudilast&rank=7 [cited 2016 April 19].

[120] Comer SD. Effects of ibudilast on oxycodone self-administration in Opioid Abusers. Available from: https://clinicaltrials.gov/ct2/show/NCT01740414?term=ibudilast&rank=8 [cited 2016 April 19].

[121] Abrams DI. Vaporized cannabis for chronic pain associated with sickle cell disease (Cannabis-SCD). ClinicalTrials.gov. Available from: https://clinicaltrials.gov/ct2/show/NCT01771731?term=sickle+pain&rank=40 [cited 2016 February 27].

[122] Morris CR, Kuypers FA, Lavrisha L, Ansari M, Sweeters N, Stewart M, et al. A randomized, placebo-controlled trial of arginine therapy for the treatment of children with sickle cell disease hospitalized with vaso-occlusive pain episodes. Haematologica. 2013;989:1375–82.

[123] Pleticha J, Maus TP, Beutler AS. Future directions in pain management. Mayo Clin Proc. 2016;914:522–33.

Section 4

Chronic Complications of Sickle Cell Disease-Management Strategies

Chapter 6

The Cardiomyopathy of Sickle Cell Disease

Omar Niss and Charles T. Quinn

Additional information is available at the end of the chapter

http://dx.doi.org/10.5772/64321

Abstract

Cardiac morbidity, early mortality, and sudden death are the major consequences of sickle cell disease (SCD) in patients surviving into adulthood. Pulmonary hypertension (PH), elevated tricuspid regurgitant jet velocity (TRV), and diastolic dysfunction have all been identified to correlate with early mortality in adults with SCD. However, the unifying pathophysiology behind these abnormalities and its connection with early mortality and sudden death have not been recognized previously. We have found that SCD patients have a unique cardiomyopathy characterized by restrictive physiology (diastolic dysfunction, left atrial dilation and normal systolic function) superimposed on features of hyperdynamic circulation (left ventricular [LV] enlargement and eccentric LV hypertrophy. The restrictive cardiomyopathy of SCD causes pulmonary congestion and post-capillary PH. This can be detected by a mild elevation in TRV, which is likely a marker of the SCD-related cardiomyopathy rather than pulmonary arterial disease. Similar to other restrictive cardiomyopathies, the SCD cardiomyopathy predisposes to arrhythmias and sudden death, even when pulmonary pressures are not severely elevated. We have also found that diffuse myocardial fibrosis is common in SCD and may underlie the diastolic dysfunction, but more studies are needed to understand the mechanisms of SCD-related cardiomyopathy and to identify new therapies to decrease cardiac morbidity and improve the life expectancy of SCD patients.

Keywords: sickle cell, cardiomyopathy, restrictive physiology, pulmonary hypertension

1. Introduction

Improvements in the medical care of sickle cell disease (SCD) in the last few decades have led to a significant decrease in childhood mortality in developed countries [1]. As more patients live into adulthood, the cumulative burden of acute and chronic organ damage has become an important determinant of quality of life, morbidity, and life expectancy. Although definitive data are lacking, the life expectancy of SCD patients does not appear to have improved in the last 15 years, and adult SCD-related mortality may have increased [2, 3]. Cardiopulmonary complications, including heart failure and arrhythmias, are the main causes of death in adults with SCD [4]. Sudden unexplained death is reported in 25–30% of SCD patients, and these are likely cardiopulmonary events [4, 5]. A number of studies conducted in the last two decades have examined the cardiac pathology and cardiac mortality in SCD and have identified risk factors for early mortality in SCD; however, a global understanding of the cardiac dysfunction in SCD is still lacking. Of the known adverse cardiac risk factors, elevation of the tricuspid regurgitant jet velocity (TRV) measured by echocardiography, pulmonary hypertension (PH), and diastolic dysfunction are the most consistent predictors of early mortality in adults with SCD [6–9]. The mechanisms and pathophysiology that link these risk factors to the cardiac phenotype of SCD, and that underlie unexplained complications such as arrhythmias and sudden death, are not clearly understood.

2. Pulmonary hypertension in SCD

PH has been recognized as a complication of SCD and a predictor of early mortality. Although the causes of PH in SCD are not fully known, several factors have been suggested to play a part in its pathogenesis, including endothelial dysfunction due to chronic hemolysis and secondary nitric oxide depletion, hypoxia, and chronic thromboembolic disease [10–12]. Hemodynamically, PH can be pre-capillary or pulmonary arterial hypertension (PAH) or post-capillary or pulmonary venous hypertension (PVH). PH is defined by a mean pulmonary artery pressure (PAP) ≥ 25 mmHg as measured by right heart catheterization [13]. Patients with PAH have a pulmonary capillary wedge pressure (PCWP) or left ventricular (LV) end-diastolic pressure ≤ 15 mmHg, while patients with PVH have PCWP > 15 mmHg [13]. The echocardiographic measurement of TRV, in combination with an estimated right atrial pressure, can be used to estimate the systolic PAP.

Multiple studies have shown that the prevalence of elevated PAP as estimated by echocardiography using a TRV value ≥ 2.5 m/s is 20–30% in SCD [8, 14, 15]. In addition, elevated TRV in SCD is associated with increased risk of early mortality in adults [8]. Although TRV measurements correlate with PAP, the use of TRV as a sole criterion results in overdiagnosis of PH [16]. Studies of right-sided heart catheterization, the gold standard to diagnose PH, have shown that only about 30% of SCD patients with elevated TRV have PH [17, 18]. When PH is present in SCD, PAP is usually only mildly elevated, and the pulmonary vascular resistance is not increased compared to other patient populations with PH [7, 18, 19], and this does not readily explain the associated risk of early mortality. Importantly, most SCD patients in these studies with confirmed PH actually had PVH, which is caused by left-sided heart disease, rather than PAH, which could be caused by endothelial dysfunction (**Figure 1**). In addition, therapeutic trials of PAH-directed therapy in SCD were not successful and currently these therapies are not recommended for treatment of PH in SCD [20, 21].

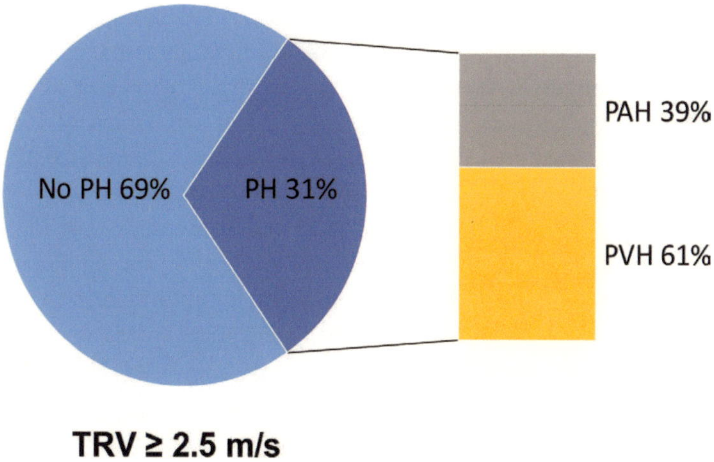

Figure 1. The percentage of SCD patients with TRV ≥2.5 m/s who had confirmed PH (PAH or PVH) by right-sided heart catheterization. Data are pooled from four different studies [7, 18, 22, 23].

These hemodynamic studies of SCD-related PH have improved our understanding of this complication. PH is less prevalent in SCD than was suggested by echocardiographic screening alone. It is also less severe and may be of a mixed origin, but most cases are caused by left-sided heart disease as evidenced by the higher frequency of PVH rather than pulmonary arterial disease. As a result, in 2013, The Fifth World Symposium on Pulmonary Hypertension changed the classification of SCD-related PH from "Group 1," which indicates pulmonary arterial hypertension to "Group 5," which refers to pulmonary hypertension with unclear or multifactorial mechanisms [13, 24]. Despite the poor diagnostic accuracy of TRV for PH, TRV is still a predictor of early mortality in adults with SCD; however, the exact cause of elevated TRV in the absence of PH and the mechanisms by which it confers increased mortality risk are poorly understood. However, elevated TRV is not associated with early mortality in children.

3. Diastolic dysfunction in SCD

Recently, diastolic dysfunction has also been recognized as an independent risk factor for mortality in SCD [9]. Diastolic dysfunction is common in SCD and was found in nearly all studies that evaluated diastolic function [17]. The prevalence and severity of diastolic dysfunction vary across studies, ranging from 11 to 77% depending on the criteria used to define diastolic dysfunction in each study. This wide range also reflects the challenges of diagnosing diastolic dysfunction and the lack of agreement on diagnostic criteria and classification of diastolic dysfunction in SCD. Nonetheless, common echocardiographic estimates of diastolic function are clearly abnormal in SCD. The ratio of early to late mitral flow velocities (E/A ratio), tissue Doppler annular velocities (e.g.; E/e' and e'/a' ratios), and left atrial (LA) volumes are significantly abnormal in SCD, and some of these measures correlate with early mortality in SCD [9, 14, 25, 26]. Diastolic dysfunction can be detected early in life in SCD patients, and even children may have severe diastolic dysfunction [25, 27–29]. This suggests that diastolic dysfunction likely precedes other non–anemia-related hemodynamic changes in SCD [17]. Diastolic dysfunction ranges in severity from an impaired relaxation of the ventricles to irreversible restrictive ventricular filling [30]. Progressive worsening of diastolic function eventually causes an increase in LV filling pressures and LA pressures. The elevated LA pressure, which correlates with chronic LA enlargement and an elevation in the diastolic estimate E/e′ ratio, leads to an increase in PCWP and some degree of PH [31]. Diastolic dysfunction is the major cause of PVH in SCD [32]. Despite the significance of diastolic dysfunction in SCD, there is still a need to define diastolic dysfunction and identify diastolic function parameters that are least affected by the hyperdynamic state of SCD. There is also a lack of understanding of the mechanisms that predispose to diastolic dysfunction in SCD. Cardiac iron overload, which plays a major part in cardiac pathology and diastolic dysfunction in thalassemia [33], is rare in SCD [34, 35] and unlikely to be a major cause of diastolic dysfunction in most individuals. More studies are needed to identify the underlying cause of diastolic dysfunction in SCD [36].

4. Anemia-related hyperdynamic features

The complex effects of chronic anemia on the heart are the result of various compensatory cardiovascular mechanisms to anemia. Altered blood viscosity, tissue hypoxia, and increased sympathetic tone are some of the factors that drive cardiovascular hemodynamic changes in anemia [37]. Chronic anemia causes arteriolar dilation and decreased afterload, while the decreased venous tone increases the preload. The increased preload, coupled with increased sympathetic tone, leads to increased stroke volume and cardiac output. Together, these changes lead to a state of volume overload [38–40]. Chronic volume overload and increased cardiac load over time leads to cardiac enlargement and left ventricular hypertrophy (LVH) [41]. LVH is an adaptive mechanism to prolonged volume or pressure overload. In states of volume overload, LVH is eccentric and defined by increased LV internal dimension with a normal ratio of wall thickness to cavity diameter (a proportionate increase in wall thickness and LV internal diameter). In contrast, concentric hypertrophy, which results from pressure overload (e.g., aortic stenosis), is characterized by increased wall thickness without a change in the ventricular chamber radius [42]. Unlike the adaptive eccentric hypertrophy of volume overload, concentric hypertrophy can become maladaptive and may lead to ventricular stiffening and heart failure over time. Typical features of volume overload characterize the hearts of SCD patients: increased stroke volume and cardiac output, increased LV end-diastolic dimensions, and eccentric LVH [17]. It is also important to note that LV dilation in SCD is associated with an increased ejection fraction and stroke volume and is different from LV dilation of "failing" ventricles, typically seen in dilated cardiomyopathies, where LV dilation is associated with LV systolic dysfunction. While anemia-related hyperdynamic features are prominent in SCD, it is difficult to differentiate fully the effects of anemia from the effects of other pathologic processes of SCD, such as vaso-occlusion and inflammation, in the heart. The

http://dx.doi.org/10.5772/64321

contribution of anemic-hyperdynamic features to other pathologic cardiac features (i.e., diastolic dysfunction, elevated TRV, and PH) has yet to be established.

5. The cardiomyopathy of SCD

Until recently, there has not been a unifying cardiac pathophysiology identified to explain the cardiac features of SCD: mild PH, elevated TRV, diastolic dysfunction, LA dilation, and LV dilation with normal systolic function. We have reported that patients with SCD have a unique cardiomyopathy with restrictive physiology that is superimposed on hyperdynamic features [17]. This cardiomyopathy with restrictive physiology provides an explanation for most cardiac features of SCD.

5.1. Restrictive cardiac physiology

Restrictive physiology is essentially defined by a stiff myocardium that causes the ventricular pressure to rise precipitously with only small increases in volume [43]. It is primarily a disease of the heart muscle that causes decreased myocardial compliance and, therefore, diastolic dysfunction, resulting in elevation in ventricular filling pressures and LA pressures and restricted filling. Restrictive cardiomyopathies (RCM) can be primary, which constitutes 5% of primary cardiomyopathies [44], or secondary to infiltrative diseases (e.g., sarcoidosis or amyloidosis), radiation, or chemotherapy [45]. Progressive fibrosis of the myocardium leading to impaired ventricular relaxation and progressive diastolic dysfunction is the primary mechanism underlying the different forms of RCM. RCM is defined by diastolic dysfunction, atrial enlargement, normal systolic function, and ventricles of normal size [44]. Unlike systolic cardiomyopathies, e.g., dilated cardiomyopathy, which is characterized by enlarged ventricles with decreased systolic function, RCM is a primary diastolic cardiomyopathy and the ventricular volumes are normal or small in primary RCM. The outcome of primary RCM is poor without heart transplantation. Age and LA size are the strongest predictors of mortality in RCM [46]. PH, venous and arterial, is a well-known consequence of RCM that is associated with a worse outcome [47]. In addition, ischemia and arrhythmias, likely from fibrosis encasing the conducting pathways, are the most common causes of death in RCM [48]. Indeed, sudden unexpected death happens in about 30% of patients with RCM [44].

5.2. Cardiomyopathy with restrictive physiology in SCD

We reviewed the echocardiographic data on SCD patients at Cincinnati Children's Hospital Medical Center and conducted a meta-analysis of reported cardiac studies in SCD. Across all the studies, we observed a pattern consistent with a cardiomyopathy with combined features of restrictive physiology and hyperdynamic circulation. The primary features of the SCD-related cardiomyopathy are (1) diastolic dysfunction, (2) LA dilation, and (3) LV enlargement with normal systolic function [17]. One main difference between primary RCM and the restrictive cardiomyopathy of SCD is LV enlargement, which is not seen in primary RCM. Indeed, formal criteria for RCM exclude enlarged ventricles, but this distinction is made to differentiate RCM from dilated cardiomyopathy. While small- or normal-size ventricles define primary RCM, which distinguishes it from the dilated cardiomyopathies with systolic dysfunction, the LV enlargement in SCD is associated with normal or even increased systolic function in SCD. Therefore, LV dilation is one of the hyperdynamic features that coexists with the features of restrictive physiology in the hearts of SCD patients.

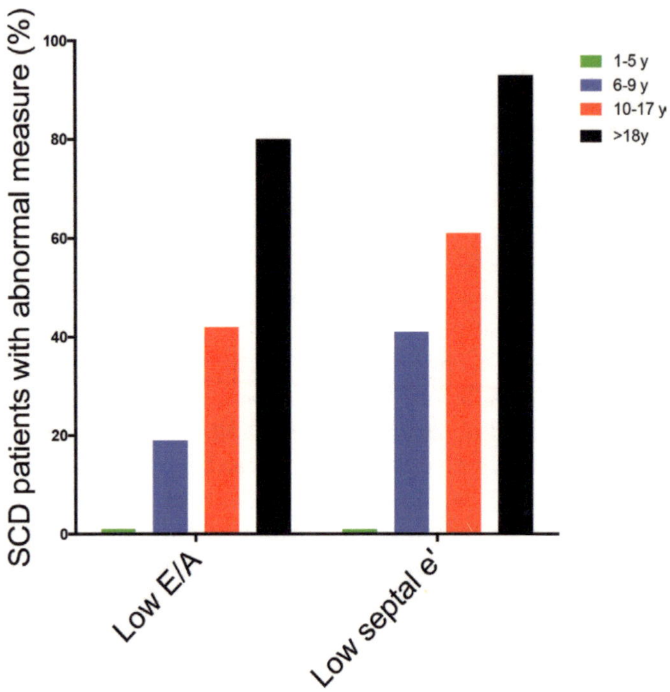

Figure 2. The percentage of SCD patients with low E/A ratio and septal e' (z-score less than −1) in the following age groups: 1–5 years, 6–9 years, 10–17 years, and older than 18 years.

In our echocardiographic study of 134 patients with SCD (age range from 3 to 22 years), diastolic dysfunction and LA enlargement were common [17]. Impaired relaxation, as reflected by abnormal tissue Doppler early velocity e' and decreased E/A ratio, worsened with age (**Figure 2**), while severe diastolic dysfunction, defined by severely abnormal E/e' ratio, was seen in up to 14% of this group of young patients. In addition, LA enlargement was observed in 62% of patients and was the most enlarged heart chamber. While LV enlargement and eccentric LVH were also observed, LA enlargement was more common and disproportionate to LV enlargement, reflecting the different mechanisms underlying LV and LA enlargement. Similar to other studies in SCD, the systolic function was normal in our study [49].

The same cardiac pattern was observed in a meta-analysis of the published cardiac studies in SCD, combining data on more than 5000 patients from 68 different studies [17]. LV enlargement was more pronounced in the meta-analysis as it included older patients with more severe anemia. Consistent with previous studies, we confirmed that LA enlargement is an early

http://dx.doi.org/10.5772/64321

cardiac feature that precedes the enlargement of other cardiac chambers in SCD [27, 50–52]. Over time, LV enlargement and LVH become more prominent because of chronic volume overload [41, 49]. At that later stage, the SCD cardiomyopathy can be described by 4-chamber enlargement, diastolic dysfunction, and normal systolic function [36]. However, the restrictive physiology remains an important and an early hemodynamic feature of the SCD cardiomyopathy that can be masked by the 4-chamber enlargement in adults with SCD. Increased LV filling and LA pressures characterize restrictive physiology, which subsequently leads to mild PVH and TRV elevation. Indeed, TRV was significantly associated with the restrictive component of the SCD cardiomyopathy (diastolic dysfunction and LA enlargement), suggesting that TRV is likely a marker of the restrictive cardiomyopathy of SCD [17].

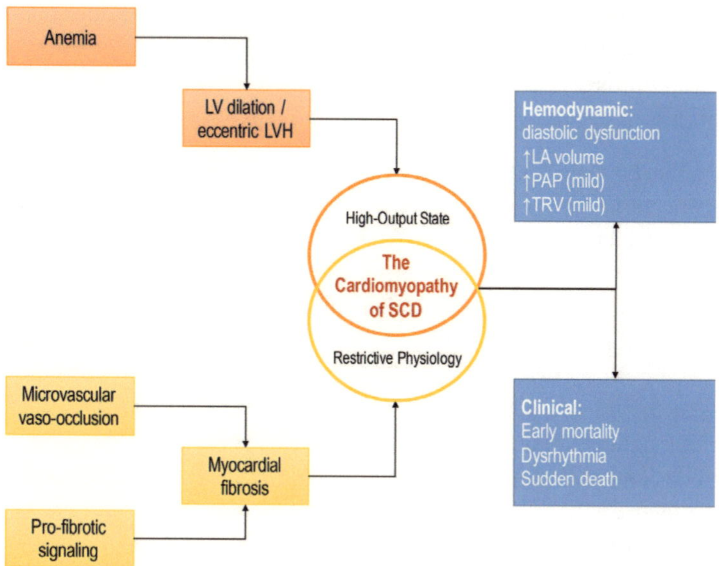

Figure 3. Schema of the proposed pathophysiologic construct of the cardiomyopathy of SCD.

In summary, the SCD-related cardiomyopathy is a restrictive cardiomyopathy, defined by diastolic dysfunction and LA enlargement, superimposed on hyperdynamic features of LV enlargement with normal systolic function. The SCD cardiomyopathy causes passive pulmonary congestion and mild PVH, which is common in SCD, and causes mild elevation in TRV that is detected by echocardiography (**Figure 3**). Interestingly, both PVH and PAH can result from diastolic failure and restrictive physiology [32]. This unique cardiomyopathy seen in most patients with SCD may coincide with PAH (confirmed by right heart catheterization with low PCWP and elevated pulmonary vascular resistance), possibly caused by endothelial dysfunction, in a small group of patients. However, the majority of SCD patients with cardiac dysfunction lack hemodynamic evidence of PAH, and most of their cardiac pathology can be explained by this unique SCD-related cardiomyopathy. The similarities in the patterns and frequency of mortality between SCD patients and patients with primary RCM are notable. The high rate of arrhythmias and sudden death, especially at times of stress, are common consequences of restrictive physiology in RCM and are complications of SCD that have not been explained and can likely be attributed to the restrictive cardiomyopathy of SCD.

5.3. Myocardial tissue characterization in SCD: cardiac MRI and autopsy studies

The cause of diastolic dysfunction and restrictive physiology in SCD is unclear. Cardiac MRI (CMR) studies have shown that cardiac iron overload is rare in SCD patients, even when systemic iron overload is present [36, 53, 54], and is unlikely to be a primary mechanism underlying cardiac dysfunction in SCD. The small number of autopsy studies in SCD provided the earliest insight into cardiac histopathology in SCD. Some of the findings in autopsy specimens include chamber enlargement and increased heart weight, pulmonary vascular changes [55, 56], and myocardial fibrosis [36, 56, 57]. Different myocardial fibrosis patterns were noted: transmural fibrosis/scarring without evidence of atherosclerosis, patchy fibrosis, diffuse myocardial fibrosis, and fibrotic foci involving the conduction system predisposing to arrhythmias [36, 58].

Recent CMR studies have provided further information about the tissue characteristics of the sickle hearts using non-invasive techniques. One technique, late gadolinium enhancement (LGE), is useful in detecting scar tissue or focal macroscopic fibrosis based on differences in the volumes of distribution of the extracellular contrast agent, gadolinium [59]. In SCD, LGE detection has been variable. Most CMR studies detected LGE in a subset of patients, reaching up to 25% of evaluated patients in one study [36, 54, 60–63]. However, because this technique is based on detecting differences in enhancement between the affected area and surrounding myocardial tissue, it will not detect diffuse myocardial fibrosis, which was also seen in the autopsies of SCD patients [36]. These autopsy and CMR studies suggest that fibrosis is probably an overlooked pathology that contributes to cardiac dysfunction in SCD. Studies are ongoing using novel CMR techniques to better characterize myocardial tissue and assess myocardial fibrosis non-invasively in SCD. Indeed, early findings from our ongoing CMR study indicate that diffuse myocardial fibrosis is common in SCD [64]. This and future studies may shed some light on the pathogenic mechanisms that underlie the cardiomyopathy of SCD.

6. Screening, diagnosis, and treatment of cardiac dysfunction in SCD

Based on the high prevalence of abnormal TRV and its correlation with PH, echocardiographic screening for PH in SCD was adopted by some groups [8]. However, because of the low predictive value of TRV in diagnosing PH in SCD and the lack of interventions that have been shown to change the outcome, if PH is detected early, echocardiographic screening for PH in SCD has become controversial. The 2014 National Heart, Lung and Blood Institute (NHLBI) Expert Panel's report on evidence-based management of SCD patients did not find sufficient evidence to make a recommendation for echocardiographic screening of asymptomatic SCD patients [65]. On the other hand, The American Thoracic Society Clinical Practice Guidelines suggested performing echocardiography every 1–3 year and increasing the frequency of screening depending on the presence of adverse risk factors (high TRV and elevated serum NT-pro-BNP or confirmed PH) [21]. However, these are experts' opinions that are not supported by strong evidence at this point. Despite incomplete information about its different causes, an elevated TRV is an adverse prognostic marker in adults with SCD, irrespective of PH, and this finding should prompt increased clinical vigilance. Although it is not clear when to begin screening and how often to continue it, at our pediatric institution, we perform a screening echocardiogram and electrocardiogram on asymptomatic individuals with SCD starting between the ages of 15 and 18 years. We screen for chamber enlargement, especially of the LA, systolic function, and diastolic abnormalities using mitral inflow and tissue Doppler annular velocities, and elevated TRV. If cardiac abnormalities are identified, the need for follow-up imaging and referral to a cardiologist is determined individually.

Similar to the difficulties in diagnosis and screening strategies, there is no proven treatment for cardiac dysfunction or PH in SCD. Few, small observational studies showed a potential effect of PAH-directed therapy in SCD-related PH [66–68], but randomized controlled trials did not demonstrate any benefit for these therapies in SCD. Small randomized controlled trials using the endothelin receptor antagonist bosentan in SCD patients with PH were terminated early due to slow enrollment [20], and a trial comparing sildenafil to placebo in SCD patients with elevated TRV was also terminated early because of adverse events [69]. Experts' guidelines recommend against the use of PAH-directed therapy in SCD [21, 65]. The role of disease-modifying therapies (i.e., hydroxyurea and transfusions) in the treatment of PH or SCD-related cardiomyopathy is also undetermined. Limited available data suggest that hydroxyurea may be beneficial in improving TRV elevation in young patients with SCD [70, 71]. However, transfusion therapy has not been studied in PH or cardiomyopathy. The American Thoracic Society expert's panel recommends using hydroxyurea for patients with increased mortality risk or chronic transfusions for patients who cannot take or were unresponsive to hydroxyurea. However, these recommendations are based on the overall beneficial effects of these disease-modifying therapies in ameliorating other aspects of SCD and not based on a demonstrated cardiopulmonary benefit [21]. Understanding the mechanisms underlying the SCD-related cardiomyopathy and different forms of PH in SCD will be important to identify directed therapies to slow or reverse cardiac dysfunction in SCD. Until then, optimizing general SCD care (e.g., beginning or optimizing hydroxyurea or chronic transfusion therapy) is the only therapeutic option with established benefits for SCD patients.

7. Conclusions

The SCD-related cardiomyopathy is a unique restrictive cardiomyopathy superimposed on LV enlargement and LVH due to hyperdynamic circulation. SCD-related cardiomyopathy is characterized by diastolic dysfunction, LA enlargement, and normal systolic function with LV enlargement. This restrictive cardiomyopathy leads to mild PH and mild elevation in TRV. Similar to other restrictive cardiomyopathies, the SCD-related cardiomyopathy may predispose to arrhythmias and sudden death. Diffuse myocardial fibrosis may be an underlying mechanism of the restrictive cardiac physiology of SCD. Definitively establishing the mechanisms underlying diastolic dysfunction and the SCD-related cardiomyopathy may lead to specific, targeted therapy to slow or reverse the cardiomyopathy and decrease the morbidity and early mortality of SCD.

Author details

Omar Niss and Charles T. Quinn*

*Address all correspondence to: Charles.Quinn@cchmc.org

Cincinnati Children's Hospital Medical Center, Cincinnati, Ohio, United States

References

[1] Quinn, CT, Rogers, ZR, McCavit, TL, et al. Improved survival of children and adolescents with sickle cell disease. Blood. 2010;115:3447–3452. DOI: 10.1182/blood-2009-07-233700.

[2] Platt, OS, Brambilla, DJ, Rosse, WF, et al. Mortality in sickle cell disease. Life expectancy and risk factors for early death. The New England Journal of Medicine. 1994;330:1639–1644. DOI: 10.1056/NEJM199406093302303.

[3] Lanzkron, S, Carroll, CP, Haywood, C, Jr. Mortality rates and age at death from sickle cell disease: U.S., 1979–2005. Public Health Reports. 2013;128:110–116.

[4] Fitzhugh, CD, Lauder, N, Jonassaint, JC, et al. Cardiopulmonary complications leading to premature deaths in adult patients with sickle cell disease. American Journal of Hematology. 2010;85:36–40. DOI: 10.1002/ajh.21569.

[5] Manci, EA, Culberson, DE, Yang, YM, et al. Causes of death in sickle cell disease: An autopsy study. British Journal of Haematology. 2003;123:359–365.

[6] Castro, O, Hoque, M, Brown, BD. Pulmonary hypertension in sickle cell disease: Cardiac catheterization results and survival. Blood. 2003;101:1257–1261. DOI: 10.1182/blood-2002-03-0948.

[7] Fonseca, GH, Souza, R, Salemi, VM, et al. Pulmonary hypertension diagnosed by right heart catheterisation in sickle cell disease. The European Respiratory Journal. 2012;39:112–118. DOI: 10.1183/09031936.00134410.

[8] Gladwin, MT, Sachdev, V, Jison, ML, et al. Pulmonary hypertension as a risk factor for death in patients with sickle cell disease. The New England Journal of Medicine. 2004;350:886–895. DOI: 10.1056/NEJMoa035477.

[9] Sachdev, V, Machado, RF, Shizukuda, Y, et al. Diastolic dysfunction is an independent risk factor for death in patients with sickle cell disease. Journal of the American College of Cardiology. 2007;49:472–479. DOI: 10.1016/j.jacc.2006.09.038.

[10] Gladwin, MT, Barst, RJ, Castro, OL, et al. Pulmonary hypertension and no in sickle cell. Blood. 2010;116:852–854. DOI: 10.1182/blood-2010-04-282095.

[11] Fijalkowska, I, Xu, W, Comhair, SA, et al. Hypoxia inducible-factor1alpha regulates the metabolic shift of pulmonary hypertensive endothelial cells. American Journal of Pathology. 2010;176:1130–1138. DOI: 10.2353/ajpath.2010.090832.

[12] Anthi, A, Machado, RF, Jison, ML, et al. Hemodynamic and functional assessment of patients with sickle cell disease and pulmonary hypertension. American Journal of Respiratory and Critical Care Medicine. 2007;175:1272–1279. DOI: 10.1164/rccm. 200610-1498OC.

[13] Galie, N, Hoeper, MM, Humbert, M, et al. Guidelines for the diagnosis and treatment of pulmonary hypertension: The task force for the diagnosis andtreatment of pulmonary hypertension of the european society of cardiology (esc) and the european respiratory society (ers), endorsed by the international society of heart and lung transplantation (ishlt). European Heart Journal. 2009;30:2493–2537. DOI: 10.1093/ eurheartj/ehp297.

[14] Cabrita, IZ, Mohammed, A, Layton, M, et al. The association between tricuspid regurgitation velocity and 5-year survival in a North West London population of patients with sickle cell disease in the United Kingdom. British Journal of Haematology. 2013;162:400–408. DOI: 10.1111/bjh.12391.

[15] Caughey, MC, Hinderliter, AL, Jones, SK, et al. Hemodynamic characteristics and predictors of pulmonary hypertension in patients with sickle cell disease. The American Journal of Cardiology. 2012;109:1353–1357. DOI: 10.1016/j.amjcard.2011.11.067.

[16] Arcasoy, SM, Christie, JD, Ferrari, VA, et al. Echocardiographic assessment of pulmonary hypertension in patients with advanced lung disease. American Journal of Respiratory and Critical Care Medicine. 2003;167:735–740. DOI: 10.1164/rccm. 200210-1130OC.

[17] Niss, O, Quinn, CT, Lane, A, et al. Cardiomyopathy with restrictive physiology in sickle cell disease. JACC Cardiovascular Imaging. 2016;9:243–252. DOI: 10.1016/j.jcmg. 2015.05.013.

[18] Parent, F, Bachir, D, Inamo, J, et al. A hemodynamic study of pulmonary hypertension in sickle cell disease. The New England Journal of Medicine. 2011;365:44–53. DOI: 10.1056/NEJMoa1005565.

[19] D'Alonzo, GE, Barst, RJ, Ayres, SM, et al. Survival in patients with primary pulmonary hypertension. Results from a national prospective registry. Annals of Internal Medicine. 1991;115:343–349.

[20] Barst, RJ, Mubarak, KK, Machado, RF, et al. Exercise capacity and haemodynamics in patients with sickle cell disease with pulmonary hypertension treated with bosentan: Results of the asset studies. British Journal of Haematology. 2010;149:426–435. DOI: 10.1111/j.1365-2141.2010.08097.x.

[21] Klings, ES, Machado, RF, Barst, RJ, et al. An official american thoracic society clinical practice guideline: Diagnosis, risk stratification, and management of pulmonary hypertension of sickle cell disease. American Journal of Respiratory and Critical Care Medicine. 2014;189:727–740. DOI: 10.1164/rccm.201401-0065ST.

[22] Fitzgerald, M, Fagan, K, Herbert, DE, et al. Misclassification of pulmonary hypertension in adults with sickle hemoglobinopathies using Doppler echocardiography. Southern Medical Journal. 2012;105:300–305. DOI: 10.1097/SMJ.0b013e318256b55b.

[23] Sharma, S, Efird, J, Kadali, R, et al. Pulmonary artery occlusion pressure may overdiagnose pulmonary artery hypertension in sickle cell disease. Clinical Cardiology. 2013;36:524–530. DOI: 10.1002/clc.22153.

[24] Simonneau, G, Gatzoulis, MA, Adatia, I, et al. Updated clinical classification of pulmonary hypertension. Journal of the American College of Cardiology. 2013;62:D34–D41. DOI: 10.1016/j.jacc.2013.10.029.

[25] Hankins, JS, McCarville, MB, Hillenbrand, CM, et al. Ventricular diastolic dysfunction in sickle cell anemia is common but not associated with myocardial iron deposition. Pediatric Blood & Cancer. 2010;55:495–500. DOI: 10.1002/pbc.22587.

[26] Sachdev, V, Kato, GJ, Gibbs, JS, et al. Echocardiographic markers of elevated pulmonary pressure and left ventricular diastolic dysfunction are associated with exercise intolerance in adults and adolescents with homozygous sickle cell anemia in The United States and United Kingdom. Circulation. 2011;124:1452–1460. DOI: 10.1161/CIRCULATIONAHA.111.032920.

[27] Blanc, J, Stos, B, de Montalembert, M, et al. Right ventricular systolic strain is altered in children with sickle cell disease. Journal of the American Society of Echocardiography: Official Publication of the American Society of Echocardiography. 2012;25:511–517. DOI: 10.1016/j.echo.2012.01.011.

[28] Eddine, AC, Alvarez, O, Lipshultz, SE, et al. Ventricular structure and function in children with sickle cell disease using conventional and tissue Doppler echocardiography. The American Journal of Cardiology. 2012;109:1358–1364. DOI: 10.1016/j.amjcard.2012.01.001.

[29] Zilberman, MV, Du, W, Das, S, et al. Evaluation of left ventricular diastolic function in pediatric sickle cell disease patients. American Journal of Hematology. 2007;82:433–438. DOI: 10.1002/ajh.20866.

[30] Nagueh, SF, Appleton, CP, Gillebert, TC, et al. Recommendations for the evaluation of left ventricular diastolic function by echocardiography. Journal of the American Society

of Echocardiography: Official Publication of the American Society of Echocardiography. 2009;22:107–133. DOI: 10.1016/j.echo.2008.11.023.

[31] Lam, CS, Roger, VL, Rodeheffer, RJ, et al. Pulmonary hypertension in heart failure with preserved ejection fraction: A community-based study. Journal of the American College of Cardiology. 2009;53:1119–1126. DOI: 10.1016/j.jacc.2008.11.051.

[32] Gordeuk, VR, Castro, OL, Machado, RF. Pathophysiology and treatment of pulmonary hypertension in sickle cell disease. Blood. 2016;127:820–828. DOI: 10.1182/blood-2015-08-618561.

[33] Kremastinos, DT, Farmakis, D, Aessopos, A, et al. Beta-thalassemia cardiomyopathy: History, present considerations, and future perspectives. Circulation: Heart Failure. 2010;3:451–458. DOI: 10.1161/CIRCHEARTFAILURE.109.913863.

[34] Meloni, A, Puliyel, M, Pepe, A, et al. Cardiac iron overload in sickle-cell disease. American Journal of Hematology. 2014;89:678–683. DOI: 10.1002/ajh.23721.

[35] Wood, JC. Cardiac iron across different transfusion-dependent diseases. Blood Reviews. 2008;22(Suppl 2):S14–S21. DOI: 10.1016/S0268-960X(08)70004-3.

[36] Desai, AA, Patel, AR, Ahmad, H, et al. Mechanistic insights and characterization of sickle cell disease-associated cardiomyopathy. Circulation Cardiovascular Imaging. 2014;7:430–437. DOI: 10.1161/CIRCIMAGING.113.001420.

[37] Metivier, F, Marchais, SJ, Guerin, AP, et al. Pathophysiology of anaemia: Focus on the heart and blood vessels. Nephrology Dialysis Transplantion. 2000;15(Suppl 3):14–18.

[38] London, GM, Guerin, AP, Marchais, SJ, et al. Cardiac and arterial interactions in end-stage renal disease. Kidney International. 1996;50:600–608.

[39] Muller, R, Steffen, HM, Brunner, R, et al. Changes in the alpha adrenergic system and increase in blood pressure with recombinant human erythropoietin (rhuepo) therapy for renal anemia. Clinical and Investigative Medicine. 1991;14:614–622.

[40] Varat, MA, Adolph, RJ, Fowler, NO. Cardiovascular effects of anemia. American Heart Journal. 1972;83:415–426.

[41] Lester, LA, Sodt, PC, Hutcheon, N, et al. Cardiac abnormalities in children with sickle cell anemia. Chest. 1990;98:1169–1174.

[42] Katz, AM. Maladaptive growth in the failing heart: The cardiomyopathy of overload. Cardiovascular Drugs Therapy. 2002;16:245–249.

[43] Kushwaha, SS, Fallon, JT, Fuster, V. Restrictive cardiomyopathy. The New England Journal of Medicine. 1997;336:267–276. DOI: 10.1056/NEJM199701233360407.

[44] Webber, SA, Lipshultz, SE, Sleeper, LA, et al. Outcomes of restrictive cardiomyopathy in childhood and the influence of phenotype: A report from the pediatric cardiomy-

opathy registry. Circulation. 2012;126:1237–1244. DOI: 10.1161/CIRCULATIONAHA. 112.104638.

[45] Nihoyannopoulos, P, Dawson, D. Restrictive cardiomyopathies. European journal of echocardiography: The Journal of the Working Group on Echocardiography of the European Society of Cardiology. 2009;10:iii23–iii33. DOI: 10.1093/ejechocard/jep156.

[46] Rivenes, SM, Kearney, DL, Smith, EO, et al. Sudden death and cardiovascular collapse in children with restrictive cardiomyopathy. Circulation. 2000;102:876–882.

[47] Murtuza, B, Fenton, M, Burch, M, et al. Pediatric heart transplantation for congenital and restrictive cardiomyopathy. The Annals of Thoracic Surgery. 2013;95:1675–1684. DOI: 10.1016/j.athoracsur.2013.01.014.

[48] Walsh, MA, Grenier, MA, Jefferies, JL, et al. Conduction abnormalities in pediatric patients with restrictive cardiomyopathy. Circulation: Heart Failure. 2012;5:267–273. DOI: 10.1161/CIRCHEARTFAILURE.111.964395.

[49] Poludasu, S, Ramkissoon, K, Salciccioli, L, et al. Left ventricular systolic function in sickle cell anemia: A meta-analysis. Journal of Cardiac Failure. 2013;19:333–341. DOI: 10.1016/j.cardfail.2013.03.009.

[50] Caldas, MC, Meira, ZA, Barbosa, MM. Evaluation of 107 patients with sickle cell anemia through tissue doppler and myocardial performance index. Journal of the American Society of Echocardiography: Official Publication of the American Society of Echocardiography. 2008;21:1163–1167. DOI: 10.1016/j.echo.2007.06.001.

[51] Colombatti, R, Maschietto, N, Varotto, E, et al. Pulmonary hypertension in sickle cell disease children under 10 years of age. British Journal of Haematology. 2010;150:601–609. DOI: 10.1111/j.1365-2141.2010.08269.x.

[52] Simmons, BE, Santhanam, V, Castaner, A, et al. Sickle cell heart disease. Two-dimensional echo and Doppler ultrasonographic findings in the hearts of adult patients with sickle cell anemia. Archives of Internal Medicine. 1988;148:1526–1528.

[53] Wood, JC, Tyszka, JM, Carson, S, et al. Myocardial iron loading in transfusion-dependent thalassemia and sickle cell disease. Blood. 2004;103:1934–1936. DOI: 10.1182/blood-2003-06-1919.

[54] Westwood, MA, Shah, F, Anderson, LJ, et al. Myocardial tissue characterization and the role of chronic anemia in sickle cell cardiomyopathy. Journal of Magnetic Resonance Imaging : JMRI. 2007;26:564–568. DOI: 10.1002/jmri.21018.

[55] Haque, AK, Gokhale, S, Rampy, BA, et al. Pulmonary hypertension in sickle cell hemoglobinopathy: A clinicopathologic study of 20 cases. Human Pathology. 2002;33:1037–1043.

[56] Martin, CR, Johnson, CS, Cobb, C, et al. Myocardial infarction in sickle cell disease. Journal of the National Medical Association. 1996;88:428–432.

[57] Darbari, DS, Kple-Faget, P, Kwagyan, J, et al. Circumstances of death in adult sickle cell disease patients. American Journal of Hematology. 2006;81:858–863. DOI: 10.1002/ajh.20685.

[58] James, TN, Riddick, L, Massing, GK. Sickle cells and sudden death: Morphologic abnormalities of the cardiac conduction system. Journal of Laboratorty Clincal Medicine. 1994;124:507–520.

[59] Doltra, A, Amundsen, BH, Gebker, R, et al. Emerging concepts for myocardial late gadolinium enhancement mri. Current Cardiology Reviews. 2013;9:185–190.

[60] Bratis, K, Kattamis, A, Athanasiou, K, et al. Abnormal myocardial perfusion-fibrosis pattern in sickle cell disease assessed by cardiac magnetic resonance imaging. International Journal of Cardiology. 2013;166:e75–76. DOI: 10.1016/j.ijcard.2013.01.055.

[61] Junqueira, FP, Fernandes, JL, Cunha, GM, et al. Right and left ventricular function and myocardial scarring in adult patients with sickle cell disease: A comprehensive magnetic resonance assessment of hepatic and myocardial iron overload. Journal of Cardiovascular Magnetic Resonance: Official Journal of the Society for Cardiovascular Magnetic Resonance. 2013;15:83. DOI: 10.1186/1532-429X-15-83.

[62] Raman, SV, Simonetti, OP, Cataland, SR, et al. Myocardial ischemia and right ventricular dysfunction in adult patients with sickle cell disease. Haematologica. 2006;91:1329–1335.

[63] Nguyen, KL, Tian, X, Alam, S, et al. Elevated transpulmonary gradient and cardiac magnetic resonance-derived right ventricular remodeling predict poor outcomes in sickle cell disease. Haematologica. 2016;101:e40–43. DOI: 10.3324/haematol.2015.125229.

[64] Niss, O, Taylor, MD, Moore, R, Fleck, R, Malik, P, Towbin, JA, Quinn, CT. 2015 Aspho abstracts. Pediatric Blood & Cancer. 2015;62:S21–S119. DOI: 10.1002/pbc.25540.

[65] Yawn, BP, Buchanan, GR, Afenyi-Annan, AN, et al. Management of sickle cell disease: Summary of the 2014 evidence-based report by expert panel members. The Journal of the American Medical Association. 2014;312:1033–1048. DOI: 10.1001/jama.2014.10517.

[66] Machado, RF, Martyr, S, Kato, GJ, et al. Sildenafil therapy in patients with sickle cell disease and pulmonary hypertension. British Journal of Haematology. 2005;130:445–453. DOI: 10.1111/j.1365-2141.2005.05625.x.

[67] Minniti, CP, Machado, RF, Coles, WA, et al. Endothelin receptor antagonists for pulmonary hypertension in adult patients with sickle cell disease. British Journal of Haematology. 2009;147:737–743. DOI: 10.1111/j.1365-2141.2009.07906.x.

[68] Morris, CR. New strategies for the treatment of pulmonary hypertension in sickle cell disease : The rationale for arginine therapy. Treatments in Respiratory Medicine. 2006;5:31–45.

[69] Machado, RF, Barst, RJ, Yovetich, NA, et al. Hospitalization for pain in patients with sickle cell disease treated with sildenafil for elevated TRV and low exercise capacity. Blood. 2011;118:855–864. DOI: 10.1182/blood-2010-09-306167.

[70] Olnes, M, Chi, A, Haney, C, et al. Improvement in hemolysis and pulmonary arterial systolic pressure in adult patients with sickle cell disease during treatment with hydroxyurea. American Journal of Hematology. 2009;84:530–532. DOI: 10.1002/ajh.21446.

[71] Pashankar, FD, Carbonella, J, Bazzy-Asaad, A, et al. Longitudinal follow up of elevated pulmonary artery pressures in children with sickle cell disease. British Journal of Haematology. 2009;144:736–741. DOI: 10.1111/j.1365-2141.2008.07501.x.

Chapter 7

Pulmonary Complications and Lung Function Abnormalities in Children with Sickle Cell Disease

Anne Greenough

Additional information is available at the end of the chapter

http://dx.doi.org/10.5772/64365

Abstract

The pulmonary complications of sickle cell disease (SCD) have a high morbidity and mortality. Fatal pulmonary complications occur in 20% of adults; those with sickle chronic lung disease (SCLD) and pulmonary hypertension have a significantly increased mortality. Treatment of SCLD is only supportive. Recurrent acute chest syndrome (ACS) episodes are the major risk factor for SCLD, and ACS is the leading cause of death. Adults with SCD tend to have restrictive lung function abnormalities, whereas, in children, obstructive abnormalities are more frequent. Lung function abnormalities are common even in young children and may reflect their chronic anaemia and increased pulmonary capillary blood volume, which increases airway obstruction and may be responsible for their increased wheezing. Whether more aggressive treatment of anaemia would improve lung function and long-term outcomes merits testing. Children with SCD experience a decline in lung function, which is most rapid in younger children in whom ACS episodes are most common highlighting the importance of identifying effective strategies to prevent and optimally treat ACS.

Keywords: Sickle cell disease, Acute chest syndrome, Obstructive lung function abnormalities, Restrictive lung function abnormalities

1. Introduction

The pulmonary complications of sickle cell disease (SCD) have a high morbidity and mortality with fatal pulmonary complications occurring in 20% of adults. Despite significant improvements in life expectancy in individuals with SCD, the median age of death for women is 48 years and for men 42 years. Young adults can develop sickle chronic lung disease (SCLD), which consists of restrictive lung disease, abnormal diffusing capacity and hypoxaemia. Those with SCLD and pulmonary hypertension have a significantly increased mortality. Treatment of SCLD is only supportive. Recurrent acute chest syndrome (ACS) episodes are the major risk factor for SCLD and ACS is the leading cause of death. Prevention and optimum management of ACS episodes then should reduce SCLD occurrence. ACS episodes occur most frequently in young children with SCD and lung function abnormalities are common in childhood. In this chapter, the aetiology, pathogenesis and management of acute chest syndrome are discussed. The presentation of SCLD is briefly summarised as this occurs in adults, but included here as it is an important adverse outcome of ACS episodes. Pulmonary hypertension is discussed elsewhere (see Chapter x), but the impact on those with lung function abnormalities is emphasised in this chapter. Lung function abnormalities in children associated with SCD are described as the factors influencing the deterioration in lung function suffered by children with SCD. Recommendations are made with regard to routine respiratory monitoring.

2. Acute chest syndrome (ACS)

2.1. Presentation

The overall incidence of ACS as indicated by the Cooperative Study of Sickle Cell Disease (CSSCD) is 10.5 per 100 patient years [1]. ACS episodes occur more commonly in children than adults. Fifty percent of SCD children will have an ACS episode prior to the age of 10 years and the highest incidence of ACS occurs in children aged between 2 and 4 years of age [2]. ACS episodes are characterised by fever, chest pain and respiratory symptoms and essential to making the diagnosis with a new pulmonary infiltrate on chest radiograph. Fever and cough are more common in young children who, compared to adults, are more likely to have isolated upper lobe disease. Adults tend to suffer chest pain, haemoptysis and shortness of breath; their middle and lower lobes are more frequently affected than the upper lobes. Severe respiratory failure, necessitating mechanical ventilation, occurs in approximately 10–15% of affected patients. Recurrence is common, occurring in 80% of those who have had a prior episode. Follow-up of 293 patients aged between 3 and 20 years for 21 months demonstrated that a history of acute pulmonary events and younger age were independently associated with developing a new ACS episode [3]. In children less than 4 years of age who had had an ACS episode, one study demonstrated that the majority were hospitalised for ACS or severe pain within 1 year, emphasising the need for an effective therapeutic intervention in that high risk group [4].

2.2. Risk factors

The incidence of ACS varies according to the haemoglobin genotype being commonest in those with HbSS and much less common in those with HbSC [2]. In a retrospective review, ACS episodes also appeared less severe in children with HbSC compared to those with HbSS as indicated by a significantly shorter hospital stay [5]. The sickle cell mutation has arisen on at least five separate occasions, on four occasions in Africa and one occasion in

Saudi Arabia or India [2]. The prevalence and recurrence of ACS episodes in Saudi Arabia are relatively low as compared to patients in Africa; this may be due to the interaction between SCD and the 'Asian' haplotype [6], which is known to be associated with a higher fetal haemoglobin (HbF) level. ACS hospitalisation has been shown to be associated with a single nucleotide polymorphism (SNP)-defined beta globin cluster [7]. The risk for ACS is increased by certain endothelin NO synthase gene polymorphisms [8]. A heme oxygenase-1 gene promoter was associated with a reduced incidence of ACS hospitalisation [9]. A gene-centric association study found an association between ACS and rs6141803, the SNP located 8.2 kb upstream of COMMD7, a gene highly expressed in the lung that interacts with nuclear factor-kB signalling [10].

High haemoglobin levels predispose to vascular obstruction and increase the risk of complications, such as ACS. High HbF levels inhibit the polymerisation of HbS and hence the higher the HbF level the lower the occurrence of ACS episodes [2]. Leucocytes release free radicals, elastase, pro-inflammatory mediators and cytokines, hence the occurrence of ACS episodes are directly proportional to the steady-state white blood cell count [11].

In approximately 10% of patients, an ACS is precipitated by a pulmonary fat embolism; affected patients tend to be older, have a lower mean oxygen saturation at presentation and have a more severe clinical course. Typically, the pulmonary signs and symptoms are preceded by bone pain. Affected individuals may have systemic signs of a fat embolism, including changes in their mental state, thrombocytopaenia and petechiae. Infarction of the bone marrow may result in fat embolisation. This can activate pulmonary secretory phospholipase A2 liberating free fatty acids. Arachidonic acid causes vasoconstriction and oleic acid upregulation of the vascular cell adhesion molecule (VCAM-1). Splinting resulting from bony thorax infarction leads to hypoventilation and atelectasis with accompanying hypoxia and hence sickling. The hypoventilation can be compounded by suppression of respiration by opoid administration. Infection causes approximately 30% of ACS episodes. The seasonal variation in ACS episodes in young children likely reflects the increase in viral infections in young children during the winter months. Children presenting with fever have an increased risk of developing an ACS episode if they have had a previous ACS episode, upper respiratory tract infection symptoms, non-compliance to penicillin, an absolute neutrophil count greater than $9 \times 10(9)/l$ and haemoglobin less than 8.6 g/dl [12]. In a multicentre study, 27 different pathogens were identified, but *Chlamyidia pneumoniae* was the most frequent pathogen, followed by *Mycoplasma pneumoniae* and respiratory syncytial virus. Parvovirus B10 has been associated with marrow necrosis and a particularly severe form of ACS.

In the Cooperative Study for Sickle Cell Disease before 6 months of age in which patients were followed beyond 5 years of age, a clinical diagnosis of asthma was made in 17% of the cohort. Asthma was associated with more frequent ACS episodes [13]. In a retrospective review of inpatient episodes for ACS, a previous history of asthma or wheezing was more common in children with HbSC than in those with HBSS causing the authors to speculate that asthma and wheezing may be more significant risk factors for ACS episodes [5].

2.3. Risk factors for recurrent ACS episodes

In a cohort of 159 children followed from birth to a median of 14.7 years, an ACS episode prior to 4 years, female gender, wheezing with shortness of breath and two or more positive skin prick tests were associated with future ACS episodes, but airway obstruction and a bronchodilator response were not [14]. Asthma has been reported to be a risk factor for recurrent ACS episodes in SCD children in Jamaica [15].

2.4. Pathogenesis

The levels of inflammatory cytokines are increased in ACS. Nitric oxide (NO) levels, however, are reduced; this is due to a number of reasons. 'Free' haemoglobin in the plasma scavenges NO. Hypoxia reduces NO production by inhibition of NO synthase and activated macrophages and leuocytes release free radical species that inactivate NO. Adhesion is increased when there are low NO levels as NO inhibits the upregulation of VCAM-1. NO also inhibits endothelin-1 production. In addition, there is a lack of inhibition of platelet activation and further potentiation of microvascular occlusion and the release of vasoconstrictor metabolites such as thromboxane A2. Sickle red blood cells, due to the greater auto-oxidation of HbS compared to HbA, produce greater levels of oxygen-related radicals including superoxide, hydrogen peroxide and peroxynitrite. There are also lower levels of antioxidant enzyme systems, e.g. superoxide dismutase, catalyse and glutathione peroxidate. The sickle cells occlude vessels causing vascular injury, especially to organs with sluggish circulation such as atelectatic areas of the lung. Neutrophils are more adherent to endothelin cells in SCD patients and this has been associated with ACS episodes.

2.5. Management

Broad spectrum antibiotics should be given, including macrolides or quinolones to treat atypical organisms. The choice of antibiotics should be guided by the patient's clinical condition and the 'local' pathogens. Oxygen therapy should be used to treat any hypoxaemia. There may, however, be a poor correlation of pulse oximetry readings with arterial oxygen tensions (see below) and hence blood gas analysis should be undertaken if there is suspicion of hypoxia. Indications for escalation of respiratory support, which is most likely in those with extensive, pulmonary involvement, are increasing hypoxia and dyspnoea and the pH following below 7.35. In such patients, non-invasive ventilation has been demonstrated to improve oxygenation and reduce heart rate [16], but may be poorly tolerated. Patients should be carefully rehydrated as SCD patients are susceptible to fluid overload; hydration should be limited to 1.5 times the maintenance fluid volume to avoid further impairment of lung function by aggravating vascular leak in the lungs. In ACS patients with hypoxia, simple or exchange transfusion can rapidly increase oxygenation [17]. An alveolar-arterial oxygen gradient >30 mmHg has been associated with a worse severity score and higher need for transfusion [17]. To improve the oxygen-carrying capacity of the blood and reduce the proportion of sickle haemoglobin a transfusion is given. In those patients with a relatively high haematocrit an exchange transfusion is administered, as a simple transfusion under such circumstances would increase the viscosity of the blood. Non-randomised trials have not shown any benefit of exchange transfusion over simple transfusion [18, 19]; nevertheless in more severe cases requiring mechanical ventilation, particularly if a simple transfusion has not improved the patient, exchange transfusion is recommended [2]. Indications to proceed to an exchange transfusion include increasing hypoxia, increasing respiratory rate, reducing platelet count and multilobar disease. The aim being to keep the haemoglobin level at 10–11 g/dl. Analgesia should be given to control pain, but the amount limited to avoid respiratory depression. Patient controlled analgesia devices may reduce the risk of narcotic-induced hypoventilation [20]. Intercostal nerve block with a long acting local anaesthetic can alleviate chest wall pain and has the advantage of reducing the amount of systemic analgesia needed to control pain [2]. Inhaled NO (20–80 ppm) in patients with ACS and pulmonary hypertension has been reported to result in rapid and significant pulmonary vasodilation and improvement in oxygenation [21, 22]. Inhaled NO increases the oxygen affinity of HbS. A large prospective randomised trial, however, failed to show any significant differences in the time to resolution of crisis, length of hospitalisation, pain scores, cumulative opioid usage and rate of ACS between the nitric oxide and the placebo groups [23]. Approximately 25% of patients wheeze during an ACS episode and may benefit from bronchodilator administration [18], but the effect of bronchodilators on long-term outcome has not been investigated in randomised controlled trials. In a small Randomised controlled trial, dexamethasone administered to children with mild to moderately severe ACS was associated with a 40% reduction in the length of hospitalisation, a shorter duration of supplementary oxygen requirement and less need for analgesia [24]. Such outcomes are biologically plausible, as corticosteroids modulate endothelin cell adhesion molecule expression including VCAM-1 and have an inhibitory effect on phospholipase A2. Readmission after an ACS episode, however, has been demonstrated to be more common in those who reported use of an inhaler or a nebuliser at home or had received corticosteroids for the ACS episode [25].

2.6. Prevention

Fetal haemoglobin (HbF) inhibits polymerisation of deoxyhaemoglobin S and the level of HbF predicts the severity of the condition being inversely related to the mortality. There are a number of agents that raise HbF levels. One such is hydroxyurea that is a ribonuclease reductase inhibitor blocking DNA synthesis. The HbF level is raised due to the resultant bone marrow suppression. Additionally, hydroxyurea as an NO donor reduces VCAM-1 production and hence decreases sickle cell adhesion to the vascular endothelin. In an RCT involving adults, hydroxyurea reduced the incidence of ACS [26]. The systematic review of studies to date concluded that hydroxyurea is effective and safe in adults severely affected by sickle cell anaemia. The Pediatric Hydroxyurea Phase 3 Clinical Trial (BABY HUG) was an RCT of daily oral hydroxurea in children with sickle cell anaemia aged 9–18 months. The trial failed to achieve its primary aim which was to determine whether daily hydroyurea would reduce spleen and renal damage by at least 50%. There were, however, significantly fewer sickle cell disease related events in the hydroxurea group, including ACS episodes [27]. Hydoxyurea, however, may cause cytopaenias and patients must be carefully monitored, especially early in the administration of therapy, which may explain why some physicians are reluctant to prescribe it [28]. The summary of the 2014 evidence-based report by expert panel members gave a recommendation of moderate strength regarding offering treatment with hydroxyurea without regard to the presence of symptoms for infants, children and adolescents [29]. Chronic transfusion in patients with a history of recurrent or severe episodes has been demonstrated by both retrospective review [30] and randomised trial [31] to reduce the frequency of ACS episodes. Routine use of incentive spirometry is recommended in SCD patients admitted to hospital with chest or bone pain. Such management in a randomised trial was associated with a lower rate of pulmonary complications (atelectasis or infiltrates) as seen on a subsequent chest radiograph [32]. A retrospective review demonstrated that introduction of an evidence-based guideline initiating mandatory incentive spirometry in children with SCD admitted for non-respiratory complaints resulted in a reduced number of transfusions and ACS episodes [33]. Stem cell transplantation in adults and children has been associated with no recurrence of painful crisis in those with stable engraftment [34]. The best results were obtained in young children who have HLA-identical sibling donors and transplanted early in the course of their disease [35]. In certain paediatric populations the success rate is 85–90% [36].

2.7. Outcome

The overall mortality for ACS is 3%, but 9% in adults [18]. The primary cause of death is respiratory failure from pulmonary emboli and bronchopneumonia. In one study [37], 60% of severe ACS episodes were associated with pulmonary hypertension which is associated with a higher risk of death. The incidence of acute kidney injury is higher in patients with ACS and pulmonary hypertension and correlates with the severity of the ACS [38]. Young children with a greater number of ACS episodes have a greater decline in lung function (see below) [39]. In young adults, the greater the number of ACS episodes the greater the reduction in lung function [40].

3. Pulmonary hypertension

In a screening study, 32% of patients had a tricuspid regurgitant jet velocity (TRV) by Doppler echocardiography of greater or equal to 2.5 m/s which corresponds to a Pulmonary artery systolic pressure of 25–35 mmHg (approximately two standard deviations above the mean). Despite mildly elevated TRV values, the prospective mortality was high with a tenfold increase in the odds ratio for death [41]. Echocardiography, however, may overestimate the prevalence of pulmonary hypertension [42]. Pulmonary hypertension in SCD is characterised by progressive obliteration of the pulmonary vasculature. Possible causes include chronic hypoxic stress causing irreversible remodelling of the pulmonary vasculature, recurrent pulmonary thromboembolism, sickle cell related vasculopathy and pulmonary scarring from recurrent ACS episodes. An elevated TRV has been reported in 11–31% of children and adolescents with SCD [43, 44]. The clinical significance is not known although an elevated TRV in children has been associated with a decline in exercise capacity [45].

http://dx.doi.org/10.5772/64365

4. Sickle chronic lung disease (SCLD)

SCLD is a progressive disease with an insidious onset progressing to end-stage respiratory failure, characterised by hypoxemia, restrictive lung disease, cor pulmonale and chest radiograph evidence of diffuse interstitial fibrosis. Recurrent ACS episodes result in damage to the lung parenchyma resulting in restrictive lung disease. In a study of 319 adults with SCD, 74% had restrictive lung function abnormalities [46]. The mean survival of SCD patients with chronic lung disease and elevated pulmonary artery pressures can be as short as 2 years. Sudden death in SCLD patients with pulmonary hypertension is common due to pulmonary thromboembolism, systemic hypotension and cardiac arrhythmia. Adult SCD patients, therefore, should be screened for pulmonary hypertension with echocardiography as, although initially the patients may be asymptomatic, their condition progresses and they suffer worsening hypoxia and chest pain with impaired exercise tolerance.

5. Asthma and outcomes of SCD

Asthma has been associated with adverse outcomes in SCD patients. Asthma has been reported to be more common in those with ACS [13] and in particular with recurrent ACS episodes [15]. In one series, after controlling for established risk factors, individuals with sickle cell anaemia and asthma had more than a two fold increased risk of mortality [47]. In another series [48], after adjusting for baseline lung function, current asthma and smoking were significantly associated with mortality during a 10-year period in young adults [48]. Patients with SCD frequently wheeze and asthma may have been over diagnosed in previous studies that used a physician's diagnosis of asthma rather than more objective tests such as determination of bronchial responsiveness. In a retrospective study, asthma and wheezing were independent risk factors for increased painful episodes and only wheezing was associated with more ACS episodes [49]. In an observational study in SCD adults, the ACS rate, lung function or risk of death was not significantly related to a diagnosis of asthma. Whereas those who had recurrent severe episodes of wheezing compared to those without wheeze had twice the number of ACS episodes, poorer lung function and an increased risk of death [50].

6. Lung function abnormalities

Obstructive lung abnormalities are reported in young children [51, 52] with restrictive abnormalities becoming more prominent with advancing age [53]. Airway hyper-responsiveness (AHR) to methacholine has been reported to be more common in SCD children, but not related to signs or symptoms of allergy [54]. There is great variation reported in the response to bronchial challenges from 0% in one study [55] to 78% [56] in another. Similarly, the response to bronchodilator varies from no difference compared to controls [53], but others [15, 57] reporting a much higher response. Nocturnal desaturation episodes, possibly due to obstructive sleep apnoea, may occur in up to 40% of children and adolescents. Oxygen saturation monitoring, however, may be inaccurate as oximeters do not differentiate between oxyHb and carboxyhaemoglobin which is raised in some patients.

6.1. Exercise capacity

There have been few studies investigating the cardio-respiratory responses of patients with sickle cell anaemia to exercise. Children with SCD have been reported to have more adipose tissue with reduced fitness and exercise performance [58]. Exercise capacity has been reported to be related to the baseline degree of anaemia and be significantly lower in subjects with a history of recurrent ACS [59]. The metabolic changes imposed by exercise may initiate sickling and vaso-occlusive episodes. Patients, therefore, are advised to start exercise slowly and progressively, to maintain hydration and avoid sudden changes in temperature [60].

6.2. Longitudinal changes in lung function

A cross-sectional study suggested that restrictive abnormalities may increase with increasing age in childhood [53]. A longitudinal study of children aged 5–18 years demonstrated at baseline the children mainly had obstructive lung function abnormalities [61]. At follow up 4 years later, the number of children with obstructive or restrictive lung function abnormalities had increased, but obstructive abnormalities were more common [61]. Retrospective analysis of results from 413 SCD children aged between 8 and 18 years, however, demonstrated an increased prevalence of restrictive abnormalities with increasing age [62]. In two cohorts of SCD children, one of which was followed for 2 years and the other for 10 years, lung function deteriorated in the SCD children compared to contemporaneously studied ethnic and age matched controls. This was the first longitudinal study to include contemporaneously studied ethnic and age-matched controls [39]. In the cohort followed for 10 years restrictive abnormalities became more common. The rate of deterioration in lung function was greater in the younger children in whom ACS episodes were more common [39].

6.3. Aetiology of the lung function abnormalities

The obstructive lung function abnormalities seen in SCD children could be due to asthma. An increased prevalence of asthma was reported in one study [15], but other studies have indicated a similar incidence to that of non-SCD populations [63, 64]. Exhaled nitric oxide is elevated in asthma due to the enhanced expression of inducible nitric oxide synthase inflamed airways. Yet in prospective study of 50 SCD children and 50 controls the exhaled NO levels between the two groups were similar and airway obstruction in the SCD children was not associated with increased methacholine sensitivity or eosinophilic inflammation [55]. An alternative explanation for the airway obstruction in SCD is the hyperdynamic pulmonary circulation due to a raised cardiac output resulting from chronic anaemia [65]. Furthermore, in a study of 18 SCD children compared to 18 ethnic and age-matched controls, the SCD children had a significantly higher respiratory system resistance, alveolar NO production and pulmonary blood flow, but not airway NO flux. There was a significant correlation between alveolar NO production and pulmonary blood flow, but not between airway NO flux and respiratory system resistance [66]. SCD patients have an increased pulmonary capillary blood volume resulting from their chronic anaemia. In a study of 25 SCD children and 25 ethnic origin matched controls, the SCD children had significantly both higher airway obstruction and pulmonary capillary blood volume before and after bronchodilator. In the SCD children there was a significant correlation between the pulmonary capillary blood volume and the increased airways airway obstruction [67]. Furthermore, transfusion in SCD children has been shown to acutely increase airway obstruction and this was significantly related to an increase in pulmonary capillary blood volume [68]. Those results suggest that the airway obstruction seen in SCD children, at least in some, relates to their increased pulmonary capillary blood flow rather than bronchial hyper-reactivity. The clinical implication of those results is that SCD children with airway obstruction may have only limited benefit from bronchodilators and this should be formally tested (see below). Strategies to reduce anaemia and the increased pulmonary capillary blood volume, such as hydroxyurea, may be beneficial in those who remain symptomatic despite optimisation of bronchodilator therapy.

7. Recommendations regarding routine respiratory monitoring

The most rapid deterioration in lung function occurs in very young children [39], thus routine respiratory monitoring should begin early, that is, as soon as the child can undertake the measurements (usually from 4 years of age) on an annual basis. Such monitoring is to enable early detection of a child whose respiratory function is deteriorating and needs escalation of treatment. Equally paired lung function assessments can determine the efficacy of treatment for an individual (see below). Young children, however, have limited ability to perform lung function tests and detailed lung function testing is not available in all centres. As a consequence, in those less than 5 years of age, impulse oscillometry is recommended as this does not require volitional input by the child; in older children spirometry gives additional information. Both techniques are applicable to developed or low resource settings (if in the latter a hand-held spirometer is used). Assessment of lung volume is also additive in older children as this will identify those starting to develop restrictive abnormalities, but the relevant techniques are expensive, particularly plethysmography. Assessment of lung volume by measurement of functional residual capacity by helium gas dilution is more generalisable in developed settings. It is important that children with wheeze are not assumed to have asthma as wheeze in SCD may have other causes. It is therefore important that they undergo assessment for bronchial hyper-reactivity according to their lung function, those with airway function less than 70% of predicted should receive a bronchodilator and those with better airway function, better than 70% predicted, should receive either a cold air or exercise challenge. A methacholine challenge should not be used as this can precipitate an ACS. To ensure all children are appropriately diagnosed as having AHR undertaking both a cold air and exercise challenge should be considered, as some children respond only to one type of challenge and not the other [69]. Theoretically, any bronchial challenge could precipitate a crisis although this has only been reported with a metacholine challenge. An alternative approach in a child with recurrent wheeze, particularly if they have an atopic family history, is to give them a trial of inhaled steroids, but importantly assess whether there has been any positive effect using respiratory diary cards and preferably lung function assessments. Clinical trials are required to evaluate the effectiveness of therapy for asthma in patients with SCD and coincident asthma and whether this influences their respiratory outcomes.

Author details

Anne Greenough

Address all correspondence to: anne.greenough@kcl.ac.uk

Division of Asthma, Allergy and Lung Biology, King's College London, London, UK

References

[1] Castro O, Brambilla DJ, Thorington B, et al. The acute chest syndrome in sickle cell disease: incidence and risk factors. The cooperative study of sickle cell disease. Blood 1994;84:643–9.

[2] Paul RN, Castro OL, Aggarwal A, et al. Acute chest syndrome: sickle cell disease. Eur J Haematol 2011;87:191–207.

[3] Paul R, Minniti CP, Nouraie M, et al. Clinical correlates of acute pulmonary events in children and adolescents with sickle cell disease. Eur J Haematol 2013;91:62–8.

[4] Vance LD, Rodeghier M, Cohen RT, et al. Increased risk of severe vaso-occlusive episodes after initial acute chest syndrome in children with sickle cell anemia less than 4 years old: sleep and asthma cohort. Am J Hematol 2015;90:371–5.

[5] Poulter EY, Truszkowski P, Thompson A, et al. Acute chest syndrome is associated with history of asthma in haemoglobin SC disease. Pediatr Blood Cancer 2011;57:289–93.

[6] Alabdulaali MK. Sickle cell disease patients in eastern province of Saudi Arabia suffer less severe acute chest syndrome than patients with African haplotypes. Ann Thorac Med 2007;2:158–62.

[7] Bean CJ, Boulet SL, Yang G, et al. Acute chest syndrome is associated with single nucleotide polymorphism-defined beta globin cluster haplotype in children with sickle cell anaemia. Br J Haematol 2013;163:268–76.

[8] Sharan K, Surrey S, Ballas S, et al. Association of T-786C eNOS gene polymorphism with increased susceptibility to acute chest syndrome in females with sickle cell disease. Br J Haematol 2004;124:240–3.

[9] Bean CJ, Boulet S, Ellingsen D, et al. Heme oxygenase-1 gene promoter polymorphism is associated with reduced incidence of acute chest syndrome among children with sickle cell disease. Blood 2012;120:3822–8.

[10] Galarenau G, Coady S, Garrett ME, et al. Gene-centric association study of acute chest syndrome and painful crisis in sickle cell disease patients. Blood 2013;122:434–42.

[11] Knight-Madden J, Greenough A. Acute pulmonary complications of sickle cell disease. Paediatr Respir Rev 2014;15:13–6.

[12] Chang TP, Kriengsoontorkij W, Chan LS, et al. Clinical factors and incidence of acute chest syndrome or pneumonia among children with sickle cell disease presenting with a fever. A 17 year review. Pediatr Emer Care 2013;29:781–6.

[13] Boyd JH, Macklin EA, Strunk RC, et al. Asthma is associated with acute chest syndrome and pain in children with sickle cell anemia. Blood 2006;108:2923–7.

[14] DeBaun MR, Rodeghier M, Cohen R, et al. Factors predicting future ACS episodes in children with sickle cell anemia. Am J Hematol 2014;89:E212–7.

[15] Knight-Madden JM, Forrester TS, Lewis NA, et al. Asthma in children with sickle cell disease and its association with acute chest syndrome. Thorax 2005;60:206–10.

[16] Fartoukh M, Lefort Y, Habibi A, et al. Early intermittent noninvasive ventilation for acute chest syndrome in adults with sickle cell disease: a pilot study. Intensive Care Med 2010;36:1355–62.

[17] Emre U, Miller ST, Gutierez M, et al. Effect of transfusion in acute chest syndrome of sickle cell disease. J Pediatr 1995;127:901–4.

[18] Vichinsky EP, Neumayr LD, Earles AN, et al. Causes and outcomes of the acute chest syndrome in sickle cell disease. National Acute Chest Syndrome Study Group. N Engl J Med 2000;342:1855–65.

[19] Turner JM, Kaplan JB, Cohen HW, et al. Exchange versus simple transfusion for acute chest syndrome in sickle cell anemia adults. Transfusion 2009;49:863–8.

[20] van Beers EJ, van Tuijn CF, Nieuwkerk PT, et al. Patient-controlled analgesia versus continuous infusion of morphine during vaso-occlusive crisis in sickle cell disease, a randomized controlled trial. Am J Hematol. 2007;82:955–60.

[21] Atz AM, Wessel DL. Inhaled nitric oxide in sickle cell disease with acute chest syndrome. Anesthesiology 1997;87:988–90

[22] Sullivan KJ, Goodwin SR, Evangelist J, et al. Nitric oxide successfully used to treat acute chest syndrome of sickle cell disease in a young adolescent. Crit Care Med 1999;27:2563–8.

[23] Gladwin MT, Kato GJ, Weiner D, et al; DeNOVO Investigators. Nitric oxide for inhalation in the acute treatment of sickle cell pain crisis: a randomized controlled trial. JAMA 2011;305:893–902.

[24] Bernini JC, Rogers ZR, Sandler ES, et al. Beneficial effect of intravenous dexamethasone in children with mild to moderately severe acute chest syndrome complicating sickle cell disease. Blood 1998;92:3082–9.

[25] Strouse JJ, Takemoto CM, Keefer JR. Corticosteroids and increased risk of readmission after acute chest syndrome in children with sickle cell disease. Pediatr Blood Cancer 2008;50:1006–12.

[26] Charache S, Terrin ML, Moore RD, et al. Effect of hydroxyurea on the frequency of painful crises in sickle cell anemia. Investigators of the Multicenter Study of Hydroxyurea in sickle cell anemia. N Engl J Med 1995;332:1317–22.

[27] Wang WC, Ware RE, Miller ST, et al. Hydroxycarbamide in very young children with sickle-cell anaemia: a multicentre, randomised, controlled trial (BABY HUG). Lancet 2011;377:1663–72.

[28] Kanter J, Kruse-Jarres R. Management of sickle cell disease from childhood through adulthood. Blood Rev 2013;27:279–87.

[29] Yawn BP, Buchanan GR, Afenyi-Annan AN, et al. Management of sickle cell disease: summary of the 2014 evidence based report by expert panel members. JAMA 2014;312:1033–48

[30] Hankins J, Jeng M, Harris S, et al. Chronic transfusion therapy for children with sickle cell disease and recurrent acute chest syndrome. J Pediatr Hematol Oncol 2005;27:158–61.

[31] Miller ST, Wright E, Abboud M, et al; STOP Investigators. Impact of chronic transfusion on incidence of pain and acute chest syndrome during the Stroke Prevention Trial (STOP) in sickle-cell anemia. J Pediatr 2001;139:785–9.

[32] Bellet PS, Kalinyak KA, Shukla R, et al. Incentive spirometry to prevent acute pulmonary complications in sickle cell diseases. N Engl J Med 1995;333:699–703.

[33] Ahmad FA, Macias CG, Allen JY. The use of incentive spirometry in pediatric patients with sickle cell disease to reduce the incidence of acute chest syndrome. J Pediatr Hematol Oncol 2011;33:415–20.

[34] Khoury R, Abboud MR. Stem-cell transplantation in children and adults with sickle cell disease: an update. Expert Rev Hematol 2011;4:343–51.

[35] Oshrine B, Talano JA. Curative treatment for severe sickle cell disease: allogeneic transplantation. Clin Ad Hematol Oncol 2015;13:249–56.

[36] Oringanje C, Nemecek E, Oniyangi O. Hematopoietic stem cell transplantation for people with sickle cell disease. Cochrane Database Syst Rev 2013;5:CD007001.

[37] Mekontso Dessap A, Leon R, Habibi A, et al. Pulmonary hypertension and cor pulmonale during severe acute chest syndrome in sickle cell disease. Am J Respir Crit Care Med 2008;177:646–53.

[38] Audard V, Homs S, Habibi A, et al. Acute kidney injury in sickle patients with painful crisis or acute chest syndrome and its relation to pulmonary hypertension. Nephrol Dial Transplant 2010;25:2524–9.

[39] Lunt A, McGhee E, Sylvester K, et al. Longitudinal assessment of lung function in children with sickle cell disease. Pediatr Pulmonol 2016;51:717–23.

[40] Knight-Madden JM, Forrester TS, Lewis NA, et al. The impact of recurrent acute chest syndrome on the lung function of young adults with sickle cell disease. Lung 2010;188:499–504

[41] Gladwin MT, Sachdev V, Jison ML, et al. Pulmonary hypertension as a risk factor for death in patients with sickle cell disease. N Engl J Med 2004;350:886–95.

[42] Parent F, Bachir D, Inamo J, et al. A hemodynamic study of pulmonary hypertension in sickle cell disease. N Engl J Med 2011;365:44–53

[43] Dahoui HA, Hayek MN, Nietert PJ, et al. Pulmonary hypertension in children and young adults with sickle cell disease: evidence for familial clustering. Pediatr Blood Cancer 2010;54:398–402.

[44] Minniti CP, Sable C, Campbell A, et al. Elevated tricuspid regurgitant jet velocity in children and adolescents with sickle cell disease: association with hemolysis and hemoglobin oxygen desaturation. Haematologica 2009;94:340–7.

[45] Gordeuk VR, Minniti CP, Nouraie M, et al. Elevated tricuspid regurgitation velocity and decline in exercise capacity over 22 months of follow up in children and adolescents with sickle cell anemia. Haematologica 2011;96:33–40.

[46] Klings ES, Wyszynski DF, Nolan VG, et al. Abnormal pulmonary function in adults with sickle cell anemia. Am J Respir Crit Care Med 2006;173:1264–9.

[47] Boyd JH, Macklin EA, Strunk RC, et al. Asthma is associated with increased mortality in individuals with sickle cell anemia. Haematologica 2007;92:1115–8.

[48] Knight-Madden JM, Barton-Gooden A, Weaver SR, et al. Mortality, asthma, smoking and acute chest syndrome in young adults with sickle cell disease. Lung 2013;191:95–100.

[49] Glassberg JA, Chow A, Wisnivesky J, et al. Wheezing and asthma are independent risk factors for increased sickle cell disease morbidity. Br J Haematol 2012;159:472–9.

[50] Cohen RT, Madadi A, Blinder MA, et al. Recurrent, severe wheezing is associated with morbidity and mortality in adults with sickle cell disease. Am J Hematol 201;86:756–61.

[51] Intzes S, Kalpatthi RV, Short R, et al. Pulmonary function abnormalities and asthma are prevalent in children with sickle cell disease and are associated with acute chest syndrome. Pediatr Hematol Oncol 2013;30:726–32.

[52] Arteta M, Campbell A, Nouraie M, et al. Abnormal pulmonary function and associated risk factors in children and adolescents with sickle cell anemia. J Pediatr Hematol Oncol 2014;36:185–9.

[53] Sylvester KP, Patey RA, Milligan P, et al. Pulmonary function abnormalities in children with sickle cell disease. Thorax 2004;59:67–70.

[54] Field JF, Stocks J, Kirkham FJ, et al. Airway hyperresponsiveness in children with sickle cell anemia. Chest 2011;139:563–8.

[55] Chaudry RA, Rosenthal M, Bush A, et al. Reduced forced expiratory flow but not increased exhaled nitric oxide or airway responsiveness to methacholine characterises paediatric sickle cell airway disease. Thorax 2014;69:580–5.

[56] Ozbek OY, Malbora B, Sen AC, Yazici AC, Ozyurek E, Ozbek N. Airway hyperreactivity detected by methacholine challenge in children with sickle cell disease. Pediatr Pulmonol 2007;42:1187–92.

[57] Koumbourlis AC, Zar HJ, Hurlet-Jensen A, Goldberg MR. Prevalence and reversibility of lower airway obstruction in children with sickle cell disease. J Pediatr 2001;138:188–92.

[58] Moheeb H, Wali YA, El-Sayed MS. Physical fitness indices and anthropometrics profiles in schoolchildren with sickle cell trait/disease. Am J Hematol 2007;82:91–7.

[59] Liem RI, Nevin MA, Prestridge A, et al. Functional capacity in children and young adults with sickle cell disease undergoing evaluation for cardiopulmonary disease. Am J Hematol 2009;84:645–9.

[60] Connes P, Machado R, Hue O, et al. Exercise limitation, exercise testing and exercise recommendations in sickle cell anemia. Clin Hemorheol Microcirc 2011;49:151–63.

[61] Koumbourlis A, Lee DJ, Lee A. Longitudinal changes in lung function and somatic growth in children with sickle cell disease. Pediatr Pulmonol 2007;42:483–8.

[62] MacLean JE, Atenafu E, Kirby-Allen M, et al. Longitudinal decline in lung volume in a population of children with sickle cell disease. Am J Respir Crit Care Med 2008;178:1055–9.

[63] Boyd JH, Moinuddin A, Strunk RC, DeBaun MR. Asthma and acute chest in sickle-cell disease. Pediatr Pulmonol 2004;38:229–32.

[64] Bernaudin F, Strunk RC, Kamdem A, et al. Asthma is associated with acute chest syndrome, but not with an increased rate of hospitalization for pain among children in France with sickle cell anemia: a retrospective cohort study. Haematologica 2008;93:1917–8.

http://dx.doi.org/10.5772/64365

[65] Batra AS, Acherman RJ, Wong WY, et al. Cardiac abnormalities in children with sickle cell anemia. Am J Hematol 2002;70:306–12.

[66] Lunt A, Ahmed N, Rafferty GF, et al. Airway and alveolar nitric oxide production, lung function, and pulmonary blood flow in sickle cell disease. Pediatr Res 2016;79:313–7.

[67] Wedderburn CJ, Rees D, Height S, et al. Airways obstruction and pulmonary capillary blood volume in children with sickle cell disease. Pediatr Pulmonol 2014;49:716–22.

[68] Lunt A, McGhee E, Robinson P, et al. Lung function, transfusion, pulmonary capillary blood volume and sickle cell disease. Respir Physiol Neurobiol 2016;222:6–10.

[69] Sylvester KP, Patey RA, Rafferty GF, Rees D, Thein SL, Greenough A. Airway hyper-responsiveness and acute chest syndrome in children with sickle cell anemia. Pediatr Pulmonol 2007;42:272–6.

Chapter 8

Neurological Complications and MRI

Jamie M. Kawadler and Fenella J. Kirkham

Additional information is available at the end of the chapter

http://dx.doi.org/10.5772/64143

Abstract

Cerebrovascular diseases (cerebral infarction, intracranial haemorrhage and vasculopathy) are common manifestations of sickle cell disease (SCD) associated with significant morbidity and mortality. These neurological complications and potential corresponding neuropsychological compromise may have devastating consequences for a child with SCD. This chapter aims to review the neurological complications in SCD using magnetic resonance imaging (MRI) as both a qualitative and a quantitative tool for detecting abnormality. Advanced MRI pulse sequences, such as high-resolution 3D T1-weighted imaging for brain volumetrics, diffusion tensor imaging for white matter integrity and non-invasive perfusion MRI for cerebral blood flow (CBF) measurement, can provide additional information about the structure and function of brain tissue beyond the scope of conventional clinical imaging. These studies have set to establish quantitative biomarkers that relate to disease severity and neuropsychological sequelae.

Keywords: sickle cell anaemia, MRI, cerebrovascular disease, stroke, neuropsychology

1. Introduction

Sickle cell disease (SCD) is the commonest cause of stroke in childhood [1, 2]. Focal cerebral ischaemia due to arterial or venous compromise is rarely fatal but accounts for 70–80% of all strokes [3–5] and nearly all episodes in children younger than 15 and adults older than 30 years. Subarachnoid and intracerebral haemorrhage typically occurs between 20 and 30 years of age and has a high mortality [4, 6, 7]. Without preventative strategies, approximately 11% of patients with genotype HbSS will experience a clinically apparent stroke by age 20 and up to 24% by age 45 [6]. Silent cerebral infarction (SCI) is diagnosed only using magnetic resonance imaging (MRI) in patients with no focal neurological deficit, but is associated with cognitive difficulties [8] that families often report. SCI can develop very early in life, with rates between 11 and 15% in children less than 2 years [9–11] and progressive accrual throughout childhood and adolescence [11, 12] and into adulthood.

2. Pathophysiology of cerebrovascular ischaemic events

Clinical stroke is defined as a focal neurological event lasting more than 24 hours and is usually permanent, whereas transient ischaemic events are focal neurological events lasting less than 24 hours (i.e. there is a full clinical recovery) [13]. Reversible ischaemic neurological deficits last more than 24 hours, but recover fully. None of these clinical definitions require neuroimaging confirmation, although episodes lasting less than 24 hours but accompanied by an acute infarct in the corresponding territory should be considered as strokes. People with HbSS and HbSβ^0-thalassaemia genotypes are at highest risk, although stroke has been documented in children with HbSS and HbSβ^+-thalassaemia genotypes [6]. Stroke can occur as early as 6–12 months [14] when HbF decreases and HbS begins to be synthesised; the first decade of life, when the onset of strokes typically occurs, appears to constitute a 'critical period' for neurologic complications and subsequent neurocognitive morbidity [6, 15].

Overt stroke is usually associated with large vessel arterial disease, with evidence of stenosis in the internal carotid artery distribution [16], and pathologies are frequently seen in brain tissue within the anterior cerebral and middle cerebral artery territories [17–19]. Transcranial Doppler (TCD) may be used to screen for high cerebral blood flow (CBF) velocities consistent with stenosis or hyperaemia; although conventional angiography is rarely justified, magnetic resonance angiography may confirm focal stenosis but is not essential for management.

Risk factors for cerebral infarction include classical risk factors as in the general population: hypertension [6, 20], presence of a prior cerebral infarct [3, 21], acute low oxygen delivery associated with lower oxygen saturation [22, 23], acute drop in haemoglobin [24] and presence of cerebral vasculopathy [18, 25] compromising cerebral blood flow (CBF). Increased CBF velocity, in response to anaemia, results in adaptive vasodilation of vessels to match metabolic demand, reducing cerebrovascular reserve [26] and causing injury to the endothelial cells lining the vascular wall [5, 27]. Any further demand when metabolic rate is high (e.g. secondary to fever or seizures) or when there is an acute drop in oxygen delivery could cause large and small vessel injury/ischaemia [28], especially in 'borderzones', where blood flow may be lower [29] in the context of large vessel disease and relative hypotension [30].

More common than overt stroke, up to 35% of children will show evidence of SCI [31], diagnosed using MRI as a lesion seen in two planes of a scan with no history of stroke [9, 30, 32, 33]. In children with evidence of SCI on MRI, there is a 14-fold increase in the risk of clinical stroke [34] and further SCI [16]. Known risk factors for SCI are lower rate for pain crises, history of seizures, increased leukocyte count and Senegal beta-globin haplotype [35], but also low baseline haemoglobin [36], male sex and higher baseline systolic blood pressure [37]. The presence of acute silent cerebral infarction events (ASCIE), seen as lesions on imaging which may or may not progress to SCI, has been shown to be temporally associated with clinical events [38]. SCI by definition are clinically silent, so timing is unknown; however, it has been postulated that these lesions are the result of recurrent micro-infarctions and recurrent acute hypoxic damage [24, 39, 40] secondary to severe anaemia, diminished pulmonary function, splenic sequestration, aplastic crisis and acute chest syndrome [41, 42].

3. Primary and secondary stroke prevention

In children, transcranial Doppler (TCD) ultrasound screening to measure blood flow velocity in the intracranial vessels has become an established and effective method of primary stroke prevention. Three groups have been identified with increasing risk of stroke: normal TCD velocities (<170cm/s), conditional TCD velocities (170–200cm/s) and abnormal velocities (>200cm/s) [43]. The Stroke Prevention (STOP) trial randomised children with abnormal TCD velocities (>200 cm/s) to regular transfusion and was discontinued early as an interim analysis showed that there was a 92% reduction in the risk stroke in the transfused arm [44, 45]. The US National Heart, Lung, and Blood Institute and UK National Health Service recommend all children should have TCD screening and be transfused if their velocities are greater than 200cm/s [46]. Current guidelines state that those children should be transfused indefinitely [47], but the TCD with transfusions changing to hydroxyurea (TWiTCH) trial suggests that, for those with no MRA abnormality may be able to switch to hydroxyurea prophylaxis after a year of transfusion [48]. Hydroxyurea does appear to reduce TCD velocities even without prior blood transfusion [1]; so, in settings where TCD is available but blood transfusion is not possible or is considered hazardous, it is probably reasonable to start hydroxyurea while the results of controlled trials are awaited [49]. In adults with SCD, there are no validated methods to screen for the increased stroke risk, as TCD studies in adults with HbSS find lower velocities than in children and cannot accurately stratify the risk of stroke [50].

For secondary stroke prevention, it is important to know the nature of the primary event and any associated arterial or venous abnormality as well as the setting (e.g. 'out-of-the-blue' or in the context of acute chest or painful crisis), as estimating recurrence risk depends on these variables [21, 51]. While chronic transfusion for secondary stroke prevention is common practice, it may not fully prevent recurrent stroke [21, 51, 52] and is associated with antibody development, iron overload and significant cost. Other treatments such as hydroxyurea for primary [53] and secondary stroke prevention [54, 55] have been showing promise.

4. Sickle cell neuroradiology

In clinical settings after an acute event (e.g. hemiplegia, seizures or acute coma), MRI and MRA protocols usually consist of T2-weighted or fluid-attenuated inversion recovery (FLAIR) sequences in the axial and coronal planes, a coronal T1-weighted image, diffusion-weighted images and time-of-flight MR angiography protocols to show intravascular appearances.

4.1. MRA findings

MRA studies confirm pattern of occlusion/stenosis from vessels of the internal carotid distribution with relative sparing of the posterior circulation [56]; stroke and SCI from vertebrobasilar artery circulation occlusion are less common, but have been reported [56, 57]. Approximately 10% of children have cerebral vasculopathy [58, 59] and/or moyamoya syndrome [25], which may be asymptomatic with SCI seen on MRI [59] but renders the child at significant risk of stroke [25].

4.2. MRI findings

4.2.1. Definition of SCI

Although stroke is identified by abrupt onset of neurological deficit and does not require neuroimaging evidence, the term 'covert stroke' [60], or SCI, was first described in the Cooperative Study in Sickle Cell Disease (CSSCD) [32] and requires both a neuroimaging definition. SCI is described for the silent infarct transfusion (SIT) trial [37, 61] as an MRI lesion measuring at least 3 mm in greatest linear dimension, visible in two planes of T2-weighted images (axial and coronal), and a neurology definition of a normal neurologic exam or an abnormal exam that could not be explained by the location of the brain lesion [62]. Many studies describe a localisation of SCI to deep white matter (**Figure 1**), particularly in the arterial borderzones [11, 42, 57, 63, 64]. Infarcts in the subcortical grey matter structures (i.e. head of caudate, cerebellum) are less common [57, 63].

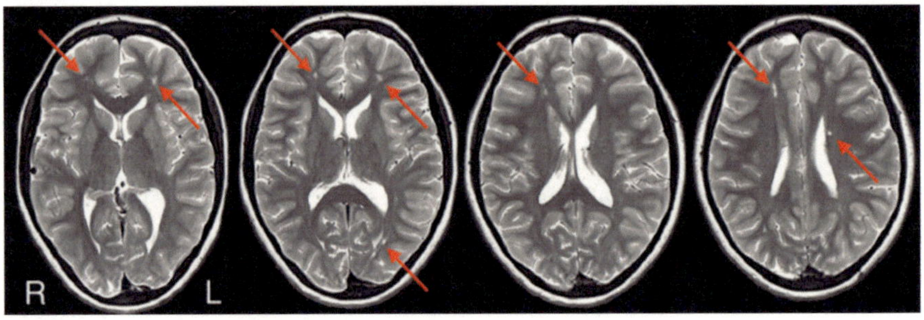

Figure 1. An example of SCI in a 12-year-old boy with HbSS.

4.2.2. Progression of SCI

Several longitudinal studies have shown the presence of SCI as a risk factor for clinical stroke and further SCI. In the CSSCD study, approximately 25% of the children with SCI, but only 2.5% of the children without SCI, had new and/or enlarging lesions on follow-up MRI scan [30], predicting a 14-fold higher risk for clinical stroke and further SCI [65].

SCI have been reported in very young children; 4/39 children (10%) with SCA and no history of stroke between 7 and 48 months of age had SCI [9]; 3/23 children (13%) at an average age of

13.7 months had SCI [10]; and 18/65 children (27.7%) with SCA who were asymptomatic had SCI [31]. A French study showed incidence of SCI as 28.2% by 8 years and 37.4% by 14 years [66]. Although it was thought that rates plateau in childhood, there is now evidence of new SCI in older adolescence and adulthood [1, 67]. In the London cohort followed from the mid-1990s [68], 30% (3/10 patients) were found to have new SCI after the age of 14, 17 and 21 years, respectively (**Figures 2** and **3**).

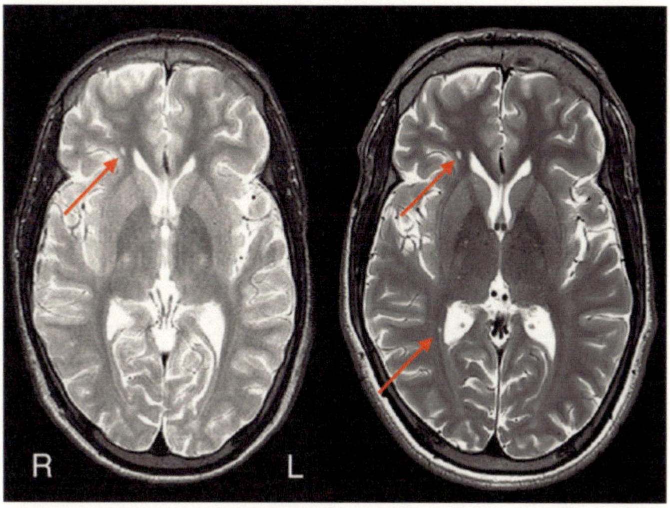

Figure 2. Serial imaging of a male with HbSS. Patient was 17 years old on T2-weighted image from 2001 (left)—showing a small right frontal SCI. Patient was 28 years old on T2-weighted image from 2013 (right)—showing no progression in size of original right frontal SCI but evidence of new SCI in the right peritrigonal region.

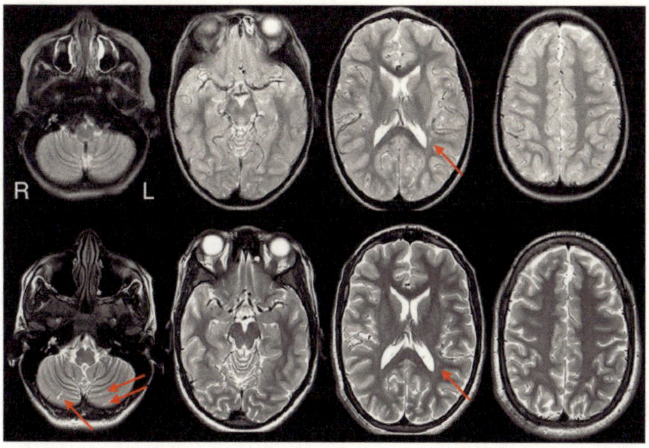

Figure 3. Serial imaging of a male with HbSS. Patient was 14 years old on T2-weighted image from 2002 (top panel)—showing a small left peritrigonal SCI. Patient was 26 years old on T2-weighted image from 2013 (bottom panel)—showing no progression in size of original SCI, but evidence of new SCI in both cerebellar hemispheres.

The SIT trial showed that in children aged 5–14 years with SCI, regular blood transfusion reduced the risk of reinfarction, both overt (clinical stroke) and silent [62]. Preliminary observational data from the Hydroxyurea Study of Long-Term Effects (HUSTLE-NCT00305175) study suggest that progressive SCI are less likely to accumulate in children taking hydroxyurea to maximum tolerated dose [69], but no randomised controlled trials are available yet.

4.2.3. Acute silent cerebral ischemic events (ASCIE)

It has been argued that categorically dividing ischaemic events between clinical stroke and SCI may be an oversimplification of the spectrum of brain injury in SCD [38]. ASCIE [38, 40], following acute severe anaemia [24, 35, 70, 71], can be detectable in the first few days after the clinical event using diffusion-weighted imaging (DWI), in which the 'apparent' diffusion coefficient (ADC) is measured within each voxel and representing an index of the mobility of water molecules inside biological tissues. In acute ischaemia, an area of oedema in the brain has a rapid decline in proton density and appears hyperintense on DWI and decreased on an ADC map, persisting for 10–14 days post-event [72], which can differentiate acute stroke from more remote events [24]. Not all children with evidence of ASCIE progress to SCI on MRI [1, 62], which strongly suggests acute ischaemia may be reversible.

4.2.4. Other acute pathologies on MRI

Imaging abnormality in the occipito-parietal or thalamic region suggests cerebral venous sinus thrombosis but there may be no parenchymal change and this diagnosis should always be excluded with a venogram in patients with SCD presenting in coma or with seizures or acute psychiatric symptoms as well as focal neurology [73]. Subarachnoid and intracerebral haemorrhage also occur [74], as a result of sinovenous thrombosis, rupture of aneurysms (usually located at the bifurcations of major vessels, particularly in the vertebrobasilar circulation) [75], or of fragile moyamoya vessels. Risk factors include recent trauma, transfusion in the past fortnight, corticosteroid or non-steroidal anti-inflammatory use and intermittent hypertension [76]. Posterior reversible encephalopathy syndrome (**Figure 4**, left) has also been reported in the context of hypertension and cyclosporine use for nephrotic syndrome [77], as well as after acute chest syndrome [78, 79]. Acute bilateral border-zone ischaemia may also occur secondary to inadequate global CBF to supply the tissue's demand for oxygen (e.g. during acute chest crisis or seizures; **Figure 4**, middle, right). Management along the lines of the current guidelines for the diagnosed condition in the general paediatric population should be considered, e.g. acute anticoagulation with heparin for cerebral venous sinus thrombosis, neurosurgery for drainage of haematoma and surgery or interventional neuroradiology for removal of aneurysm after intracranial haemorrhage, and steady slow reduction of any associated high blood pressure associated with PRES [80, 81].

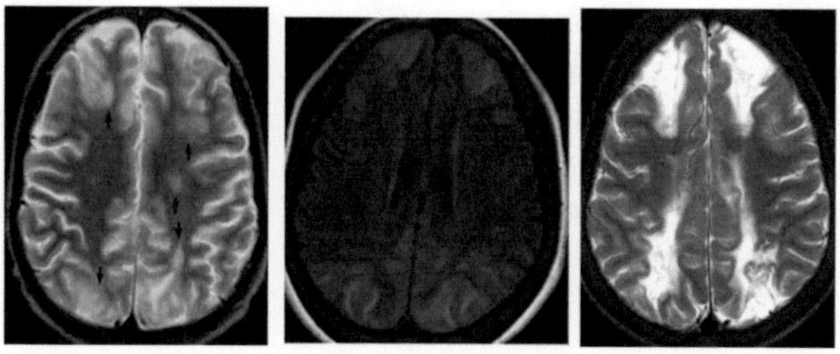

Figure 4. Left: Signal change in the grey and white matter (arrows; posterior reversible encephalopathy syndrome) in a 9-year-old boy with HbSS and nephrotic syndrome who had seizures after cyclosporin therapy. Middle: Bilateral borderzone ischaemia in a 25-year-old woman with HbSS who collapsed with seizures soon after discharge after acute chest crisis. Right: Infarction in both anterior and posterior borderzones in an 8-year-old boy with previously uncomplicated sickle cell anaemia who developed seizures and coma after surgery to drain a painful swelling of his left cheek associated with fever.

5. Quantitative MRI findings: cross-sectional and longitudinal case control studies

Since the 1990s when MRI was used routinely in clinical practice, vast improvements in MRI hardware, software, sequence design and processing techniques have allowed for quantitative measurement of neurological abnormality in SCD. Beyond conventional MRI protocols for acute CNS event detection, only in the last 10–15 years advanced MRI sequences for quantitative analyses have been published, providing further insight into the pathophysiology and progression of neurological complications.

5.1. Morphometric studies using T1-weighted MRI

High-resolution T1-weighted data, with good contrast between grey and white matter, can give valuable insight into volumetrics of the brain. An earlier report showed significant reduction in total subcortical grey matter volume (i.e. basal ganglia volume) as compared to cortical grey matter volume [82]. Decrease in volume of specific subcortical structures (e.g. hippocampus, amygdala, globus pallidus, caudate and putamen) follows parallel to increasing burden of SCI: those with evidence of SCI in white matter have decreased volumes of deep grey matter structures compared to those without SCI and controls [83].

Morphometric studies give a quantitative approach to brain tissue volumes. In a surface-based morphometric study, older children without SCI showed significant thinning of cortex compared to younger patients in the posterior medial surfaces of both hemispheres [84]. A whole-brain voxel-based morphometry (VBM) study found in children without evidence of SCI, decreased grey matter volume in bilateral frontal, temporal and parietal lobes was found to correlate with low IQ [85]. Also using VBM, Baldeweg et al. [86] found that in a group with existing SCI, there were significant decreases in white matter density extending bilaterally from the anterior frontal lobes along the ventricles to parieto-occipital lobes, as well as along the corpus callosum. In those without evidence of SCI, smaller but similar significant decreases in white matter density were found, suggesting patients may have compromised white matter even with normal conventional imaging (**Figure 5**). The only longitudinal morphometric study to date has found different trajectories for brain tissue growth during childhood, with a significant decline in total grey matter volume distributed broadly across the brain compared to healthy controls (HC) [87].

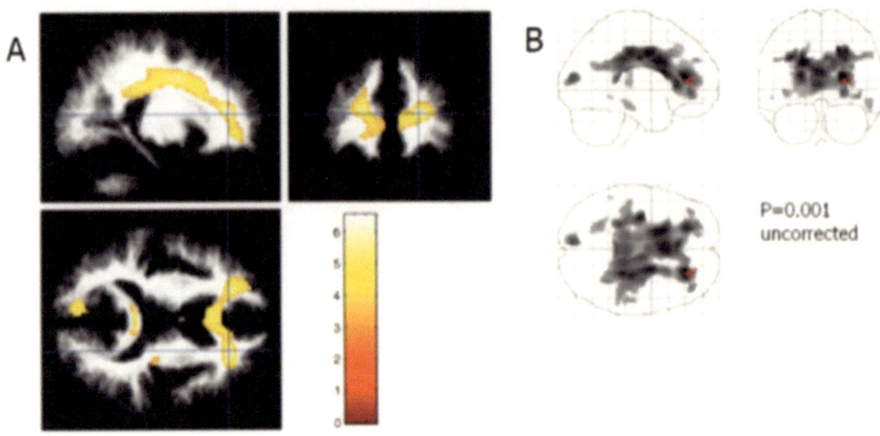

Figure 5. Voxel-based morphometry study showing decreased white matter density extending bilaterally from the anterior frontal lobes along the ventricles to parieto-occipital lobes (image taken with permission from Baldeweg et al. [86]).

5.2. Diffusion tensor imaging

Diffusion tensor imaging (DTI) relies on the properties of the diffusion of water molecules to show directionality (anisotropy) of the underlying tissue. Anisotropy can be quantified by measuring at least six directions [88], unlike ADC maps from DWI data that only require three directions, by a diffusion tensor, a mathematical model usually visualised as an ellipsoid (**Figure 6**). From the diffusion tensor model, several quantitative metrics can be calculated: fractional anisotropy (FA), or the degree of anisotropy ranging from 0 to 1 representing the coherence, organisation and/or density of the underlying tissue, and mean diffusivity (MD), or the average water molecular displacement which is equivalent to ADC. MD can also be divided into axial diffusivity (AD), the magnitude of diffusion along the principal direction of diffusion, and radial diffusivity (RD), or the average magnitude of diffusion along the two perpendicular directions of diffusion. These metrics may provide additional information related to demyelination [89] and axonal damage [90]. There are two main approaches to analyse diffusion data: a voxel-based approach using regions-of-interest (ROIs) or whole-brain data, or tractography (**Figure 6**), where reconstruction of major white matter tracts can be performed by following the continuity and direction of maximum diffusion from contiguous voxels [91].

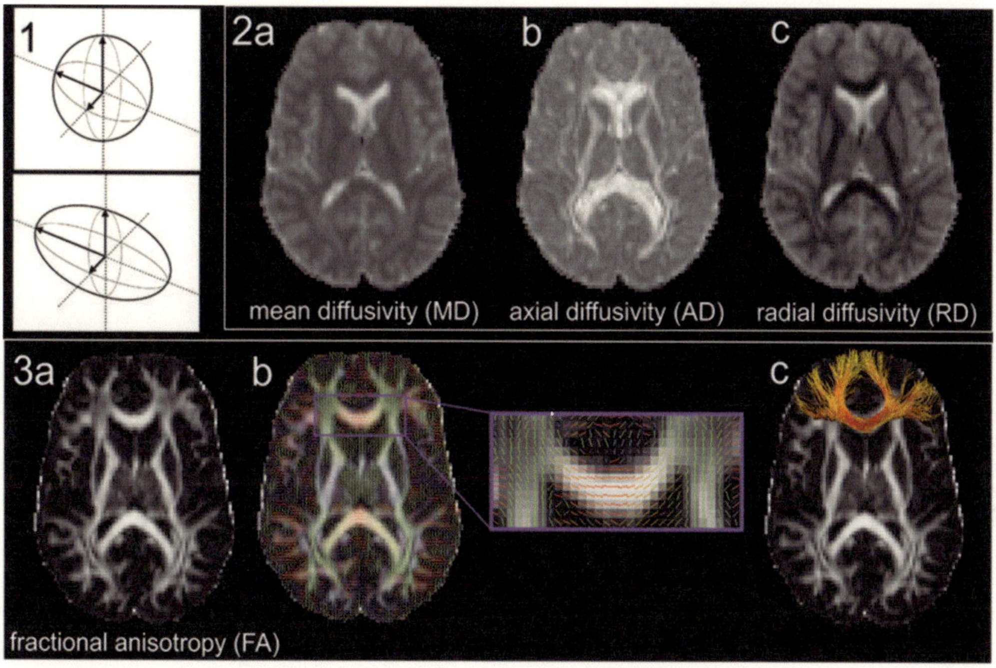

Figure 6. Diffusion tensor imaging. (1) The diffusion tensor model showing ellipsoids representing voxel with isotropic diffusion (top) and anisotropic diffusion (bottom). (2) Diffusivity maps showing (a) mean diffusivity (b) axial diffusivity and (c) radial diffusivity. (3) (a) Fractional anisotropy maps with (b) directions of principal diffusion overlaid (c) tractography of anterior corpus callosum overlaid.

A DWI study showed significant increases in mean regional ADC of patients relative to controls in six large ROIs (left and right frontal lobe, left and right cerebellum, pons and vermis), and in patients with no evidence of infarct, there was increased ADC in four regions (excluding pons and vermis) [92]. These widespread differences in diffusion have been confirmed by DTI studies. In a combined ROI and tractography study of 16 patients with SCD aged 16–45, reduced FA was found in the corpus callosum, centrum semiovale, periventricular areas and ROIs in the subcortical white matter. Tractography of the corpus callosum showed reduced fibre count (i.e. streamlines) and reduced FA in the anterior body [93]. Two studies have used a whole-brain analysis technique known as tract-based spatial statistics (TBSS) [94], in which a 'skeleton' of white matter is investigated to reduce partial volume effects. In a study of two groups of children with SCA, some of whom had mild gliosis although none had SCI, patients with mild gliosis had increased diffusivity and reduced FA in the body of the corpus callosum, whereas the no-SCI group had reduced FA in the centrum semiovale compared to controls [95]. Another TBSS study in 25 patients with no evidence of SCI showed FA significantly lower in cerebral peduncles and cerebellar white matter, whereas there were widespread increases in MD and RD across frontal and parietal lobes, corpus callosum and subcortical white matter. Furthermore, significant negative correlations were found between daytime peripheral oxygen saturation (SpO_2) and haemoglobin and RD in the anterior corpus callosum [96] (**Figure 7**).

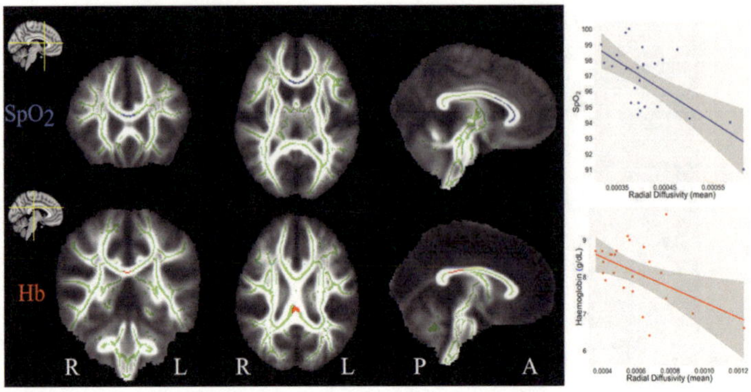

Figure 7. Results from a recent DTI-TBSS study [96], showing the white matter 'skeleton' (green) and significant correlations between RD and daytime peripheral oxygen saturation (blue) and haemoglobin (red).

5.3. Perfusion MRI

Perfusion MRI, either through traditional imaging after injection of a paramagnetic contrast agent (e.g. Gadolinium) or non-invasive arterial-spin labelling (ASL) techniques, has the longest history in quantitative MRI in SCD. In patients with chronic cerebrovascular pathology and stroke, dynamic susceptibility contrast MRI (DSC-MRI) has shown *focal* areas of reduced CBF and prolonged mean transit time in the affected corresponding to stroke-like lesions [29, 97]. Studies have consistently shown elevated *global* cerebral blood flow (CBF) [98–104], in association with the elevated cerebral blood flow velocity [28], which may be both a response to and a risk factor for cerebral hypoxia [98, 99] and related to low haematocrit [98] and haemoglobin and haemoglobin F [103]. Strouse et al. [99] found a strong inverse correlation with CBF and both full-scale IQ and performance IQ, which may be more sensitive than CBF velocity measured by TCD [105].

ASL protocols have become more popular as they do not require intravenous injection; however, they have widely differed in acquisition, CBF quantification and arterial territory segmentation techniques [103], leading to discrepancies in interpretation. CBF quantification depends on the T1 value of blood, which is assumed in some studies [99, 101] but might be more accurate if it were corrected for haematocrit [100]. An ASL acquisition with multiple inflow times [106] does not require prior assumptions about the necessary delay for the fully labelled bolus of blood to arrive and may characterise the full haemodynamic behaviour within a voxel. Unpublished data from a London cohort (n=39 patients) with multiple inflow time data confirms global elevated CBF compared to a previously published reference range for healthy children [1]. This study also shows significant correlations with oxygen saturation and haematocrit with CBF in the anterior, middle and posterior cerebral arteries.

5.3.1. Combined diffusion and perfusion studies

Kirkham et al. [29] found perfusion/diffusion mismatch in areas seen as normal on T2-weighted images, suggesting CBF was reduced but not enough for cytotoxic oedema and tissue

http://dx.doi.org/10.5772/64143

death. Similarly, a combined perfusion/diffusion study [102] found abnormal appearing white matter, described as leukoencephalopathy as well as SCI, had decreased CBF and also decreased FA.

6. Cognitive outcome and relationship to brain imaging findings

Chronic disease (e.g. conditions secondary to anaemia such as diminished pulmonary function and chronic hypoxic damage resulting in brain damage), potentially accumulating over time [107], could explain compromised cognitive functioning in children with SCD [41]. Recurrent micro-infarctions of the central nervous system, possibly undetected by screening measures, may affect general neuropsychological function [108].

6.1. General intelligence

Full-scale intelligence quotient (IQ) is the most commonly reported and widely studied standardised measure of general cognitive ability in SCD. Chodorkoff and Whitten [2] (1963) published the first study investigating IQ between patients with SCD and controls—finding no differences; however from the 1980s/early 1990s there were many studies suggesting that patients have lowered global intelligence scores than matched controls, even when excluding those with history of stroke or abnormal neurological examination [109–114]. Results from studies at that time were mixed; some reported no differences in full-scale IQ (FSIQ) between patients and controls [115–117], whereas others found patients had lowered intelligence scores than matched controls [109–112].

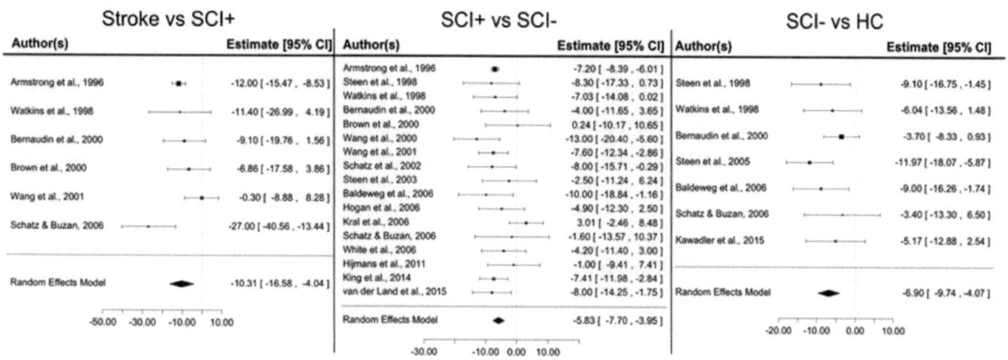

Figure 8. Forest plots of mean differences between SCD patients categorised by MRI status: stroke, silent cerebral infarct (SCI+), no evidence of SCI (SCI−) and healthy controls. Mean differences (estimates) were significant between patients with history of stroke vs. SCI+ (left panel), SCI+ vs. SCI− (middle panel) and SCI− vs. HC (right panel). CI: confidence interval [3].

With the routine use of MRI added in the mid-1990s, patients were classed into groups based on history of stroke and presence or absence of SCI [42]; since then, several studies have confirmed that children with SCI generally have lower IQ scores than those without evidence of SCI [86, 92, 118–121]. Recent meta-analyses have found children with history of stroke perform significantly worse than those with SCI by 10 IQ points, children with SCI perform significantly worse than children with normal MRI by 5–6 IQ points [122] and children with normal MRI perform significantly worse than healthy controls by approximately 7 IQ points [8] (**Figure 8**).

6.1.1. SCI and IQ

Although children with normal MRI have lowered IQ than healthy controls, these findings may link presence of SCI and size of SCI with IQ. Differences in T2-weighted/FLAIR protocols and lesion quantification methods have varied, and are difficult to interpret. Results are mixed; where one study did not provide any correlation result with IQ [86], two studies found volume of SCI to be a significant predictor of IQ [123, 124] and one study found only patients with larger lesions had lower IQ [125].

6.2. Executive functioning

Due to the localisation of SCI primarily in the frontal lobe white matter, much work has focused on deficits in executive functioning, an umbrella term for frontal lobe functions such as inhibition, planning, organisation, processing, decision-making, mental flexibility and working memory. A comprehensive systematic review published in 2007 [126] found that 11 out of 13 studies showed executive function and attention were impaired in children with SCD, in domains such as sustained attention [127–129], cognitive flexibility [68, 130] and working memory [64, 68, 123, 127, 131–133]. Some executive function deficits have been linked specifically to the presence of frontal lobe lesions [127, 129, 134], including one cognitive screening study finding the Test of Variables of Attention task was sensitive and specific in identifying 86% of children with SCI [135]. Patients with no evidence of SCI were found to have deficits in visuomotor functions compared to siblings [127, 129], whereas other studies found no differences in sustained visual attention [92], working memory [123] or set-shifting [68]. A study of neurologically intact adults with SCD showed deficits in processing speed, working memory and other executive functions compared to controls [136].

6.3. Non-imaging biomarkers of function

Anaemia is a major mediator of cognitive function in neurologically intact children (i.e. without cerebrovascular abnormalities). Anaemia severity has shown moderate to large correlations with IQ [41, 119, 137, 138]. Severely anaemic patients (i.e. haematocrit <20%) have shown poorer performance on both verbal and performance aspects of IQ [119], and have accounted for a significant proportion of variance in FSIQ [64, 138] and executive functions [64].Low nocturnal peripheral oxygen saturation was associated with reduced performance on the Tower of London test, which measures strategic planning and rule learning [139]. In the baseline data from the Silent Infarct Trial, a 1% reduction in daytime oxygen saturation was associated with a reduction in 0.75 full scale IQ points [122].

http://dx.doi.org/10.5772/64143

Anaemia and hypoxia may also interact with social/environmental factors such as socioeconomic status [140]. Large cohort studies have found socioeconomic status and parent education as major predictors of cognitive function, rather than SCI [122, 141].

7. Impact of therapeutic interventions

Although primary stroke prevention with prophylactic blood transfusions is effective [45], with post-RCT epidemiological evidence for reduction in the number of strokes in children with sickle cell disease [142, 143], treatment is expensive [144], the number needed to treat to prevent one stroke is 7 and lifelong regular blood transfusion [145] is a heavy burden for the child and the family, with risk of allo-immunisation and infection. Regular blood transfusion also prevents reinfarction in those with SCI, but the number needed to treat to prevent one reinfarction was even higher; the outcomes for the SIT trial included overt strokes and it is not clear whether this treatment can halt or reverse the progression of SCI while there was no benefit in terms of IQ [61, 62]. Longer term clinical and imaging follow-up is required as blood transfusion does not prevent all recurrent infarcts, worsening vasculopathy [51] or progressive atrophy [146].

Hydroxyurea does appear to reduce TCD velocities and the TWiTCH trial supports its use for primary prevention in those with abnormal TCD velocities who have normal MRA and have been transfused for a year. There is now a little observational evidence suggesting prevention of progression of SCI [69] and intellectual decline [147] but RCTs are needed.

Daytime and nocturnal desaturation is associated with higher TCD velocities [39] as well as predicting increased stroke risk [22, 23]. Hydroxyurea may reduce stroke risk by improving oxygen saturation [148] and other strategies, e.g. to prevent the development of or to treat obstructive sleep apnoea, are under investigation. The SIT trial was the first to use MRI as an imaging endpoint; the new techniques such as volumetric analysis and DTI may be useful intermediate endpoints in RCTs of complex interventions, such as the Prevention of morbidity in Sickle Cell Disease (POMS) randomised trials of auto-adjusting continuous positive airways pressure [149, 150].

8. Conclusion

In SCD, neurological complications secondary to chronic anaemia and hypoxia are prevalent from an early age. The research is mounting that stroke and SCI, as well as other pathologies, can have marked impact on neuropsychological outcome of the child. In clinical settings, MRI and MRA have been considered valuable tools for diagnosis and management of acute CNS events, but only relatively recently the role of quantitative neuroimaging has emerged for establishing potential biomarkers of SCD severity. Cross-sectional studies using high-resolution 3D T1-weighted images, diffusion tensor imaging and perfusion imaging have found pertinent tissue characteristics beyond the detection of conventional, clinical MRI/MRA. These studies open the way for use of quantitative MRI as endpoints in clinical trials.

Author details

Jamie M. Kawadler* and Fenella J. Kirkham

*Address all correspondence to: jamie.kawadler.11@ucl.ac.uk

Developmental Neurosciences, UCL Institute of Child Health, University College London, London, UK

References

[1] Hales PW, Kawadler JM, Aylett SE, Kirkham FJ, Clark CA. Arterial spin labeling characterization of cerebral perfusion during normal maturation from late childhood into adulthood: normal "reference range" values and their use in clinical studies. J Cereb blood flow Metab. Nature Publishing Group; 2014 Feb 5;34(5):776–84.

[2] Chodorkoff J, Whitten CF. Intellectual status of children with sickle cell anemia. J Pediatr. 1963 Jul;63:29–35.

[3] Kawadler JM, Clayden JD, Clark CA, Kirkham FJ. Intelligence Quotient in Paediatric Sickle Cell Disease: a Systematic Review and Meta-Analysis. Dev Med Child Neurol. 2016; [Epub ahead of print].

[4] Ohene-Frempong K. Stroke in sickle cell disease: demographic, clinical, and therapeutic considerations. Semin Hematol. 1991 Jul;28(3):213–9.

[5] Pavlakis SG, Prohovnik I, Piomelli S, DeVivo DC. Neurologic complications of sickle cell disease. Adv Pediatr. 1989 Jan;36:247–76.

[6] Ohene-Frempong K, Weiner SJ, Sleeper LA, Miller ST, Embury S, Moohr JW, et al. Cerebrovascular accidents in sickle cell disease: rates and risk factors. Blood. 1998 Jan; 91(1):288–94.

[7] Powars DR, Schroeder WA. Progress in the natural history studies of the clinical severity of sickle cell disease: epidemiologic aspects. In: Caughey WA, editor. Biochemical and Clinical Aspects of Hemoglobin Abnormalities. New York: Academic Press; 1978. pp. 151–64.

[8] Kawadler JM, Clayden JD, Clark CA, Kirkham FJ. Intelligence quotient in paediatric sickle cell disease: a systematic review and meta-analysis. Dev Med Child Neurol. 2016; [Epub ahead of print]

[9] Wang WC, Langston JW, Steen RG, Wynn LW, Mulhern RK, Wilimas JA, et al. Abnormalities of the central nervous system in very young children with sickle cell anemia. J Pediatr. 1998 Jun;132(6):994–8.

[10] Wang WC, Pavlakis SG, Helton KJ, Mckinstry RC, Casella JF, Adams RJ, et al. MRI abnormalities of the brain in one-year-old children with sickle cell anemia. Pediatr Blood Cancer. 2008;51:643–6.

[11] Kwiatkowski JL, Zimmerman RA, Pollock AN, Seto W, Smith-Whitley K, Shults J, et al. Silent infarcts in young children with sickle cell disease. Br J Haematol. 2009 Aug;146(3): 300–5.

[12] Bernaudin F, Verlhac S, Coïc L, Lesprit E, Brugières P, Reinert P. Long-term follow-up of pediatric sickle cell disease patients with abnormal high velocities on transcranial Doppler. Pediatr Radiol. 2005 Mar;35(3):242–8.

[13] Lindsay P, Furie KL, Davis SM, Donnan GA, Norrving B. World stroke organization global stroke services guidelines and action plan. Int J Stroke. 2014 Oct;9 Suppl A1:4–13.

[14] Tarazi RA, Grant ML, Ely E, Barakat LP. Neuropsychological functioning in preschool-age children with sickle cell disease: the role of illness-related and psychosocial factors. Child Neuropsychol. 2007 Mar;13(2):155–72.

[15] Balkaran B, Char G, Morris JS, Thomas PW, Serjeant BE, Serjeant GR. Stroke in a cohort of patients with homozygous sickle cell disease. J Pediatr. 1992 Mar;120(3):360–6.

[16] Pegelow CH, Wang W, Granger S, Hsu LL, Vichinsky E, Moser FG, et al. Silent infarcts in children with sickle cell anemia and abnormal cerebral artery velocity. Arch Neurol. 2001 Dec;58(12):2017–21.

[17] Russell MO, Goldberg HI, Hodson A, Kim HC, Halus J, Reivich M, et al. Effect of transfusion therapy on arteriographic abnormalities and on recurrence of stroke in sickle cell disease. Blood. 1984 Jan;63(1):162–9.

[18] Stockman JA, Nigro MA, Mishkin MM, Oski FA. Occlusion of large cerebral vessels in sickle-cell anemia. N Engl J Med. 1972 Oct 26;287(17):846–9.

[19] Gerald B, Sebes JI, Langston JW. Cerebral infarction secondary to sickle cell disease: arteriographic findings. AJR Am J Roentgenol. 1980 Jun;134(6):1209–12.

[20] Strouse JJ, Lanzkron S, Urrutia V. The epidemiology, evaluation and treatment of stroke in adults with sickle cell disease. Expert Rev Hematol. 2011;4(6):597–606.

[21] Scothorn DJ, Price C, Schwartz D, Terrill C, Buchanan GR, Shurney W, et al. Risk of recurrent stroke in children with sickle cell disease receiving blood transfusion therapy for at least five years after initial stroke. J Pediatr. 2002 Mar;140(3):348–54.

[22] Kirkham FJ, Hewes DK, Prengler M, Wade A, Lane R, Evans JP. Nocturnal hypoxaemia and central-nervous-system events in sickle-cell disease. Lancet. 2001 May 26;357(9269):1656–9.

[23] Quinn CT, Sargent JW. Daytime steady-state haemoglobin desaturation is a risk factor for overt stroke in children with sickle cell anaemia. Br J Haematol. 2008 Feb;140(3): 336–9.

[24] Dowling MM, Quinn CT, Plumb P, Rogers ZR, Rollins NK, Koral K, et al. Acute silent cerebral ischemia and infarction during acute anemia in children with and without sickle cell disease. Blood. 2012 Nov 8;120(19):3891–7.

[25] Dobson SR, Holden KR, Nietert PJ, Cure JK, Laver JH, Disco D, et al. Moyamoya syndrome in childhood sickle cell disease: a predictive factor for recurrent cerebrovascular events. Blood. 2002 May 1;99(9):3144–50.

[26] Prohovnik I, Pavlakis SG, Piomelli S, Bello J, Mohr JP, Hilal S, et al. Cerebral hyperemia, stroke, and transfusion in sickle cell disease. Neurology. 1989;39:344–8.

[27] Hess DC, Adams RJ, Nichols FT. Sickle cell anemia and other hemoglobinopathies. Semin Neurol. 1991 Dec;11(4):314–28.

[28] Prohovnik I, Hurlet-Jensen A, Adams R, De Vivo D, Pavlakis SG. Hemodynamic etiology of elevated flow velocity and stroke in sickle-cell disease. J Cereb Blood Flow Metab. 2009 Apr;29(4):803–10.

[29] Kirkham FJ, Calamante F, Bynevelt M, Gadian DG, Evans JP, Cox TC, et al. Perfusion magnetic resonance abnormalities in patients with sickle cell disease. Ann Neurol. 2001 Apr;49(4):477–85.

[30] Pegelow CH. Longitudinal changes in brain magnetic resonance imaging findings in children with sickle cell disease. Blood. 2002 Apr 15;99(8):3014–8.

[31] DeBaun MR, Armstrong FD, McKinstry RC, Ware RE, Vichinsky E, Kirkham FJ. Silent cerebral infarcts: a review on a prevalent and progressive cause of neurologic injury in sickle cell anemia. Blood. 2012 May 17;119(20):4587–96.

[32] Moser FG, Miller ST, Bello JA, Pegelow CH, Zimmerman RA, Wang WC, et al. The spectrum of brain MR abnormalities in sickle-cell disease: a report from the Cooperative Study of Sickle Cell Disease. AJNR Am J Neuroradiol. 1996 May;17(5):965–72.

[33] Steen RG, Fineberg-Buchner C, Hankins G, Weiss L, Prifitera A, Mulhern RK. Cognitive deficits in children with sickle cell disease. J Child Neurol. 2005 Feb; 20(2):102–7.

[34] Miller ST, Wright E, Abboud M, Berman B, Files B, Scher CD, et al. Impact of chronic transfusion on incidence of pain and acute chest syndrome during the Stroke Prevention Trial (STOP) in sickle-cell anemia. J Pediatr. 2001 Dec;139(6):785–9.

[35] Kinney TR, Sleeper LA, Wang WC, Zimmerman RA, Pegelow CH, Ohene-Frempong K, et al. Silent cerebral infarcts in sickle cell anemia: a risk factor analysis. The Cooperative Study of Sickle Cell Disease. Pediatrics. 1999 Mar;103(3):640–5.

[36] Quinn CT, Miller ST. Risk factors and prediction of outcomes in children and adolescents who have sickle cell anemia. Hematol Oncol Clin North Am. 2004 Dec;18(6):1339–54, ix.

[37] DeBaun MR, Sarnaik S a, Rodeghier MJ, Minniti CP, Howard TH, Iyer RV, et al. Associated risk factors for silent cerebral infarcts in sickle cell anemia: low baseline hemoglobin, sex, and relative high systolic blood pressure. Blood. 2012 Apr 19;119(16): 3684–90.

[38] Dowling MM, Quinn CT, Rogers ZR, Buchanan GR. Acute silent cerebral infarction in children with sickle cell anemia. Pediatr Blood Cancer. 2010;54:461–4.

[39] Quinn CT, Variste J, Dowling MM. Haemoglobin oxygen saturation is a determinant of cerebral artery blood flow velocity in children with sickle cell anaemia. Br J Haematol. 2009 May;145(4):500–5.

[40] Quinn CT, McKinstry RC, Dowling MM, Ball WS, Kraut MA, Casella JF, et al. Acute silent cerebral ischemic events in children with sickle cell anemia. JAMA Neurol. 2013 Oct 29;70(1):58–65.

[41] Brown RT, Armstrong FD, Eckman JR. Neurocognitive aspects of pediatric sickle cell disease. J Learn Disabil. 1993 Jan;26(1):33–45.

[42] Armstrong FD, Thompson RJ, Wang W, Zimmerman R, Pegelow H, Miller S, et al. Cognitive functioning and brain magnetic resonance imaging in children with sickle cell disease. Pediatrics. 1996;97(6):864–70.

[43] Adams RJ, Nichols FT, Figueroa R, McKie V, Lott T. Transcranial Doppler correlation with cerebral angiography in sickle cell disease. Stroke. 1992 Aug;23(8):1073–7.

[44] Adams RJ, McKie VC, Carl EM, Nichols FT, Perry R, Brock K, et al. Long-term stroke risk in children with sickle cell disease screened with transcranial Doppler. Ann Neurol. 1997 Nov;42(5):699–704.

[45] Adams RJ, McKie VC, Hsu L, Files B, Vichinsky E, Pegelow C, et al. Prevention of a first stroke by transfusions in children with sickle cell anemia and abnormal results on transcranial Doppler ultrasonography. N Engl J Med. 1998 Jul;339(1):5–11.

[46] Goldstein LB, Adams R, Becker K, Furberg CD, Gorelick PB, Hademenos G, et al. Primary prevention of ischemic stroke: a statement for healthcare professionals from the Stroke Council of the American Heart Association. Stroke. 2001 Jan;32(1):280–99.

[47] Wang WC, Kovnar EH, Tonkin IL, Mulhern RK, Langston JW, Day SW, et al. High risk of recurrent stroke after discontinuance of five to twelve years of transfusion therapy in patients with sickle cell disease. J Pediatr. 1991 Mar;118(3):377–82.

[48] Ware RE, Davis BR, Schultz WH, Brown RC, Aygun B, Sarnaik S, et al. Hydroxycarbamide versus chronic transfusion for maintenance of transcranial doppler flow velocities in children with sickle cell anaemia-TCD With Transfusions Changing to Hydroxyurea (TWiTCH): a multicentre, open-label, phase 3, non-inferiority trial. Lancet (London, England). 2016 Feb;387(10019):661–70.

[49] Galadanci NA, Abdullahi SU, Tabari MA, Abubakar S, Belonwu R, Salihu A, et al. Primary stroke prevention in Nigerian children with sickle cell disease (SPIN): challenges of conducting a feasibility trial. Pediatr Blood Cancer. 2015 Mar;62(3):395–401.

[50] Valadi N, Silva GS, Bowman LS, Ramsingh D, Vicari P, Filho AC, et al. Transcranial Doppler ultrasonography in adults with sickle cell disease. Neurology. 2006 Aug 22;67(4):572–4.

[51] Hulbert ML, McKinstry RC, Lacey JL, Moran CJ, Panepinto JA, Thompson AA, et al. Silent cerebral infarcts occur despite regular blood transfusion therapy after first strokes in children with sickle cell disease. Blood. 2011 Jan;117(3):772–9.

[52] Hulbert ML, Scothorn DJ, Panepinto JA, Scott JP, Buchanan GR, Sarnaik S, et al. Exchange blood transfusion compared with simple transfusion for first overt stroke is associated with a lower risk of subsequent stroke: a retrospective cohort study of 137 children with sickle cell anemia. J Pediatr. 2006 Nov;149(5):710–2.

[53] DeBaun MR, Kirkham FJ. New option for primary stroke prevention in sickle cell anaemia. Lancet (London, England). Elsevier Ltd; 2015;387(10019):626–7.

[54] Ware RE, Zimmerman SA, Schultz WH. Hydroxyurea as an alternative to blood transfusions for the prevention of recurrent stroke in children with sickle cell disease. Blood. 1999 Nov;94(9):3022–6.

[55] Lagunju IA, Brown BJ, Sodeinde OO. Stroke recurrence in Nigerian children with sickle cell disease treated with hydroxyurea. Niger Postgrad Med J. 2013 Sep;20(3):181–7.

[56] Pavlakis SG, Bello J, Prohovnik I, Sutton M, Ince C, Mohr JP, et al. Brain infarction in sickle cell anemia: magnetic resonance imaging correlates. Ann Neurol. 1988 Mar;23(2): 125–30.

[57] Adams RJ, Nichols FT, McKie V, McKie K, Milner P, Gammal TE. Cerebral infarction in sickle cell anemia: mechanism based on CT and MRI. Neurology. 1988 Jul 1;38(7):1012.

[58] Abboud MR, Cure J, Granger S, Gallagher D, Hsu L, Wang W, et al. Magnetic resonance angiography in children with sickle cell disease and abnormal transcranial Doppler ultrasonography findings enrolled in the STOP study. Blood. 2004 Apr;103(7):2822–6.

[59] Thangarajh M, Yang G, Fuchs D, Ponisio MR, McKinstry RC, Jaju A, et al. Magnetic resonance angiography-defined intracranial vasculopathy is associated with silent cerebral infarcts and glucose-6-phosphate dehydrogenase mutation in children with sickle cell anaemia. Br J Haematol. 2012 Nov;159(3):352–9.

[60] Hindmarsh PC, Brozovic M, Brook CG, Davies SC. Incidence of overt and covert neurological damage in children with sickle cell disease. Postgrad Med J. 1987 Sep; 63(743):751–3.

[61] Casella JF, King AA, Barton B, White DA, Noetzel MJ, Ichord RN, et al. Design of the silent cerebral infarct transfusion (SIT) trial. Pediatr Hematol Oncol. 2010 Mar;27(2):69–89.

[62] DeBaun MR, Gordon M, McKinstry RC, Noetzel MJ, White DA, Sarnaik S a, et al. Controlled trial of transfusions for silent cerebral infarcts in sickle cell anemia. N Engl J Med. 2014 Aug;371(8):699–710.

[63] Pavlakis SG, Bello J, Prohovnik I, Sutton M, Ince C, Mohr JP, et al. Brain infarction in sickle cell anemia: magnetic resonance imaging correlates. Ann Neurol. 1988 Mar;23(2): 125–30.

[64] Kral MC, Brown RT, Connelly M, Curé JK, Besenski N, Jackson SM, et al. Radiographic predictors of neurocognitive functioning in pediatric sickle cell disease. J Child Neurol. 2006;21(1):37–44.

[65] Miller ST, Macklin EA, Pegelow CH, Kinney TR, Sleeper LA, Bello JA, et al. Silent infarction as a risk factor for overt stroke in children with sickle cell anemia: a report from the Cooperative Study of Sickle Cell Disease. J Pediatr. 2001 Sep;139(3):385–90.

[66] Bernaudin F, Verlhac S, Arnaud C, Kamdem A, Chevret S, Hau I, et al. Impact of early transcranial Doppler screening and intensive therapy on cerebral vasculopathy outcome in a newborn sickle cell anemia cohort. Blood. 2011 Jan;117(4):1130–40; quiz 1436.

[67] Kassim AA, Pruthi S, Day M, Rodeghier M, Gindville MC, Brodsky MA, et al. Silent cerebral infarcts and cerebral aneurysms are prevalent in adults with sickle cell disease. Blood. 2016 Apr;127(16):2038–40.

[68] Watkins KE, Hewes DK, Connelly A, Kendall BE, Kingsley DP, Evans JE, et al. Cognitive deficits associated with frontal-lobe infarction in children with sickle cell disease. Dev Med Child Neurol. 1998 Aug;40(8):536–43.

[69] Nottage KA, Ware RE, Smeltzer MP, Dowdy J, Wang WC, Hankins JS, et al. Brain MRI/MRA Findings after Hydroxyurea Treatment in Children with Sickle Cell Anemia. Blood. American Society of Hematology; 2014;124(21):89–89.

[70] Steen RG, Emudianughe T, Hankins GM, Wynn LW, Wang WC, Xiong X, et al. Brain imaging findings in pediatric patients with sickle cell sisease. Radiology. 2003;228:216–25.

[71] Enninful-Eghan H, Moore RH, Ichord R, Smith-Whitley K, Kwiatkowski JL. Transcranial Doppler ultrasonography and prophylactic transfusion program is effective in preventing overt stroke in children with sickle cell disease. J Pediatr. 2010 Sep;157(3): 479–84.

[72] Muir KW, Buchan A, von Kummer R, Rother J, Baron J-C. Imaging of acute stroke. Lancet Neurol. 2006 Sep;5(9):755–68.

[73] Sébire G, Tabarki B, Saunders DE, Leroy I, Liesner R, Saint-Martin C, et al. Cerebral venous sinus thrombosis in children: risk factors, presentation, diagnosis and outcome. Brain. 2005 Mar;128(Pt 3):477–89.

[74] Kossorotoff M, Brousse V, Grevent D, Naggara O, Brunelle F, Blauwblomme T, et al. Cerebral haemorrhagic risk in children with sickle-cell disease. Dev Med Child Neurol. 2015 Feb;57(2):187–93.

[75] Nabavizadeh SA, Vossough A, Ichord RN, Kwiatkowski J, Pukenas BA, Smith MJ, et al. Intracranial aneurysms in sickle cell anemia: clinical and imaging findings. J Neurointerv Surg. 2016 Apr;8(4):434–40.

[76] Strouse JJ, Hulbert ML, DeBaun MR, Jordan LC, Casella JF. Primary hemorrhagic stroke in children with sickle cell disease is associated with recent transfusion and use of corticosteroids. Pediatrics. 2006 Nov;118(5):1916–24.

[77] Coley SC, Porter DA, Calamante F, Chong WK, Connelly A. Quantitative MR diffusion mapping and cyclosporine-induced neurotoxicity. AJNR Am J Neuroradiol. 1999 Sep; 20(8):1507–10.

[78] Solh Z, Taccone MS, Marin S, Athale U, Breakey VR. Neurological PRESentations in Sickle Cell Patients Are Not Always Stroke: A Review of Posterior Reversible Encephalopathy Syndrome in Sickle Cell Disease. Pediatr Blood Cancer. 2016 Jun;63(6):983–9.

[79] Henderson JN, Noetzel MJ, McKinstry RC, White DA, Armstrong M, DeBaun MR. Reversible posterior leukoencephalopathy syndrome and silent cerebral infarcts are associated with severe acute chest syndrome in children with sickle cell disease. Blood. 2003 Jan;101(2):415–9.

[80] Roach ES, Golomb MR, Adams R, Biller J, Daniels S, Deveber G, et al. Management of stroke in infants and children: a scientific statement from a Special Writing Group of the American Heart Association Stroke Council and the Council on Cardiovascular Disease in the Young. Stroke. 2008 Sep;39(9):2644–91.

[81] Monagle P, Chan AKC, Goldenberg NA, Ichord RN, Journeycake JM, Nowak-Göttl U, et al. Antithrombotic therapy in neonates and children. Chest J. 2012 Feb;141(2 Suppl):e737S.

[82] Steen RG, Emudianughe T, Hunte M, Glass J, Wu S, Xiong X, et al. Brain volume in pediatric patients with sickle cell disease: Evidence of volumetric growth delay? AJNR Am J Neuroradiol. 2005 Mar;26(3):455–62.

[83] Kawadler JM, Clayden JD, Kirkham FJ, Cox TC, Saunders DE, Clark CA. Subcortical and cerebellar volumetric deficits in paediatric sickle cell anaemia. Br J Haematol. 2013 Nov;163(3):373–6.

[84] Kirk GR, Haynes MR, Palasis S, Brown C, Burns TG, McCormick M, et al. Regionally specific cortical thinning in children with sickle cell disease. Cereb Cortex. 2009 Jul; 19(7):1549–56.

[85] Chen R, Pawlak MA, Flynn TB, Krejza J, Herskovits EH, Melhem ER. Brain morphometry and intelligence quotient measurements in children with sickle cell disease. J Dev Behav Pediatr. 2009 Dec;30(6):509–17.

[86] Baldeweg T, Hogan AM, Saunders DE, Telfer P, Gadian DG, Vargha-Khadem F, et al. Detecting white matter injury in sickle cell disease using voxel-based morphometry. Ann Neurol. 2006 Apr;59(4):662–72.

[87] Chen R, Arkuszewski M, Krejza J, Zimmerman RA, Herskovits EH, Melhem ER. A Prospective longitudinal brain morphometry study of children with sickle cell disease. Am J Neuroradiol. 2015;36:403–10.

[88] Basser PJ, Mattiello J, LeBihan D. MR diffusion tensor spectroscopy and imaging. Biophys J. 1994 Jan;66(1):259–67.

[89] Ciccarelli O, Catani M, Johansen-Berg H. Diffusion-based tractography in neurological disorders: concepts, applications, and future developments. Lancet Neurol. 2008;7(August):715–27.

[90] Song S-K, Sun S-W, Ramsbottom MJ, Chang C, Russell J, Cross AH. Dysmyelination revealed through MRI as increased radial (but unchanged axial) diffusion of water. Neuroimage. 2002 Nov;17(3):1429–36.

[91] Basser PJ, Pajevic S, Pierpaoli C, Duda J, Aldroubi A. In vivo fiber tractography using DT-MRI data. Magn Reson Med. 2000 Oct;44(4):625–32.

[92] Scantlebury N, Mabbott D, Janzen L, Rockel C, Widjaja E, Jones G, et al. White matter integrity and core cognitive function in children diagnosed with sickle cell disease. J Pediatr Hematol Oncol. 2011 Apr;33(3):163–71.

[93] Balci A, Karazincir S, Beyoglu Y, Cingiz C, Davran R, Gali E, et al. Quantitative brain diffusion-tensor MRI findings in patients with sickle cell disease. AJR Am J Roentgenol. 2012 May;198(5):1167–74.

[94] Smith SM, Jenkinson M, Johansen-Berg H, Rueckert D, Nichols TE, Mackay CE, et al. Tract-based spatial statistics: voxelwise analysis of multi-subject diffusion data. Neuroimage. 2006 Jul;31(4):1487–505.

[95] Sun B, Brown R, Hayes L, Burns T, Huamani J, Bearden D, et al. White matter damage in asymptomatic patients with sickle cell anemia: screening with dIffusion tensor imaging. AJNR Am J Neuroradiol. 2012;33(11):2043–9.

[96] Kawadler JM, Kirkham FJ, Clayden JD, Hollocks MJ, Seymour EL, Edey R, et al. White matter damage relates to oxygen saturation in children with sickle cell anemia without silent cerebral infarcts. Stroke. 2015;1793–800.

[97] Tzika AA, Massoth RJ, Ball WS, Majumdar S, Dunn RS, Kirks DR. Cerebral perfusion in children: detection with dynamic contrast-enhanced T2*-weighted MR images. Radiology. 1993 May;187(2):449–58.

[98] Oguz KK, Golay X, Pizzini FB, Freer CA, Winrow N, Ichord R, et al. Sickle cell disease: continuous arterial spin-labeling perfusion MR imaging in children. Radiology. 2003 May;227(2):567–74.

[99] Strouse JJ, Cox CS, Melhem ER, Lu H, Kraut M a, Razumovsky A, et al. Inverse correlation between cerebral blood flow measured by continuous arterial spin-labeling (CASL) MRI and neurocognitive function in children with sickle cell anemia (SCA). Blood. 2006 Jul;108(1):379–81.

[100] Gevers S, Nederveen AJ, Fijnvandraat K, van den Berg SM, van Ooij P, Heijtel DF, et al. Arterial spin labeling measurement of cerebral perfusion in children with sickle cell disease. J Magn Reson Imaging. 2012 Nov;35(4):779–87.

[101] van den Tweel XW, Nederveen AJ, Majoie CBLM, van der Lee JH, Wagener-Schimmel L, Van Walderveen MAA, et al. Cerebral blood flow measurement in children with sickle cell disease using continuous arterial spin labeling at 3.0-Tesla MRI. Stroke. 2009 Mar;40(3):795–800.

[102] Helton KJ, Paydar A, Glass J, Weirich EM, Hankins J, Li C, et al. Arterial spin-labeled perfusion combined with segmentation techniques to evaluate cerebral blood flow in white and gray matter of children with sickle cell anemia. Pediatr Blood Cancer. 2009;52:85–91.

[103] Helton KJ, Glass JO, Reddick WE, Paydar A, Zandieh AR, Dave R, et al. Comparing segmented ASL perfusion of vascular territories using manual versus semiautomated techniques in children with sickle cell anemia. J Magn Reson Imaging. 2014 Jan;41(2): 439–46.

[104] Hales PW, Kawadler JM, Aylett SE, Kirkham FJ, Clark CA. Arterial spin labeling characterization of cerebral perfusion during normal maturation from late childhood into adulthood: normal "reference range" values and their use in clinical studies. J Cereb Blood Flow Metab. Nature Publishing Group; 2014 Feb; 34(5):776–84.

[105] Kral MC, Brown RT, Nietert PJ, Abboud MR, Jackson SM, Hynd GW. Transcranial Doppler ultrasonography and neurocognitive functioning in children with sickle cell disease. Pediatrics. Am Acad Pediatrics; 2003;112(2):324–31.

[106] Buxton RB, Frank LR, Wong EC, Siewert B, Warach S, Edelman RR. A general kinetic model for quantitative perfusion imaging with arterial spin labeling. Magn Reson Med. 1998 Sep;40(3):383–96.

[107] Logothetis J, Haritos-Fatouros M, Constantoulakis M, Economidou J, Augoustaki O, Loewenson RB. Intelligence and behavioral patterns in patients with Cooley's anemia

(homozygous beta-thalassemia); a study based on 138 consecutive cases. Pediatrics. 1971 Nov;48(5):740–4.

[108] Chapar GN. Chronic diseases of children and neuropsychologic dysfunction. J Dev Behav Pediatr. 1988 Aug;9(4):221–2.

[109] Swift A V, Cohen MJ, Hynd GW, Wisenbaker JM, McKie KM, Makari G, et al. Neuropsychologic impairment in children with sickle cell anemia. Pediatrics. 1989 Dec;84(6): 1077–85.

[110] Hariman LM, Griffith ER, Hurtig AL, Keehn MT. Functional outcomes of children with sickle-cell disease affected by stroke. Arch Phys Med Rehabil. 1991 Jun;72(7):498–502.

[111] Wasserman ALL, Wilimas JAA, Fairclough DLL, Mulhern RKK, Wang W. Subtle neuropsychological deficits in children with sickle cell disease. Am J Pediatr Hematol Oncol. 1991;13(1):14–20.

[112] Knight S, Singhal A, Thomas P, Serjeant G. Factors associated with lowered intelligence in homozygous sickle cell disease. Arch Dis Child. 1995;73(4):316–20.

[113] Noll RB, Stith L, Gartstein MA, Ris MD, Grueneich R, Vannatta K, et al. Neuropsychological functioning of youths with sickle cell disease: comparison with non-chronically ill peers. J Pediatr Psychol. 2001 Mar;26(2):69–78.

[114] Hijmans CT, Fijnvandraat K, Grootenhuis MA, van Geloven N, Heijboer H, Peters M, et al. Neurocognitive deficits in children with sickle cell disease: a comprehensive profile. Pediatr Blood Cancer. 2011 May;56(5):783–8.

[115] Fowler M, Whitt J, Lallinger R, Nash K, Atkinson S, Wells R, et al. Neuropsychologic and academic functioning of children with sickle cell anemia. Dev Behav Pediatr. 1988;9(4):213–20.

[116] Goonan BT, Goonan LJ, Brown RT, Buchanan I, Eckman JR. Sustained attention and inhibitory control in children with sickle cell syndrome. Arch Clin Neuropsychol. 1994 Jan;9(1):89–104.

[117] Midence K, McManus C, Fuggle P, Davies S. Psychological adjustment and family functioning in a group of British children with sickle cell disease: preliminary empirical findings and a meta-analysis. Br J Clin Psychol. 1996 Sep;35:439–50.

[118] Steen RG, Reddick WE, Mulhern RK, Langston JW, Ogg RJ, Bieberich AA, et al. Quantitative MRI of the brain in children with sickle cell disease reveals abnormalities unseen by conventional MRI. J Magn Reson Imaging. 1998;8(3): 535–43.

[119] Bernaudin F, Verlhac S, Freard F, Roudot-Thoraval F, Benkerrou M, Thuret I, et al. Multicenter prospective study of children with sickle cell disease: radiographic and psychometric correlation. J Child Neurol. 2000 May;15(5):333–43.

[120] Wang W, Enos L, Gallagher D, Thompson R, Guarini L, Vichinsky E, et al. Neuropsychologic performance in school-aged children with sickle cell disease: a report from the Cooperative Study of Sickle Cell Disease. J Pediatr. 2001 Sep;139(3):391–7.

[121] Steen RG, Miles MA, Helton KJ, Strawn S, Wang W, Xiong X, et al. Cognitive impairment in children with hemoglobin SS sickle cell disease: relationship to MR imaging findings and hematocrit. AJNR Am J Neuroradiol. 2003 Mar;24(3):382–9.

[122] King AA, Strouse JJ, Rodeghier MJ, Compas BE, Casella JF, McKinstry RC, et al. Parent education and biologic factors influence on cognition in sickle cell anemia. Am J Hematol. 2014 Feb;89(2):162–7.

[123] Schatz J, Buzan R. Decreased corpus callosum size in sickle cell disease: relationship with cerebral infarcts and cognitive functioning. J Int Neuropsychol Soc. 2006 Jan;12(1): 24–33.

[124] van der Land V, Hijmans CT, de Ruiter M, Mutsaerts HJMM, Cnossen MH, Engelen M, et al. Volume of white matter hyperintensities is an independent predictor of intelligence quotient and processing speed in children with sickle cell disease. Br J Haematol. 2015 Oct;168:553–6.

[125] Schatz J, White DA, Moinuddin A, Armstrong M, DeBaun MR. Lesion burden and cognitive morbidity in children with sickle cell disease. J Child Neurol. 2002 Dec;17(12): 891–5.

[126] Berkelhammer LD, Williamson AL, Sanford SD, Dirksen CL, Sharp WG, Margulies AS, et al. Neurocognitive sequelae of pediatric sickle cell disease: a review of the literature. Child Neuropsychol. 2007 Mar;13(2):120–31.

[127] Craft S, Schatz J, Glauser TA, Lee B, DeBaun MR. Neuropsychologic effects of stroke in children with sickle cell anemia. J Pediatr. 1993 Nov;123(5):712–7.

[128] Brown RT, Davis PC, Lambert R, Hsu L, Hopkins K, Eckman J. Neurocognitive functioning and magnetic resonance imaging in children with sickle cell disease. J Pediatr Psychol. 2000;25(7):503–13.

[129] Schatz J, Brown RT, Pascual JM, Hsu L, Debaun MR. Poor school performance and cognitive functioning with silent cerebral infarcts and sickle cell disease. Neurology. 2001;56:1109–11.

[130] Berg C, Edwards DF, King A. Executive function performance on the children's kitchen task assessment with children with sickle cell disease and matched controls. Child Neuropsychol. 2012 Sep;18(5):432–48.

[131] White DA, Salorio CF, Schatz J, Debaun M. Preliminary study of working memory in children with stroke related to sickle cell disease. J Clin Exp Neuropsychol. 2000;22(2): 257–64.

[132] Brandling-Bennett EM, White DA, Armstrong MM, Christ SE. Developmental neuropsychology patterns of verbal long-term and working memory performance reveal

deficits in strategic processing in children with frontal infarcts related to sickle cell disease. Dev Neuropsychol. 2003;24(1):423–34.

[133] Hijmans CT, Grootenhuis MA, Oosterlaan J, Peters M, Fijnvandraat K. Neurocognitive deficits in children with sickle cell disease are associated with the severity of anemia. Pediatr Blood Cancer. 2011;(July 2010):297–302.

[134] Christ SE, Moinuddin A, McKinstry RC, DeBaun M, White DA. Inhibitory control in children with frontal infarcts related to sickle cell disease. Child Neuropsychol. 2007 Mar;13(2):132–41.

[135] DeBaun MR, Schatz J, Siegel MJ, Koby M, Craft S, Resar L, et al. Cognitive screening examinations for silent cerebral infarcts in sickle cell disease. Neurology. 1998 Jun;50(6):1678–82.

[136] Vichinsky E, Neumayr L, Gold J. Neuropsychological dysfunction and neuroimaging abnormalities in neurologically intact adults with sickle cell anemia. JAMA. 2010;303(18):1823–31.

[137] Thompson RJ, Gustafson KE, Bonner MJ, Ware RE. Neurocognitive development of young children with sickle cell disease through three years of age. J Pediatr Psychol. 2002;27(3):235–44.

[138] Steen RG, Xiong X, Mulhern RK, Langston JW, Wang WC. Subtle brain abnormalities in children with sickle cell disease: relationship to blood hematocrit. Ann Neurol. 1999 Mar;45(3):279–86.

[139] Hollocks MJ, Kok TB, Kirkham FJ, Gavlak J, Inusa BP, DeBaun MR, et al. Nocturnal oxygen desaturation and disordered sleep as a potential factor in executive dysfunction in sickle cell anemia. J Int Neuropsychol Soc. 2012 Jan;18(1):168–73.

[140] Schatz J, Finke R, Roberts CW. Interactions of biomedical and environmental risk factors for cognitive development: a preliminary study of sickle cell disease. J Dev Behav Pediatr. 2004 Oct;25(5):303–10.

[141] King A, Rodeghier M, Panepinto J, Strouse J, Casella J, Quinn C, et al. Silent cerebral infarction, income and grade retention among students with sickle cell. Am J Hematol. 2014;2–28.

[142] Fullerton HJ, Adams RJ, Zhao S, Johnston SC. Declining stroke rates in Californian children with sickle cell disease. Blood. 2004 Jul;104(2):336–9.

[143] Telfer P, Coen P, Chakravorty S, Wilkey O, Evans J, Newell H, et al. Clinical outcomes in children with sickle cell disease living in England: a neonatal cohort in East London. Haematologica. 2007 Jul;92(7):905–12.

[144] Cherry MG, Greenhalgh J, Osipenko L, Venkatachalam M, Boland A, Dundar Y, et al. The clinical effectiveness and cost-effectiveness of primary stroke prevention in

children with sickle cell disease: a systematic review and economic evaluation. Health Technol Assess. 2012 Jan;16(43):1–129.

[145] Adams RJ, Brambilla D. Discontinuing prophylactic transfusions used to prevent stroke in sickle cell disease. N Engl J Med. 2005 Dec;353(26):2769–78.

[146] Kawadler JM, Clark CA, McKinstry RC, Kirkham FJ. Brain atrophy in paediatric sickle cell anaemia: findings from the silent infarct transfusion (SIT) trial. Br J Haematol. 2016; [Epub ahead of print].

[147] Puffer E, Schatz J, Roberts CW. The association of oral hydroxyurea therapy with improved cognitive functioning in sickle cell disease. Child Neuropsychol. 2007 Mar; 13(2):142–54.

[148] Pashankar FD, Manwani D, Lee MT, Green NS. Hydroxyurea improves oxygen saturation in children with sickle cell disease. J Pediatr Hematol Oncol. 2015 Apr;37(3): 242–3.

[149] Marshall MJ, Bucks RS, Hogan AM, Hambleton IR, Height SE, Dick MC, et al. Auto-adjusting positive airway pressure in children with sickle cell anemia: results of a phase I randomized controlled trial. Haematologica. 2009;94(7):4–8.

[150] Howard J, Inusa B, Liossi C, Jacob E, Murphy PB, Hart N, et al. Prevention of morbidity in sickle cell disease—qualitative outcomes, pain and quality of life in a randomised cross-over pilot trial of overnight supplementary oxygen and auto-adjusting continuous positive airways pressure (POMS2a): study protocol for a randomised controlled trial. Trials. 2015;16(1):376.

Chapter 9

Asthma, Airway Hyperresponsiveness, and Lower Airway Obstruction in Children with Sickle Cell Disease

Aravind Yadav, Ricardo A. Mosquera and
Wilfredo De Jesus Rojas

Additional information is available at the end of the chapter

http://dx.doi.org/10.5772/64328

Abstract

As a comorbid condition of sickle cell disease (SCD), asthma leads to increased complications and mortality. However, poor understanding of asthma phenotypes in SCD and the complex interaction with SCD-related airway inflammation, manifested by bronchial hyperresponsiveness or obstructive airway, pose a unique clinical challenge. The objective of this chapter is to provide a comprehensive review and discussion of epidemiology, pathophysiology, interactions, and clinical implications of airway hyperresponsiveness (AHR), obstructive airway, and asthma in SCD. Discussion will cover new understanding and limitations of asthma diagnosis and management in SCD. AHR, lower obstructive airway, and asthma are highly prevalent in SCD. Despite overlapping features, these entities are nonetheless distinct as demonstrated by basic science and clinical data. Diagnosis of asthma should be based on a physician assessment. We provide new unpublished data of a prospective study on diagnosing asthma in a small preschool population. Administered validated asthma-screening questionnaire to SCD children reveals good sensitivity and specificity as an asthma detection tool. It is unclear at this time if detection of bronchial lability or asthma early in life would result in better outcome of patients, or if improved control of SCD attenuates lower airway pathology. Being able to distinguish asthma from bronchial lability in the preschool age children would allow for appropriate intervention early in life.

Keywords: sickle cell disease, children, pediatrics, asthma, obstructive airway, lower airway obstruction, wheezing, hyperresponsive airway, hyperreactive airway, reactive airway disease

1. Introduction

Asthma is a heterogeneous chronic airway disease seen in 10% of children, characterized by airway hyperresponsiveness (AHR) and recurrent episodes of airway obstruction due to airway inflammation. In the general population, a physician diagnosis of asthma supported by pulmonary function testing or laboratory evidence is often sufficient to make such a diagnosis, but continues to remain an elusive topic in sickle cell disease (SCD).

As a comorbid condition of SCD, asthma may lead to increased complications and mortality. Children with SCD experience frequent concurrent wheezing, respiratory complications such as pneumonia or acute chest syndrome (ACS), airway hyper-responsiveness, and airway obstruction, attributed to SCD-related airway inflammation but not necessarily from asthma. As a result, wheezing (clinical surrogate for bronchial hyperresponsiveness), obstructive airway, and asthma are present in higher prevalence within the SCD population, with significant overlap (**Figure 1**), rendering common office procedures such as spirometry (measure of airway obstruction), methacholine challenge testing (measure of hyperresponsiveness), and exhaled nitric oxide (measure of asthma-related airway inflammation) inadequate to distinguish them apart.

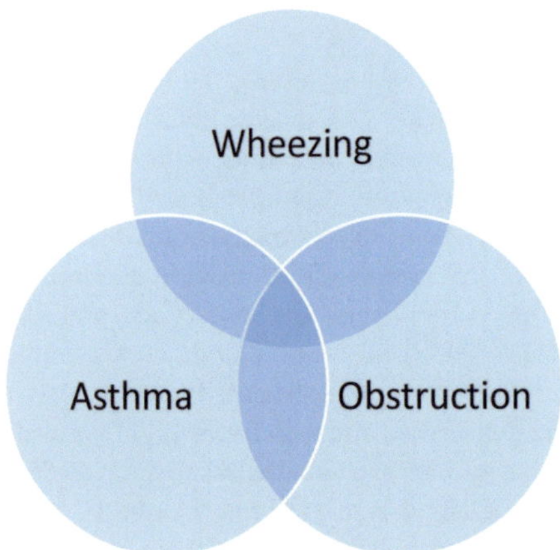

Figure 1. The relationship of asthma, wheezing, and lower airway obstruction in SCD.

2. Pathophysiology (interrelationship between wheezing, asthma, and obstruction)

The mechanism by which wheezing, obstruction, and asthma develop in SCD is poorly understood. Transgenic SCD mice demonstrate higher airway resistance via an altered immunologic pulmonary response, priming the lungs to increased inflammation, and airway hyperresponsiveness after sensitization to allergens [1]. Therefore, as an inflammatory

http://dx.doi.org/10.5772/64328

comorbid condition, asthma likely contributes to sickle hemoglobin-induced vasculopathy and in reverse, SCD attributes to airway inflammation leading to development of asthma, obstruction, or bronchial hyperresponsiveness (**Figure 2**). How SCD subtypes variably influence the lower airways is not adequately described.

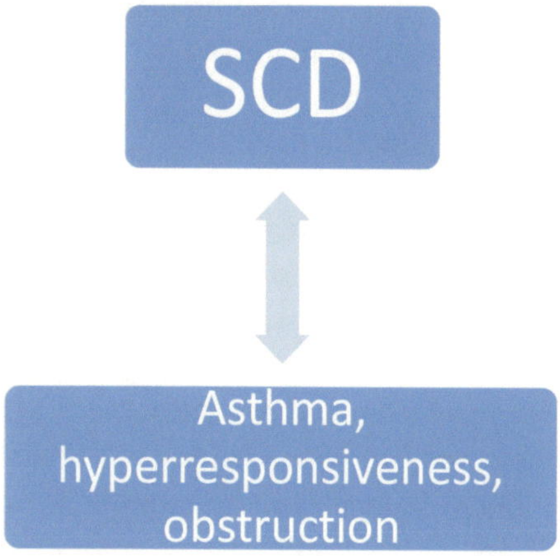

Figure 2. Interrelationship of SCD inflammation with lower airway inflammation.

Severe airway narrowing may lead to local hypoxia, promote sickling and systemic inflammation which in turn may increase airway inflammation.

2.1. Lower airway obstruction in SCD

SCD mice compared with hemoglobin A mice possess greater resistance in the airways at baseline and after allergen challenge [1]. Reversal of SCD-related inflammation through bone marrow transplant and hydroxyurea lead to improved pulmonary function, implying SCD adversely affects the lower airways. The effect of SCD on the lower airways starts early in life. Predominant lower airway obstruction (LAO) abnormality is already present in early infancy, even prior to a diagnosis of asthma [2]. Majority of older children and adolescents with SCD have either normal pattern of lung function or lower airway obstruction (LAO). Cross-sectional prevalence of lower airway obstruction estimates it being high in SCD children [3], ranging from 20 to 50%. Longitudinal studies further elaborate a tendency of lower airway obstruction development in childhood [4]. SCD LAO is not associated with increased methacholine sensitivity or eosinophilic inflammation, eluding to airway hyperresponsiveness and asthma, respectively, being distinct entities from lower airway obstruction. Increasing age, female gender, history of asthma or wheezing, tobacco smoke exposure, and high lactate dehydrogenase (LDH) are independent predictors of obstruction [5]. Clinical significance of LAO in children remains uncertain; however, some reports describe association with increased vaso-occlusive crisis [6], but not with ACS or mortality. Ongoing SCD-related airway inflammation eventually leads to LAO, which in turn increases eosinophil and collagen deposition in the lungs of SCD mice to a greater extent than control mice [1]. Whether an ongoing LAO eventually progresses into asthma remains uncertain, but SCD airway inflammation could have deleterious effect on asthma control. Clinically differentiating asthma from LAO poses a challenge, but respiratory symptoms or complications are primarily associated with the former. As asthma is poorly characterized in SCD, it isn't clear if a mild asthma evolves to a more severe form over time and how best to differentiate mild form of asthma from LAO. Management guidelines currently do not recommend monitoring pulmonary function routinely in all SCD children unless symptomatic [7].

2.2. Airway hyperresponsiveness in SCD

AHR is a cardinal feature of asthma in children without SCD; however, a high prevalence of up to 55–75% in the absence of asthma or reactive airway disease symptoms exists in SCD children, reaffirming that these entities are distinct [8–10]. Younger age, higher serum immunoglobulin E (IgE) concentration, eosinophilia, and a higher LDH level were independently associated with AHR [11]. The pro-inflammatory state of the SCD lung and its contribution to AHR is not completely understood but Nitric oxide (NO) metabolism dysregulation may possibly contribute to its etiology, independent of asthma. A lack of relationship between methacholine-induced AHR and either traditional symptoms or a physician diagnosis of asthma suggest a potential novel mechanism for AHR in SCD [12]. Clinical significance of AHR includes increased complications such as ACS and more frequent vaso-occlusive events [13]. The presence of elevated eicosanoids in SCD asthma is not associated with AHR. Hydroxyurea use may attenuate AHR, though more confirmatory studies are needed. Not enough data are available on the beneficial effects of bronchodilators or whether asthma anti-inflammatory controller medication is beneficial in preventing complications.

2.3. Asthma in sickle cell disease

Asthma is a multifactorial disease that manifests in illness as a final combination of heritability (genetics), triggers (environment), and immunologic alterations that promote hyperresponsiveness of the airway. This entity is diagnosed based on a physician assessment through the combination of medical history and physical examination.

A familial pattern of inheritance of asthma exists among first-degree relatives of probands with diagnosis of both SCD and asthma, suggesting that asthma is a distinct comorbid condition with SCD rather than a lung disease phenotype mimicking asthma [14]. Autopsy lung histological findings of a deceased SCD patient with asthma during an acute respiratory event are consistent with characteristic features of bronchial asthma. Pain crisis and ACS rates were increased in SCD children without a diagnosis of asthma but with a positive family history of asthma, compared with children without asthma and a negative family history. When adjusted to a diagnosis of asthma, individuals with family history of asthma had increased complications compared to those with asthma but without a family atopic risk [15]. Inflammatory genes and their corresponding mediators of asthma pathogenesis may therefore contribute to vascular inflammation.

Inflammatory mediators implicated in the pathogenesis of asthma and pain provide additional evidence suggesting that there is a common mechanism between asthma and SCD. Phospholipase A2 activity on cell membrane component arachidonic acid leads to production of leukotriene products (LTB4, LTC4, LT D4, and CysLT) which in the lungs have effects on asthma pathogenesis and neutrophil activation (**Figure 3**). Baseline levels of leukotrienes were significantly elevated in those with SCD compared to healthy population. Among children with SCD, levels were higher in those with asthma than those without asthma [16]. Leukotriene significantly increases during pain crisis or acute chest syndrome in children with sickle cell disease [17, 18]. Although LTB4 levels have a lesser role in the process of asthma, their actions on the activation, migration, and adhesion of neutrophils to the endothelium suggest that LTB4 could contribute to the process of vaso-occlusion. In one study, the T-lymphocyte helper cell cytokine, interleukin (IL)-4, elevation was associated with SCD rather than asthma status [19]. Consistent with SCD-triggered inflammation leading to airway changes, we previously reported preliminary data of neutrophilia and eosinophilia systemic inflammation, inversely associated with pulmonary function in asymptomatic asthmatic SCD children [20].

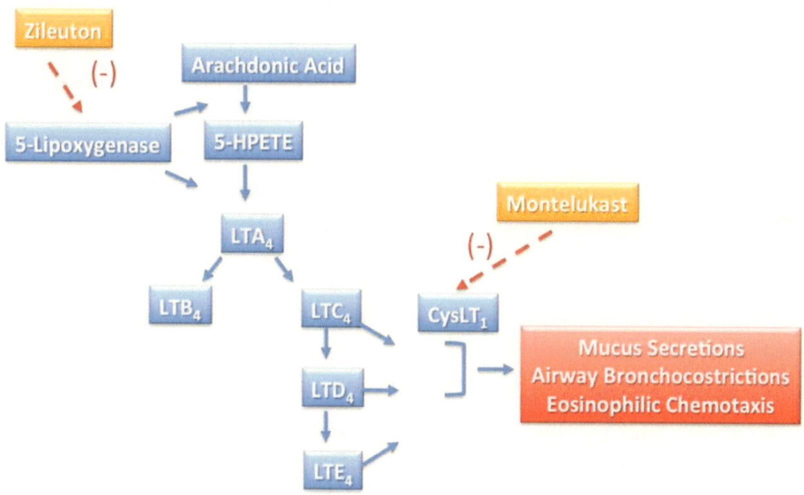

Figure 3. Eicosanoid metabolism and leukotriene biosynthesis.

Histologic findings in sickle cell mice indicate SCD independently induces a baseline lung pathology that increases large and small airway resistance and primes the lungs to increased inflammation and airway hyperresponsiveness post- sensitization. Individuals with SCD may therefore have a unique, divergent phenotype, perhaps amenable to a different therapeutic approach. Among children in the general population, an elevated IgE level and aeroallergen sensitization are among the strongest risk factors for asthma. Earlier reports of elevated IgE [21] and allergen-specific IgE [22] in physician-diagnosed asthma in SCD children were not replicated subsequently. Aeroallergen sensitization in physician-diagnosed asthma SCD children was significantly higher than the non-asthma group but was of limited clinical value in detection of asthma [23].

Asthma disproportionately affects African-American children in the United States with a prevalence of about 20%. The prevalence of comorbid asthma in patients with SCD has not been well defined, as such studies require simultaneous surveillance in the general population. In children with SCD, estimates of asthma prevalence are similar to that in children of African descent as in the general population. It is not certain if SCD imparts a modest tendency to develop asthma. Without a clear definition of asthma or understanding of asthma phenotype in SCD, the epidemiological data may vary widely. It is well described that a physician's diagnosis of asthma is not synonymous with LAO or AHR, and the prevalence of asthma in multiple SCD cohorts is much lower than LAO and AHR.

Available additional tests include spirometry, methacholine challenge, and exhaled nitric oxide, for school-aged children provide additional objective measurements to support the physician's assessment to make a diagnosis of asthma in children. Potentially, signs and symptoms suggestive of asthma, such as wheezing or an obstructive pattern on pulmonary function testing, may be related to pulmonary manifestations of SCD and thus represent a different pathophysiology than asthma. A high incidence of abnormal pulmonary function findings, including LAO or a restrictive pattern in the SCD population limit its use in the diagnosis of asthma. Bronchodilatory effect of beta agonists was appreciated in many non-asthma SCD patients [3]. Similarly for AHR in SCD, methacholine challenge is unable to differentiate those who have asthma from those without [12]. Due to dysregulation of the arginine-NO metabolic pathway in SCD, fractional exhaled nitric oxide (FeNO) levels used to assess airway eosinophilia activity could be compromised. Recently, it was shown that FeNO measures were not significantly different in SCD children with a physician diagnosis of asthma from those without asthma [23].

SCD mice with experimentally induced asthma are more susceptible to death and pulmonary inflammation compared with control mice, suggesting that asthma contributes significantly to morbidity and mortality in SCD. In children with both SCD and asthma, respiratory symptoms are a risk factor for painful episodes. Several clinical studies have since confirmed that concomitant asthma increases SCD complications of vaso-occlusive events, ACS, pneumonia, and even mortality [24–27]. Children were diagnosed as asthmatic prior to onset of their first ACS episode, suggesting that asthma exacerbations may predispose to ACS episodes. Mechanisms by which asthma predisposes to increased morbidity and mortality remain unclear.

3. Physician assessment in asthma diagnosis

To date, all studies defining asthma are based on a physician's subjective assessment. The objective criteria used to make a physician diagnosis of asthma are not well defined and may vary from one physician to another. Whether a physician diagnosis of asthma in children with SCD has the same constellation of clinical features that are recognized among children without SCD is not known.

http://dx.doi.org/10.5772/64328

3.1. Asthma-screening questionnaire in school-aged children with SCD

In 2015, we published data that demonstrated the utility of an asthma-screening questionnaire to identify physician-diagnosed asthma in SCD children. In this study, we prospectively administered a previously validated asthma-screening questionnaire to 41 SCD children on a routine clinic visit. Prevalence of obstructive airway was high at 51.2% and physician diagnosis of asthma was lower, 33.3%. The sensitivity and specificity were high in detecting physician diagnosis of asthma in this SCD population [28].

An asthma-screening questionnaire showed to be a useful tool in identifying at-risk SCD children who may benefit from further asthma management as an effective, easy-to-administer screening tool. More importantly, as the screening questionnaire had been developed and validated in the general population, it provided new evidence that a physician diagnosis of asthma in children with and without SCD was consistent. In another study, after extensive evaluation of SCD children for respiratory symptomology, atopic risk, pulmonary function measures, and inflammatory markers; parental history of asthma, wheezing causing shortness of breath, and wheezing after exercise were predictive of development of asthma [23], indicating the importance of a proper history and physical in determining an asthma diagnosis. We did not observe a difference between parental history of asthma in SCD with the asthma and non-asthma groups, but allergic rhinitis was significantly seen in the asthma group.

3.2. Wheezing and SCD

Children with SCD are more likely to wheeze than non-SCD children in the same geographical setting [29]. Wheezing likely is a clinical surrogate of SCD inflammation-related AHR, bronchial asthma airway inflammation, or both. No age association between wheezing and asthma diagnosis exists; therefore, children with wheezing were no more likely to carry an asthma diagnosis than adults [30]. Some SCD patients have recurrent wheezing without a personal or familial history of asthma. Risk factors including upper respiratory tract infection, environmental tobacco smoke exposure, maternal history of asthma, lower socioeconomic status, excessive production of inflammatory mediators such as leukotrienes, low vitamin D level, and exposure to acetaminophen in early life were found to be associated with wheezing independent of asthma [30]. Many of these risk factors are similar to early life wheezing in the general population and asthma. The International Study of Asthma and Allergies in Childhood (ISAAC) to assess current respiratory symptoms of asthma showed that recent use of acetaminophen was associated with an exposure-dependent increased risk of asthma [31]; therefore, further work is needed in SCD due to high exposure of pain medications. Recurrent, severe wheezing regardless of asthma status was associated with increased pain crisis, ACS, and mortality. Wheezing and asthma are likely independent risk factors of SCD complications [32].

The Asthma Predictive Index (API) was developed for children less than 3 years old with recurrent wheezing. This index was created as a guide for the primary physician to determine which children would likely have asthma later in life. The API takes into consideration a combination of major and minor criteria (**Table 1**) to evaluate the patient asthma risk.

Major criteria	Minor criteria
Parental asthma	Food allergies
Physician diagnosis of atopic dermatitis	Eosinophilia >4%
Sensitization to aeroallergens	Wheezing apart from colds

Table 1. Asthma predictive index: a positive API requires ≥3 episodes of wheezing a year during the first 3 years of age and one of the two major criteria or two of the three minor criteria.

In preschool children aged 3–5 years, or younger, the diagnosis of asthma sometimes is a challenge. Many times, viral respiratory illnesses may mimic early asthma symptoms. Cardinal symptoms that suggest asthma include dry cough, trouble in breathing, chest tightness or pain, and wheezing, most of them are also present in SCD. Asthma could be exacerbated by weather changes, colds, emotions, or exercise. In SCD patients, diagnosis of asthma may be even harder taking into consideration the vaso-occlusive pathophysiology involved in this disease as an additional confounding factor for asthma symptoms. It is uncertain if the API can be reliably applied to the SCD population.

3.3. Asthma in the preschool SCD population

For a primary physician, diagnosis of asthma in the preschool population may be a potential challenge notwithstanding other several comorbidities that can mask asthma symptoms like in those patients with SCD.

In our unpublished 3-years prospective study, a validated asthma-screening questionnaire was administrated to 12 preschool SCD children (aged 2–5 years) on a routine clinic visit. Prevalence of physician diagnosis of asthma at initial visit was 33.3% (n = 4). We found that the abbreviated three-question version had 100% sensitivity and 62.5% specificity in detecting asthma early in life in this subject population when followed over time. The Breathmobile Case Identification Survey (BCIS) in preschool-age children in the general population had a high sensitivity (70%) and specificity (84%) [33]. Further work is required to assess early asthma-screening approaches in SCD.

These data demonstrate that a validated asthma-screening tool intended for the general population might be relevant in preschool SCD and might be used as a screening tool for a valid asthma diagnostic approach. A validated screening tool implemented in early asthma diagnosis will help the primary physician to assess objectively and uniformly the diagnosis of asthma in preschool SCD children in order to identify individuals at risk of major complications or those with poorly controlled asthma.

It is unclear if detection of bronchial lability or asthma diagnosis earlier would result in better outcomes or if improved asthma control in SCD attenuates lower airway pathology. Identifying mild asthma would continue to remain a challenge. Previously, due to poor understanding of an asthma diagnosis in this high-risk population, clinical trials were difficult to conduct, resulting in a gap of knowledge. Future research to evaluate the impact of early asthma detection in the development of further comorbidities in SCD children should be explored.

http://dx.doi.org/10.5772/64328

4. Asthma management in SCD

Sickle cell disease is marked by high utilization of medical services. A history of asthma was associated with an increased risk of SCD emergency department (ED) utilization for both pain and ACS [34]. Recently, the patient-centered medical home (PCMH) emerged as a viable method to improve delivery of medical care. The American Academy of Pediatrics (AAP) currently defines a PCMH as care that is accessible, continuous, comprehensive, family-centered, coordinated, compassionate, and culturally effective. Children with SCD reported to experience comprehensive care had lower rates of ED encounters and hospitalizations after controlling for demographics and health status. SCD patients with asthma are anticipated to benefit the most in this setting.

Achievement of asthma control to reduce pulmonary complications and mortality are the goals of the National Asthma Education and Prevention Program (NAEPP) expert panel report 3 on 2007 guidelines. These guidelines focus on impairment and risk as key factors to assess asthma severity and control. Treatment recommendations are summarized in a stepwise approach for long-term asthma treatment taking into consideration the patient age and epidemiologic risk factors. Currently, physicians follow the NAEPP 2007 asthma guidelines in order to minimize future comorbidities and reduce asthma-related mortality in the pediatric population.

It is known that the pathophysiology of asthma involves several overlapping areas that affect the asthma phenotype in each patient. Also many comorbid factors can play a direct role in the development of asthma, SCD being one of them. Concerns regarding asthma management in SCD using the standard NAEPP 2007 approach have arisen, taking in consideration the hemolytic and chronic inflammatory state of this disease. Current consensus in the management of asthma in SCD agrees with the use of NAEPP 2007 guidelines to treat SCD asthma until new studies demonstrate a different approach.

Acute asthma exacerbations

- Rescue medications may include inhaled bronchodilators (albuterol and ipratropium) and systemic corticosteroids.
- Several cases have been described associating oral corticosteroid use with rebound pain and ACS. However, their use should not be withheld in the setting of an acute asthma exacerbation. A slow taper of systemic corticosteroids may decrease the risk for rebound pain.
- Admit all patients with acute asthma exacerbations requiring corticosteroids and consider a lower threshold to admit SCD patients with mild asthma exacerbations in view of the potential complications, such as ACS or pain crisis.

Long-term asthma control

- Physicians are encouraged to prescribe inhaled corticosteroids (ICS) as the first line for asthma-controlled medication and to consider additional controlled medications such as leukotriene inhibitors.

- Consult pulmonary specialist and hematologist when starting ICS in an SCD patient.
- Interval pulmonary function test in the outpatient setting is recommended.
- Asthma assessment on all SCD patients at least annually.
- A Doppler echocardiogram annually in SCD patient with asthma to screen for pulmonary hypertension.
- A baseline EKG should be completed before starting therapy with beta2 agonists due to increased risk of prolonged QTc complications in SCD.

In the following sections, we expand the available literature on asthma management in the SCD population and explore future areas of interest about this topic [35].

4.1. Oxygen therapy

As part of the management of acute asthma exacerbations in the general population, oxygen therapy plays an important role in the correction of asthma-induced hypoxemia, secondary to V/Q mismatch. In SCD, oxygen is also part of the initial management for acute chest syndrome. It is known that in SCD, the onset of erythrocyte sickling can be triggered by hypoxemia and, for instance, the development of acute chest syndrome. More studies are needed to evaluate the benefit of oxygen in SCD in the acute setting of asthma. Short-term oxygen in an acute asthma exacerbation should be initiated with SCD during a moderate to severe asthma exacerbation.

4.2. Bronchodilators

Acute hyper-responsiveness can be treated successfully with short-term inhaled bronchodilators that selectively stimulate the Beta-2 receptors in the airway and relax the smooth muscle. In SCD, the approach may be different if acute chest syndrome overlaps with an acute asthma exacerbation. On red blood cells, beta2-receptor stimulation was associated with cellular adhesion in vivo. This may theoretically promote vaso-occlusive episodes in SCD but clinically this phenomenon has not been described. Studies to evaluate the effectiveness in the treatment of asthma and acute chest syndrome in SCD have not been performed. Several Cochrane Reviews have shown consistently the lack of well-designed randomized controlled trials in this area. As a clinician, this information will be helpful to evaluate the risks of the use of inhaled bronchodilators in the therapy for acute chest syndrome and asthma in the SCD population [36].

Inhaled beta2 agonist has been related with life-threatening cardiac events in adults with long QT syndrome [37]. Prolonged QTc is a frequent finding in the SCD pediatric and young adult population. Considering this, evaluation for possible life-threatening events in SCD related to QTc prolongation after beta2 agonist use may be warranted [38]. An EKG prior to starting a beta2 agonist will provide useful information at initial evaluation in SCD asthma management to prevent additional comorbidities. A randomized control trial evaluating the risk of the use of beta2 agonists in SCD secondary to QTc prolongation needs to be explored.

Long-term bronchodilators (long-acting beta-agonists [LABAs]) are recommended for asthma control in those with moderate to severe persistent asthma as per NAEPP 2007 guidelines. In SCD, some concerns arise about the use considering the epidemiology of the disease. In the Salmeterol Multicenter Research Trial (SMART), African-American subgroup showed an increased risk for respiratory-related deaths [39], prompting the US Food and Drug Administration (USFDA) to issue a black box warning. The safety profile of LABA is currently being investigated in the pediatric population with the VRESTRI clinical trial and is expected to complete in 2017.

An alternative approach to address the risk of short-acting beta-agonists (SABA or LABA) use in the African-American SCD population for asthma management is the use of short-acting and long-acting anticholinergics. Ipratropium and tiotropium work as acetylcholine receptor antagonists, causing bronchodilation. A randomized clinical trial in 2015 has compared the effectiveness and safety of tiotropium versus LABAs. In this study, African-American adults with moderate to severe asthma were enrolled over 18 months. The combination of LABAs or tiotropium with ICS showed no significant differences in asthma exacerbations, forced expiratory volume in 1 s (FEV1), asthma control questionnaire (ACQ) scores, or patient reported outcomes [40].

An observational study evaluated the increased pulmonary capillary volume as a possible explanation for airway obstruction in SCD patients. They found that an increased pulmonary capillary volume contributes to increased airway obstruction and, for instance, may limit the effect of ipratropium in reducing airway obstruction in SCD [41].

4.3. Leukotriene's inhibitors

During acute asthma episodes, prolific release of inflammatory metabolites contributes to airway bronchoconstriction and acute exacerbations. Leukotrienes are arachidonic acid metabolites that contribute to airway inflammation in asthma and may have additional pathophysiologic roles in SCD. Lung leukotriene cascade activates and releases additional metabolites including LTA_4, LTB_4, LTC_4, LTD_4, and LTE_4 after activation of the 5-lipoxygenase, a key enzyme in the biosynthesis of leukotrienes (**Figure 3**).

Montelukast is an adjuvant therapy that works as a leukotriene receptor antagonist (LTRA) in the airway mast cells, eosinophils, and also in lung epithelial cells. Of all LTRAs, LTD4 is the most potent bronchoconstrictive leukotriene. Additional chemo-attractive properties have been attributed to Cyst-LTs with a direct effect on lung vascular permeability, mucous secretion, and airway narrowing. Currently, under recruitment process, a phase-2 clinical trial tries to evaluate the effect of montelukast as an adjuvant medication to hydroxyurea for SCD vaso-occlusion treatment. This trial will provide valuable information about the role of leukotrienes in the SCD inflammatory state. Additional studies are needed to evaluate efficacy of LTRA inhibitors in SCD and asthma.

Zileuton is a specific 5-lipoxygenase inhibitor with a direct activity by decreasing leukotriene production. It is suggested that zileuton could have benefits in SCD considering the structural analog of hydroxyurea, and the advantage of inducing fetal hemoglobin to improve oxygen affinity and delivery. In vitro trials have documented a potential effect in downregulating SCD inflammatory state through nitric oxide pathways in a dose-dependent effect [42]. Upregulation of IL-13 with hydroxyurea and downregulation of IL-13 with zileuton has been documented in vitro. This observation promotes the idea that zileuton is a potential drug for management of the SCD inflammatory state [43]. A phase-I trial evaluated the role and tested the safety of zileuton to reduce inflammation associated with SCD in a dose-dependent manner in children and adults [44]. Phase-II and -III clinical trials are pending to be done to explore the interactions between zileuton and hydroxyurea in SCD.

4.4. Corticosteroid

As per NAEPP 2007 guidelines, moderate to severe persistent asthma involves the introduction of an inhaled corticosteroid in order to achieve asthma control in the pediatric population. However, unclear data about the use and safety of corticosteroid in SCD children introduce challenges in the management.

Specific data regarding the use of corticosteroid in the management of asthma are needed. Some trials have evaluated systemic corticosteroids in the setting of acute chest syndrome in SCD. In a randomized trial evaluating the efficacy of dexamethasone in SCD with acute chest syndrome a beneficial effect was found [45]. Significant statistical data showed lower rates of hospitalizations, blood transfusions, duration of oxygen and analgesic medications; however, the subjects were never evaluated for pre-existing asthma diagnosis. Noteworthy here is that the rebound readmission rate in the dexamethasone group has raised some concern.

Rebound pain crisis after systemic corticosteroid use had been a concern in SCD. The potent anti-inflammatory effects of systemic corticosteroid may have a role in the management of ACS and asthma. Nevertheless, rebound pain and subsequent readmission may limit their use to an SCD sub-population [46]. It is suggested to use a longer course of systemic steroid with slow taper, but controlled clinical trials would be needed to evaluate this approach.

It is currently recommended to follow NAEPP 2007 guidelines as part of the treatment of asthma in SCD. Systemic steroid may be used in moderate to severe asthma exacerbations with a close monitoring for rebound pain. An individual approach may be considered to start inhaled corticosteroids in persistent asthma in SCD to avoid asthma-related morbidity, while upcoming clinical trials provide the clinician evidence-based guidelines about the best strategies for asthma management in SCD. However, poor understanding of asthma phenotype in SCD and additive bronchial asthma airway inflammation to underlying SCD inflammation, and its impact on asthma control has not been explored. Current clinical trials for inhaled mometasone and budesonide are being conducted to address the gap in the knowledge.

4.5. New therapy in asthma

New modes of asthma management may have beneficial effects on SCD asthma airway inflammation and asthma. However, no data are currently available on these modes of therapy. These include immunotherapy, monoclonal antibody against specific immune protein, and

http://dx.doi.org/10.5772/64328

bronchial thermoplasty. The role of hydroxyurea and other anti-inflammatory interventions of SCD in improving asthma control requires investigation.

Author details

Aravind Yadav*, Ricardo A. Mosquera and Wilfredo De Jesus Rojas

*Address all correspondence to: Aravind.yadav@uth.tmc.edu

University of Texas Health Science Center at Houston, Houston, USA

References

[1] Pritchard KA Jr, Feroah TR, Nandedkar SD, Holzhauer SL, Hutchins W, Schulte ML, Strunk RC, Debaun MR, Hillery CA. Effects of experimental asthma on inflammation and lung mechanics in sickle cell mice. Am J Respir Cell Mol Biol. 2012 Mar; 46(3), 389–96.

[2] Koumbourlis AC, Hurlet-Jensen A, Bye MR. Lung function in infants with sickle cell disease. Pediatr Pulm. 1997; 24, 277–81.

[3] Koumbourlis AC, Zar HJ, Hurlet-Jensen A, Goldberg MR. Prevalence and reversibility of lower airway obstruction in children with sickle cell disease. J Pediatr. 2001 Feb; 138(2), 188–92.

[4] Koumbourlis AC, Lee DJ, Lee A. Longitudinal changes in lung function and somatic growth in children with sickle cell disease. Pediatr Pulm. 2007; 42, 483–88.

[5] Mehari A, Klings ES. Chronic pulmonary complications of sickle cell disease. Chest. 2016 May;149(5):1313–24.

[6] Boyd JH, DeBaun MR, Morgan WJ, Mao J, Strunk RC. Lower airway obstruction is associated with increased morbidity in children with sickle cell disease. Pediatr Pulm. 2009; 44, 290–96.

[7] Yawn BP, Buchanan GR, Afenyi-Annan AN, Ballas SK, Hassell KL, James AH, Jordan L, Lanzkron SM, Lottenberg R, Savage WJ, Tanabe PJ, Ware RE, Murad MH, Goldsmith JC, Ortiz E, Fulwood R, Horton A, John-Sowah J. Management of sickle cell disease: summary of the 2014 evidence-based report by expert panel members. JAMA. 2014 Sep 10; 312(10), 1033–48.

[8] Leong MA, Dampier C, Varlotta L, Allen JL. Airway hyper-reactivity in children with sickle cell disease. J Pediatr. 1997; 131, 278–83.

[9] Strunk RC, Brown MS, Boyd JH, Bates P, Field JJ, DeBaun MR. Methacholine challenge in children with sickle cell disease: a case series. Pediatr Pulm. 2008; 43, 924–29.

[10] Ozbek OY, Malbora B, Sen N, Yazici AC, Ozyurek E, Ozbek N. Airway hyper-reactivity detected by methacholine challenge in children with sickle cell disease. Pediatr Pulm. 2007; 42, 1187–92.

[11] Field JJ, Stocks J, Kirkham FJ, Rosen CL, Dietzen DJ, Semon T, Kirkby J, Bates P, Seicean S, DeBaun MR, Redline S, Strunk RC. Airway hyperresponsiveness in children with sickle cell anemia. Chest. 2011; 139, 563–68.

[12] Shilo NR, Alawadi A, Allard-Coutu A, Robitaille N, Pastore Y, Bérubé D, Jacob SV, Abish S, Dauletbaev N, Lands LC. Airway hyperreactivity is frequent in non-asthmatic children with sickle cell disease. Pediatr Pulm. 2015 Dec 30.

[13] Sylvester KP, Patey RA, Rafferty GF, Rees D, Thein SL, Greenough A. Airway hyper-responsiveness and acute chest syndrome in children with sickle cell disease. Pediatr Pulm. 42 (2007), 272–76.

[14] Phillips KL, An P, Boyd JH, Strunk RC, Casella JF, Barton BA, DeBaun MR. Major gene effect and additive familial pattern of inheritance of asthma exist among families of probands with sickle cell anemia and asthma. Am J Hum Biol. 2008 Mar–Apr; 20(2), 149–53.

[15] Field JJ, Macklin EA, Yan Y, Strunk RC, DeBaun MR. Sibling history of asthma is a risk factor for pain in children with sickle cell anemia. Am J Hematol. 2008; 83(11), 855–57.

[16] Jennings JE, Ramkumar T, Mao J, Boyd J, Castro M, Field JJ, Strunk RC, DeBaun MR. Elevated urinary leukotriene E4 levels are associated with hospitalization for pain in children with sickle cell disease. Am J Hematol. 2008 Aug; 83(8), 640–43.

[17] Field JJ, Strunk RC, Knight-Perry JE, Blinder MA, Townsend RR, DeBaun MR. Urinary cysteinyl leukotriene E4 significantly increases during pain in children and adults with sickle cell disease. Am J Hematol. 2009 Apr; 84(4), 231–33.

[18] Field JJ, Krings J, White NL, Yan Y, Blinder MA, Strunk RC, Debaun MR. Urinary cysteinyl leukotriene E(4) is associated with increased risk for pain and acute chest syndrome in adults with sickle cell disease. Am J Hematol. 2009 Mar; 84(3), 158–60.

[19] Knight-Madden J, Vergani D, Patey R, Sylvester K, Hussain MJ, Forrester T, Greenough A. Cytokine levels and profiles in children related to sickle cell disease and asthma status. J Interferon Cytokine Res. 2012 Jan; 32(1), 1–5.

[20] Yadav A, Stark JM, Brown DL, Mosquera RA. Correlation between lung function test and blood cell count in asthmatic children with sickle cell disease. Am J Respir Crit Care Med. 2013; 187, A1788.

[21] An P, Barron-Casella EA, Strunk RC, Hamilton RG, Casella JF, DeBaun MR. Elevation of IgE in children with sickle cell disease is associated with doctor diagnosis of asthma and increased morbidity. J Allergy Clin Immunol. 2011 Jun; 127(6), 1440–46.

[22] Ross JG, Bernaudin F, Strunk RC, Kamdem A, Arnaud C, Hervé M, Delacourt C, DeBaun MR. Asthma is a distinct comorbid condition in children with sickle cell anemia with elevated total and allergen-specific IgE levels. J Pediatr Hematol Oncol. 2011 Jul; 33(5), e205–08.

[23] Strunk RC, Cohen RT, Cooper BP, Rodeghier M, Kirkham FJ, Warner JO, Stocks J, Kirkby J, Roberts I, Rosen CL, Craven DI, DeBaun MR. Wheezing symptoms and parental asthma are associated with a physician diagnosis of asthma in children with sickle cell anemia. J Pediatr. 2014; 164, 821–826.e821.

[24] Knight-Madden JM, Forrester TS, Lewis NA, Greenough A. Asthma in children with sickle cell disease and its association with acute chest syndrome. Thorax. 2005; 60, 206–10.

[25] Boyd JH, Macklin EA, Strunk RC, DeBaun MR. Asthma is associated with acute chest syndrome and pain in children with sickle cell anemia. Blood. 2006; 108, 2923–27.

[26] Boyd JH, Macklin EA, Strunk RC, DeBaun MR. Asthma is associated with increased mortality in individuals with sickle cell anemia. Haematologica. 2007; 92, 1115–18.

[27] Knight-Madden JM, Barton-Gooden A, Weaver SR, Reid M, Greenough A. Mortality, asthma, smoking and acute chest syndrome in young adults with sickle cell disease. Lung. 2013; 191(1), 95–100.

[28] Yadav A, Corrales-Medina FF, Stark JM, Hashmi SS, Carroll MP, Smith KG, Meulmester KM, Brown DL, Jon C, Mosquera RA. Application of an asthma screening questionnaire in children with sickle cell disease. Pediatr Allergy Immunol Pulmonol. 2015 Sep 1; 28(3), 177–82.

[29] Galadanci NA, Liang WH, Galadanci AA, Aliyu MH, Jibir BW, Karaye IM, Inusa BP, Vermund SH, Strunk RC, DeBaun MR. Wheezing is common in children with sickle cell disease when compared with controls. J Pediatr Hematol Oncol. 2015 Jan; 37(1), 16–19.

[30] Knight-Madden J, Greenough A. Acute pulmonary complications of sickle cell disease. Paediatr Respir Rev. 2014 Mar; 15(1), 13–16.

[31] Beasley RW, Clayton TO, Crane J, Lai CK, Montefort SR, Mutius EV, Stewart AW; ISAAC Phase Three Study Group. Acetaminophen use and risk of asthma, rhinoconjunctivitis, and eczema in adolescents: international study of asthma and allergies in childhood phase three. Am J Respir Crit Care Med. 2011 Jan 15; 183(2), 171–78.

[32] Glassberg JA, Chow A, Wisnivesky J, Hoffman R, Debaun MR, Richardson LD. Wheezing and asthma are independent risk factors for increased sickle cell disease morbidity. Br J Haematol. 2012; 159, 472–79.

[33] Berg J, Brecht ML, Morphew T, Tichacek MJ, Chowdhury Y, Galant S. Identifying preschool children with asthma in Orange County. J Asthma. 2009 Jun; 46(5), 460–64.

[34] Glassberg JA, Wang J, Cohen R, Richardson LD, DeBaun MR. Risk factors for increased ED utilization in a multinational cohort of children with sickle cell disease. Acad Emerg Med. 2012 Jun; 19(6), 664–72.

[35] Gomez E, Morris CR. Asthma management in sickle cell disease. Biomed Res Int. 2013; 2013, 604140.

[36] Knight-Madden JM, Hambleton IR. Inhaled bronchodilators for acute chest syndrome in people with sickle cell disease. Cochrane Database Syst Rev. 2014 Aug 2; 8, CD003733.

[37] Thottathil P, Acharya J, Moss AJ, Jons C, McNitt S, Goldenberg I, Zareba W, Kaufman E, Qi M, Robinson JL; International Long QT Syndrome Investigative Group. Risk of cardiac events in patients with asthma and long-QT syndrome treated with beta(2) agonists. Am J Cardiol. 2008 Oct 1; 102(7), 871–74.

[38] Liem RI, Young LT, Thompson AA. Prolonged QTc interval in children and young adults with sickle cell disease at steady state. Pediatr Blood Cancer. 2009 Jul; 52(7), 842–46.

[39] Nelson HS, Weiss ST, Bleecker ER, Yancey SW, Dorinsky PM; SMART Study Group. The salmeterol multicenter asthma research trial: a comparison of usual pharmacotherapy for asthma or usual pharmacotherapy plus salmeterol. Chest. 2006 Jan; 129(1), 15–26.

[40] Wechsler ME, Yawn BP, Fuhlbrigge AL, Pace WD, Pencina MJ, Doros G, Kazani S, Raby BA, Lanzillotti J, Madison S, Israel E; BELT Investigators. Anticholinergic vs long-acting β-agonist in combination with inhaled corticosteroids in black adults with asthma: the BELT randomized clinical trial. JAMA. 2015; 314(16), 1720–30.

[41] Wedderburn CJ, Rees D, Height S, Dick M, Rafferty GF, Lunt A, Greenough A. Airways obstruction and pulmonary capillary blood volume in children with sickle cell disease: pulmonary capillary blood volume-SCD children. Pediatr Pulm. 2014 Jul; 49(7), 716–22.

[42] Haynes J Jr, Baliga BS, Obiako B, Ofori-Acquah S, Pace B. Zileuton induces hemoglobin F synthesis in erythroid progenitors: role of the L-arginine-nitric oxide signaling pathway. Blood. 2004; 103(10), 3945–50.

[43] Kuvibidila S, Baliga BS, Gardner R, et al. Differential effects of hydroxyurea and zileuton on interleukin-13 secretion by activated murine spleen cells: implication on the expression of vascular cell adhesion molecule-1 and vasoocclusion in sickle cell anemia. Cytokine. 2005; 30(5), 213–18.

[44] Mpollo MEM, Quarmyne M, Rayes O, Gonsalves CS, Vanderah L, Canter C, Haynes Jr. J, Clavijio CF, Uwe C, Kalinyak K, Joiner CH, Vinks AA, Malik P. A phase I trial of zileuton in sickle cell disease. Blood. 2013; 122, 993–993.

http://dx.doi.org/10.5772/64328

[45] Bernini JC, Rogers ZR, Sandler ES, Reisch JS, Quinn CT, Buchanan GR. Beneficial effect of intravenous dexamethasone in children with mild to moderately severe acute chest syndrome complicating sickle cell disease. Blood. 1998 Nov 1; 92(9), 3082–89.

[46] Strouse JJ, Takemoto CM, Keefer JR, Kato GJ, Casella JF. Corticosteroids and increased risk of readmission after acute chest syndrome in children with sickle cell disease. Pediatr Blood Cancer. 2008 May; 50(5), 1006–12.

Chapter 10

Leg Ulceration in Sickle Cell Disease: An Early and Visible Sign of End-Organ Disease

Aditi P. Singh and Caterina P. Minniti

Additional information is available at the end of the chapter

http://dx.doi.org/10.5772/64234

Abstract

Introduction: Leg ulcers are a frequent and debilitating complication of sickle cell disease (SCD), particularly of the SS genotype. The prevalence of leg ulcers in patients with sickle cell disease (SCD) varies geographically ranging widely from 75% in Jamaica to as low as 1% in Saudi Arabia. The prevalence of leg ulcers in the Cooperative Study of Sickle Cell Disease (CSSCD) in the United States was 5% in SS genotype with the incidence increasing with age. As patients with SCD have increasingly improved survival, the prevalence of leg ulcers is likely to be higher. These ulcers are slow to heal, have a high rate of recurrence, and are associated with severe unremitting pain and depression, thus leading to high healthcare costs. Despite being a well-recognized complication of SCD, there are no specifically designed evidence-based guidelines to help clinicians manage these patients.

Methods: To prepare this manuscript, we searched PubMed using the search terms "sickle cell," "ulcer," "sickle cell," and "wound." We also appraised the references mentioned in the identified articles. Inclusion criteria included case reports, case series, retrospective reviews, clinical trials, randomized controlled trials, systematic reviews, and meta-analyses from 1945 to 2016. We present our extensive personal observations and expert opinion, whenever there is a lack of reliable data.

Conclusion: Our understanding of the pathophysiology of leg ulceration in sickle cell disease is improved, though still limited since the first described case in the English literature over 100 years ago. Moreover, there remains a paucity of good quality randomized clinical trials to test new and effective therapies. No evidence-based guidelines for the management of these patients are available. Currently, a holistic multidisciplinary approach is recommended with adequate systemic control of SCD as well as aggressive local therapy, with a focus on targeting pathways involved in potentiating healing of these ulcers including novel approaches like topical nitric oxide donors. SCD patients with leg ulcers represent a cohort of patients who are at an increased risk of developing other vasculopathic complications that have a potentially common mechanism including pulmonary hypertension, renal and retinal disease, and priapism. Prospective trials are needed to better evaluate the natural history of these patients in the modern era and develop preventative and therapeutic strategies for the management of this serious complication.

Keywords: leg ulcers, wounds, sickle cell disease

1. History

The first patient with SCD described in the English medical literature more than 100 years ago suffered from leg ulceration [1, 2, 4–7, 9]; however, it was not until 1939 that the causal role of SCD in leg ulceration was established [3].

2. Epidemiology

2.1. Prevalence and geographic variation

Leg ulcers are a frequent and debilitating complication of sickle cell disease, particularly of the SS genotype. The prevalence of leg ulcers in patients with sickle cell disease (SCD) varies geographically widely ranging from 75% in Jamaica to 1% in Saudi Arabia [4–5]. In the Cooperative Study of Sickle Cell Disease (CSSCD) in the United States, the overall prevalence was 2.5%, in persons 10 years of age and older and was higher in patients with SS disease (4.97%) and SS-alpha thalassemia (3.92%) compared to patients with SC disease and SS-beta thalassemia [6]. However, over 70% of the study population was under the age of 30 years, and along with improved survival of SCD patients, the prevalence of leg ulcers is likely to be much higher. In a sickle cell clinic in West Indies, 58% had a history of leg ulcers out of 102 patients who survived beyond 60 years of age [8]. About 20% of the 505 patients screened at the National Institutes of Health (NIH) recalled having had an ulcer [9]. The incidence of leg ulcers in sickle cell patients is hard to elucidate given the lack of any recent large prospective trials. The incidence of leg ulcers in patients with SS genotype was 9.97/100 persons in the Cooperative Study of Sickle Cell Disease [6]. In comparison, the prevalence of venous ulcers in the general population in the United States is approximately 600,000 annually [10] with 1% of the population is affected at any given time. Thus, the incidence of leg ulcers in patients with SCD exceeds that of the general population by more than tenfold and also occurs at a younger age.

The striking geographic differences in leg ulcer prevalence may be attributed in part to the differing age structure of the studied populations; however, there does seem to be a difference even after adjusting for age. Different SCD haplotypes differ in their clinical severity. The Bantu haplotype usually has more severe clinical manifestations compared to others; however, there exists a considerable variation within haplotypes as well [11]. Leg ulcers have been reported to be more common in carriers of the CAR beta-globin gene cluster haplotype [12]. Among patients who have the Asian haplotype, leg ulceration is rare among adults in both the eastern province of Saudi Arabia [5, 13] and central India [4, 14]. Though not yet defined, environmental, socioeconomic, and genetic factors are most likely responsible for the variations in incidence.

2.2. Age

Studies from Jamaica and personal observations indicate that leg ulcers' first occurrence is rare before 10 years of age, is most frequently seen between 10 and 25 years of age, and continues to increase in frequency after 30 years [2, 4]. In the CSSCD, incidence increased sharply after second decade of life, ranging from 14.59 to 19.17 in hemoglobin SS patients and from 7.57 to 11.13 in patients with hemoglobin SS-alpha thalassemia [6].

3. Risk factors

3.1. Gender

Some studies found a male preponderance with the rates being 15 and 5/100 person-years in men and women, respectively, in the CSSCD cohort [6]. Similar patterns were observed in Ghana [15]. However, no difference was seen in studies from Nigeria and Jamaica [4] nor in more recent reports [12].

3.2. Hematology

3.2.1. Type of SCD

The prevalence of leg ulcers is higher in patients with SS and SS-alpha thalassemia than among those with SC, SB+, or SB0 genotypes. Alpha thalassemia with two alpha gene deletions seems to be protective against development of leg ulcers in patients with sickle cell disease [6]. In CSSCD, incidence of leg ulcers was significantly lower in SS patients with two alpha gene deletions compared to patients with SS disease and SS patients with three alpha gene deletions. More recent data have shown that alpha thalassemia (one gene deletion) is not protective [12].

3.2.2. Hemoglobin and hemoglobin F level

Data from CSSCD suggest that higher hemoglobin level as well as higher fetal hemoglobin percentage is protective against development of leg ulcers in SS patients, whereas only fetal hemoglobin is protective in SS- alpha thalassemia patients [6].

Incidence of leg ulcers was 43.2 events per 100 person-years in patients with hemoglobin levels <6 g and 2.4 events per 100 person-years in patients with hemoglobin >12 g.

In both genotypes, the incidence of leg ulcers decreased with an increase in fetal hemoglobin. Incidence was 0.7/100 person-years in patients with HbF levels of >10% compared to 13/100 person-years in patients with HbF levels of <5%. Most recent series [12, 16] did not show a relationship between HbF and leg ulcers. Of note is that the latter study included individuals that received hydroxyurea (HU) therapy and whose elevated HbF levels were not constitutional, but induced by the use of this drug. Patients did not enjoy its protecting effects since birth, as in the case of the older studies. Furthermore, hydroxyurea's other (negative) effects on angiogenesis could have blunted the benefits of high hemoglobin F.

4. Pathogenesis

4.1. Mechanical obstruction of microcirculation

Sickle cell disease is characterized by vasoocclusion. The rigid deformed sickle cells get entrapped in the microcirculation leading to hyperviscosity, decreased blood flow through venules and capillaries, and chronic hemolysis resulting in anemia, ischemia-reperfusion injury, and inflammation causing end-organ damage [4]. Studies have shown that the hematocrit to viscosity ratio as well as red blood cell (RBC) deformability was reduced in sickle cell patients with leg ulcers [17, 18]. The marginal circulation of the malleoli is particularly susceptible to this obstruction of microcirculation, making them the most common site for sickle cell leg ulcers.

4.2. Hemolysis-vascular dysfunction syndrome

Nitrogen oxide (NO) is a natural occurring free radical found in plasma. Receptors for NO present on the endothelium initiate relaxation of vascular smooth muscle causing vasodilation and increased blood flow along with reduced neutrophil adhesion. Chronic hemolysis is a hallmark of SCD and results in red blood cell (RBC) membrane damage, cell breakdown, and extrusion of free hemoglobin into plasma. This free hemoglobin scavenges NO, reducing its bioavailability and thus linked to hemolysis-vascular dysfunction syndrome which is characterized by chronic vasoconstriction contributing to leg ulcers, priapism, and pulmonary hypertension [19, 20].

4.3. Venous incompetence

An early study of 16 SCD patients with leg ulcers using manometry and the Doppler studies failed to demonstrate venous insufficiency as a primary factor in development of leg ulcers in SCD [21]. However, edema and pain often precede ulceration in these patients, and numerous studies since then have linked venous stasis with sickle cell leg ulcers [7]. Venous stasis in the calf muscles was suggested by the delayed clearance of ^{99m}Tc [22] and by magnetic resonance spectroscopy studies [23] in SS patients with leg ulcers as compared with those without.

Mohan et al. described reduced venous refilling time and cutaneous red blood cell flux recovery time after exercise in patients with SS disease with leg ulcers compared to SS and AA patients without ulcers. They proposed incompetence in venous valves around the ankle resulting in venous hypertension and development as well as delayed healing of leg ulcers [24]. The Jamaican cohort study of 183 SS and 137 age- and sex-matched AA controls showed significant association of venous incompetence and leg ulcers in SCD. Contributing factors

http://dx.doi.org/10.5772/64234

were hypothesized to include sluggish circulation with dependency, turbidity and impaired linear flow at venous valves, hypoxia-induced sickling, rheological effects of high white cell counts, and activation of coagulation cascade [25]. Cummings et al. obtained similar results in 2007 with venous incompetence significantly linked to development of leg ulcers in SCD [26]. Minniti et al. used laser speckle contrast imaging (LSCI) and infrared (IR) thermography to study regional blood flow of ulcer beds. The presence of venostasis was confirmed by their finding of increased number of blood vessels with fibrin thrombi and vascular occlusion [16]. Cutaneous hemosiderosis, dermatosclerosis, and prominent superficial veins are frequently found in SCD patients and further support the role of venostasis in the pathogenesis of leg ulcers. Further clinical evidence comes from the fact that ulcers tend to worsen on prolonged standing and improve with bed rest and compression therapy [7, 16, 25, 26].

4.4. Hypercoagulability, thrombosis, and inflammation

Ischemic injury caused by microvascular occlusion by sickle cells initiates a pro-inflammatory and procoagulant cascade that is initiated by the upregulation of RBC integrins. This is

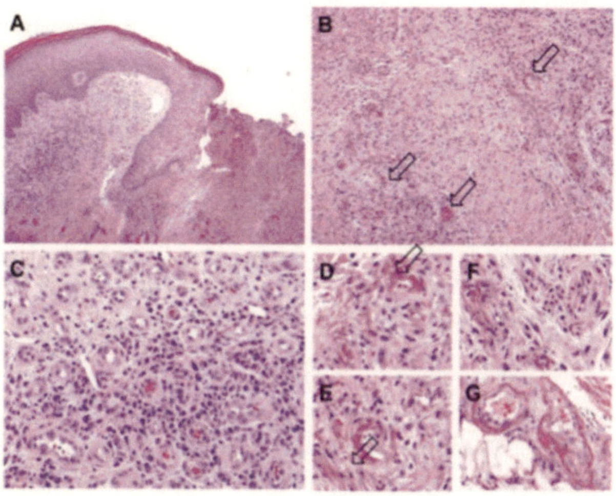

Figure 1. Microscopic analysis of skin biopsies. Evidence of increase in vascularity, chronic inflammation, vasculopathy with blood vessels occlusion, fibrin deposition in the intima, and microthrombi. *Panel A*: Scanning magnification view of the skin punch biopsy showing edge of an ulcer from the right ankle of patient MD. The epidermal changes adjacent to the ulcer are characterized by acanthosis, hyperkeratosis, and attenuated rete ridges. There are increased vascularity and inflammation in the dermis (H&E, 100× original magnification). *Panel B*: The histological changes subjacent to the ulcer bed are characterized by chronically inflamed granulation tissue with vasculopathic changes involving some of the small blood vessels (H&E, 200× original magnification). *Panel C*: High magnification view of the superficial dermal vessels peripheral to the ulcer shows proliferation of thick-walled capillaries and venules, consistent with chronic stasis. There is a lymphoplasmacytic inflammatory infiltrate in the dermis (H&E, 400× original magnification). *Panels D–F*: Very high magnification view of involved vessels subjacent to the ulcer bed reveals eosinophilic fibrin deposits within the vessel wall and partial occlusion of the vascular lumen (H&E, 600× original magnification). *Panel G*: Scanning magnification view of the skin punch biopsy obtained from the right dorsal foot of patient DD shows vasculopathic changes involving a cluster of small blood vessel in the deep dermis (H&E, 40× original magnification). *Panel H*: High magnification view of the involved vessels reveals eosinophilic fibrin deposits within the vessel wall associated with intimal hyperplasia and narrowing of the vascular lumen (H&E, 400× original magnification). Reproduced with permission from Minniti et al. [16].

followed by RBC adhesion to the endothelium, platelet aggregation, and granulocyte recruitment with the release of pro-inflammatory cytokines [27]. The cycle of vessel obstruction and ischemic injury is hence perpetuated, culminating in further end-organ damage. Minniti et al. provided histopathologic evidence of vasculopathy characterized by mural fibrin thrombi causing luminal narrowing and progressive vascular occlusion in small vessels in ulcer beds of SCD patients with leg ulcers [16] (**Figure 1**). Earlier studies also alluded to the procoagulant state in SCD patients including elevated levels of factor VIII and low levels of antithrombin III and prothrombin complexes [28, 29]. SCD ulcer patients have higher levels of soluble ICAM-1 and the key inflammatory cytokine IL-1 beta [30]. Oxidative stress has been shown to play a role in leg ulcer pathogenesis in sickle cell patients, and patients with glutathione S-transferase polymorphism (GSTM1 and GSTT1 null phenotypes) have been shown to have a high risk of developing ulcers [31].

4.5. Autonomic dysfunction

Cardiac output is increased in patients with SS disease, and this may affect the distribution of peripheral blood flow and reflex vascular responses [4]. Normal microcirculation of the lower extremity (LE) is characterized by the venoarteriolar vasoconstriction reflex and the disappearance of vasomotion in the dependent position. It was noted that the venoarteriolar reflex was abolished and vasomotion preserved in the dependent position of the leg in SCD patients [32]. In addition to a high resting perfusion in patients with SCD to maintain normal integrity of cutaneous tissue, there occurs a pronounced vasoconstriction on dependency that exacerbates ischemia and pain, delays healing, and promotes recurrence of leg ulcers [7, 33].

4.6. Bacterial colonization

The role of bacteria in the pathogenesis of leg ulcers is uncertain. Secondary bacterial colonization is inevitable and usually not considered to be clinically significant. Commonly isolated bacteria in African reports include *Staphylococcus aureus*, beta-hemolytic *Streptococci*, *Pseudomonas aeruginosa*, and *Salmonella*. Anaerobes comprised >50% of isolated bacteria in an African series, whereas bacterial flora is predominantly aerobic and polymicrobial in Jamaican reports. Bacterial colonization although unlikely to initiate ulceration may contribute to persistent inflammation of surrounding tissue that results in delayed healing [7]. Baum et al. reported improved healing with topical antibiotics; however, this carries the risks of bacterial resistance, contact sensitization, and disruption of wound moisture balance [7]. Researchers no longer rely solely on culture for identification of bacteria and are utilizing sophisticated sequencing techniques to elucidate the full diversity of microbial communities on the human body [34]. The ulcer skin microbiome, which has been thought only as a commensal on healthy skin, can contribute to delayed healing of ulcers in patients with sickle cell disease by causing excessive activation of both the innate and adaptive immune systems [35]. Emerging data from the study of diabetic wounds shows that the diversity of the skin microbiome correlates with ulcer characteristics [36], and it is likely that similar mechanisms are at play in sickle cell leg ulcers that may explain the variability in their occurrence.

http://dx.doi.org/10.5772/64234

4.7. Genetic factors

Studies suggest that the expression of certain genes may contribute to the development of leg ulcers in SCD; however, the data on genetic associations with leg ulcers remains limited [12].

4.7.1. Candidate gene studies

Ofusu et al. published a study of 9 cases and 29 controls in 1987 suggesting a possible association of HLA-B35 and CW14 alleles, with carriers of both alleles having a 17-fold increased risk of developing leg ulcers. This study was limited due to its small size as well as the identified region being hard to study due to long-range disequilibrium [12, 37].

Another candidate gene study of 243 cases and 516 controls from the CSSCD by Nolan et al. identified associations with single nucleotide polymorphisms (SNPs) in Klotho (promotes endothelial NO production), TEK (involved in angiogenesis), and numerous genes in the transforming growth factor-β (TGF-β)/BMP pathway (modulates angiogenesis and wound healing) [38].

Some of the same SNPs have been reported to be associated with risk of stroke, pulmonary hypertension, and priapism, further supporting the observation that leg ulcers are often associated with other sickle cell sub-phenotypes [12].

4.7.2. Genome-wide association studies

Preliminary results from genome-wide association studies of 219 cases and 1180 controls from the CSSCD identified 30 SNPs associated with leg ulcer. It also showed that a cluster of genes in the MHC III region of chromosome 6 to be highly associated with leg ulcers [12]. A cross-sectional study identified that an SNP in IL-6, a pro-inflammatory cytokine, was associated with higher likelihood of leg ulcer and retinopathy [39].

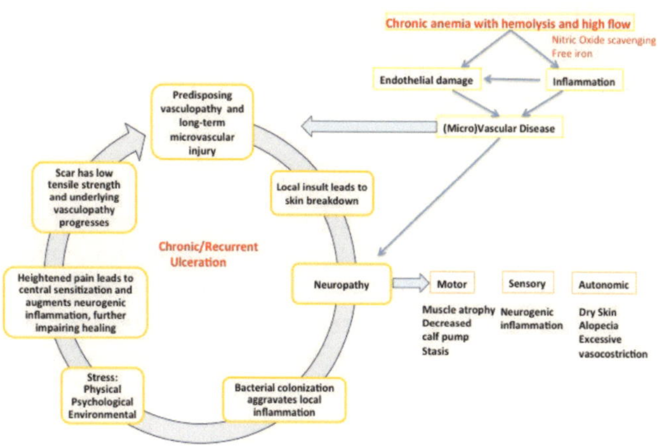

Figure 2. Proposed simplified mechanism of sickle cell ulcer pathogenesis. Reproduced and modified with permission from Minniti et al. [2].

4.7.3. Summary

Minniti and Kato proposed a stepwise, multifactorial model for SCD ulcer pathogenesis (see **Figure 2**) that depicts an interplay between poor nutrition, low BMI, skin injury, inflammation, thrombosis, hemolysis, vasculopathy, neuropathy, and poor socioeconomic status [2, 9, 16, 29, 33, 40].

5. Characteristics of ulceration

5.1. Mode and age of onset

Ulcer onset can be traumatic or spontaneous. Trauma accounts for approximately half the cases, which are incited by relatively insignificant physical damage such as scratches, abrasions, and animal or insect bites. In spontaneous ulcers, there is no history of trauma, but a lesion develops within the dermis often with surrounding induration and hyperpigmentation [7]. Initially, lesions may be covered by an intact epidermis, which then breaks down forming small, deep, and painful ulcers. Spontaneous ulcers are thought to originate from skin infarction. Ulcers occur initially in the second decade of life, around 18–20 years of age. The occurrence of a de novo ulcer in older patients is not common, unless the patient had an ulcer before.

5.2. Site

Leg ulcers most frequently affect the skin around the medial or lateral malleoli but can also occur on the anterior shin or dorsum of the foot [4] and occasionally in the digits [Minniti, personal observation]. The predilection for the malleoli is likely multifactorial due to marginal blood flow at the site, high venous pressure, less subcutaneous fat, thin skin, and lymphedema [12, 27]. This is similar to other hematologic conditions including hereditary spherocytosis, β-thalassemia intermedia, and Felty's syndrome. While medial involvement was more common in two studies [41, 42], there was no such difference found for the medial, lateral, left, or right legs in the CSSCD [6].

5.3. Size

In the CSSCD, ulcers ranged between 0.5, 5–10, 10–15, and >15 cm with equal frequency. Most Jamaican studies had ulcers <10 cm in size. However, large circumferential ulcers portend a poor prognosis due to inevitable damage to vessels and lymphatics [4]. Pain is not related to wound size, and often initial, small ulcers are extremely painful (see **Figure 3**). Purulence, poor granulation tissue, and nonhealing are frequently reported in ulcers >10 cm.

5.4. Appearance

Ulcers in individuals with sickle cell disease usually have a punched appearance with well-defined margins and slightly raised edges. The base comprises granulation tissue, often

http://dx.doi.org/10.5772/64234

covered by yellow slough. More than half of patients will have more than two ulcers that are present at the same time, and multiple small ulcers may then coalesce to form a large ulcer.

Histology of an early leg ulcer shows neovascularization, chronic inflammation, vasculopathy with blood vessel occlusion, fibrin deposition in the intima, and microthrombi [16] (see **Figure 1**). The epidermis adjacent to the ulcer reveals acanthosis, hyperkeratosis, and attenuated rete ridges. There is increased vascularity and inflammation in the dermis with a lymphoplasmacytic inflammatory infiltrate. Chronically inflamed granulation tissue with vasculopathic changes in small blood vessels is found subjacent to the ulcer bed [2, 4].

5.5. Staging and severity of leg ulcers

Ulcers may be staged according to their depth as follows [12]:

Stage 1: Nonblanchable erythema of intact skin, which may present as skin discoloration, warmth, edema, or induration in darker skinned patients.

Stage 2: Partial-thickness skin loss involving epidermis, dermis, or both, presenting as an abrasion, blister, or shallow crater.

Stage 3: Full-thickness skin loss involving damage to or necrosis of subcutaneous tissue that may extend down to, but not through, underlying fascia. The ulcer presents clinically as a deep crater with or without undermining of adjacent tissue.

Stage 4: Full-thickness skin loss with extensive tissue destruction or damage to muscle, bone, or supporting structures (tendon, joint capsule).

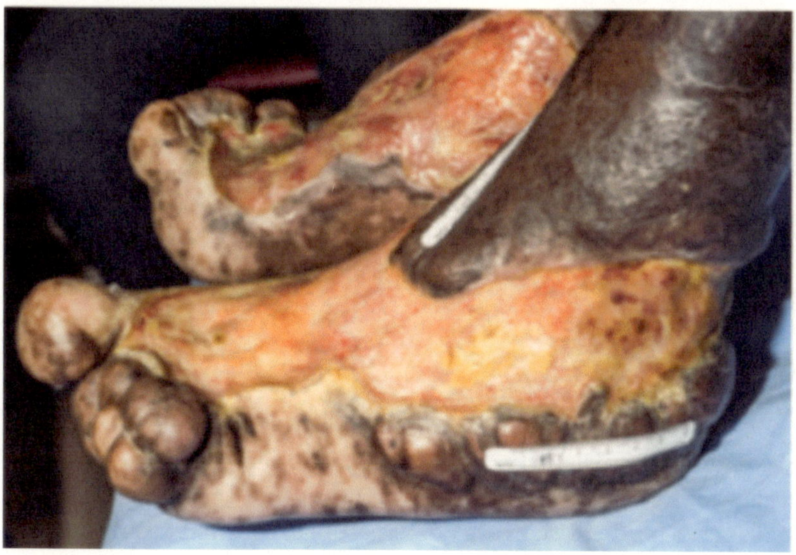

Figure 3. Large sickle cell leg ulcers associated with foot deformities (from author's personal collection).

5.6. Healing and recurrence

Leg ulcers can be classified as acute or chronic although there is no consensus as to a specific length of time to define chronicity. An acute ulcer usually heals in less than a month. Chronic ulcers usually persist for at least 6 months and may last for several years. As described above, ulcer healing is typically slow as the ulcer fills in with granulation tissue, and a bluish epithelium may be seen growing in from the ulcer margin. Healing rates of 3.3–8.1 mm2/d have been reported in SS disease [43, 44] compared with rates of 400 mm2/d in other types of leg ulcer [45]. Even after satisfactory healing, 25–52% recurred in the CSSCD [6]. It is generally accepted, and it is the author's experience that if an ulcer does not heal within 6 months, its chances of ever healing are slim.

Minniti et al. have proposed three patterns of leg ulcers in SCD [2]:

- *One-time ulcer*

One half of patients with SCDs will develop only one ulcer in their lifetime. It usually occurs in the second decade of life, heals within several months, and may recur during periods of stress. These patients often have infrequent pain crisis and have renal and pulmonary complications.

- *Stuttering ulcer*

Twenty-five percent of SCD patients develop small ulcers that recur every 6–12 months for several years.

- *Chronic, recurrent ulcer*

Approximately 1% SCD patients in the United States develop an ulcer that persists for years or even decades and/or ulcers that recur in the same or nearby sites. These patients experience the most disabling chronic pain, unemployment, and depression. Amputation may need to be considered in rare cases to improve quality of life [2, 46]. These patients are often tall, undernourished, and severely anemic with high hemolytic rate. They may have nephropathy, have rare vasoocclusive crisis, and often have trouble with employment, social interaction, and depression.

6. Diagnosis

6.1. History

Leg ulcer pain may be severe, excruciating, penetrating, sharp, and stinging. Patients often report a crescendo of localized pain just before new ulcers develop [2]. About 40–50% of patients recall prior trauma [15, 16], often trivial or pruritus that incites scratching and skin breakdown. The pain is often exacerbated by exposure to cold and to air. The size of the ulcer does not necessarily correlate with intensity of the pain, and very small ulcerations can be extremely painful as well. Most patients require opioids for pain control.

Patients should be specifically asked about history of ulcers, since many patients will report having leg ulcers at some point in their lifetime and may not volunteer the information themselves. History should also document prior ulcer therapies and other complications associated with leg ulcers in SCD including pulmonary hypertension, stroke, priapism, acute chest syndrome [38, 45], lower extremity venous thrombosis, and retinopathy [2].

6.2. Physical examination

Physical exam should assess the wound size with ruler measurement as well as digital photography for greater accuracy [47]. Surrounding skin hypo- or hyperpigmentation, edema, and muscle atrophy should be noted. Although serous discharge and fibrinous material are common, periwound erythema, purulent discharge, and worsening pain may be signs of acute infection. Inguinal lymph nodes are often enlarged, especially during ulcer exacerbations and do not necessarily signify infection. Pulse oximetry as well as blood pressure may be low. Attention should be paid to the nutritional status of patients as many are malnourished [2].

6.3. Lab testing and imaging

Sickle cell individuals with ulcers often have infrequent pain crises and may not have sought regular medical care prior to their presentation. Occasionally, this will be the first time a physician has evaluated them for end-organ diseases. Complete blood count and chemistry panel often reveal markers of severe chronic hemolysis. A significant increase in LDH may be seen [48]. Urinalysis may show microalbuminuria. Serum C-reactive protein (CRP) and erythrocyte sedimentation rate (ESR) are often elevated. Patients may have low levels of antithrombin III, protein C or S, high level of factor VIII, or positive lupus anticoagulant. Wound cultures usually reveal only superficial colonizing bacteria and are rarely helpful. Nutritional status and exercise tolerance with 6-minute walk test (6MWT) should be recorded. When interpreting 6MWT, be aware that shorter distances secondary to physical impairment and pain can be caused by the ulcer. Echocardiography should be obtained to evaluate tricuspid regurgitant velocity to screen for pulmonary hypertension. Imaging studies of bones commonly show demineralization and bone infarcts. MRI should be obtained when osteomyelitis is suspected, but the gold standard for diagnosis remains bone biopsy. Osteomyelitis in the underlying bone is a rare occurrence, but if not diagnosed and treated appropriately will prevent healing [2]. A Doppler ultrasound of the lower extremities should be obtained to rule out the presence of a DVT.

7. Treatment

The management of leg ulcers in SCD involves a multipronged and multidisciplinary approach (see **Table 1**) with involvement of the primary hematologist, wound care specialist, nutritionist, surgeon, and social worker [2]. There remains a paucity of data from randomized controlled trials to guide treatment [49]. Current practice relies mostly on data from small case reports and case series along with expert opinion.

Local therapies	Systemic therapies
Topical antibiotics	Zinc sulfate
Skin grafts (autologous or bioengineered)	Pentoxifylline
RGD peptide matrix	L-Carnitine
Moist wound dressing	Arginine butyrate
Growth factors	Endothelin antagonists: bosentan
Medical honey	Hydroxyurea
Allogeneic keratinocytes	Red blood cell transfusions
Collagen matrix	Systemic antibiotics
Autologous or allogeneic platelet gel	Hyperbaric oxygen therapy
Synthetic heparan sulfate	
Topical sodium nitrite	
Energy-based modalities	
Negative-pressure wound therapy	
Leg compression and leg elevation	
Topical analgesics	
MIST™	
Transdermal oxygen	
Maggots	
Surgical debridement	

Table 1. Treatment modalities that have been used in patients with sickle cell disease and leg ulcers.

7.1. Topial treatment

7.1.1. Role of topical antibiotics

A randomized controlled trial of a topical antibiotic preparation (neomycin, bacitracin, and polymyxin B) in 30 patients with SS disease and chronic leg ulceration showed a significant reduction in ulcer size over a period of 8 weeks in the treatment group compared to the control group [50]. However, this trial had a high risk of bias, and the majority of the literature since 1987 questions the role of bacterial infections in wound pathogenesis [7, 51].

7.1.2. Type of dressing

La Grenade et al. conducted a randomized controlled trial, in 32 patients with SS disease, of Solcoseryl®, DuoDerm®, and conventional therapy, cleaning with Eusol® (a mild antiseptic) followed by wet dressing. Patients were randomized to one of three therapies and monitored for 12 weeks. DuoDerm® (ConvaTec, Greensboro, NC) hydrocolloid dressing was generally unacceptable, and two-thirds of the patients defaulted from this treatment. Solcoseryl®, a deproteinized extract from calf's blood that is meant to improve the tissue utilization of oxygen, increased ulcer healing compared to the controls, but the difference was not significant [52].

7.1.3. RGD peptide matrix

A 2014 Cochrane review described single trial that used an arginine-glycine-aspartic acid matrix (RGD peptide matrix) that achieved noticeable benefit in the treatment of leg ulcers in SCD. The RGD peptide matrix is believed to act as a synthetic extracellular matrix to promote cell migration, keratinocyte layer formation, and wound strengthening. Chronic ulcers treated with RGD peptide matrix had a statistically significant decrease in surface area; however, further studies are needed to corroborate these findings [51, 53].

7.1.4. Moist wound-healing approach

A small retrospective cohort study underscored the efficacy of simple moist wound-healing approach in patients with chronic leg ulcers in SCD who had failed to heal despite treatments such as debridement, split-thickness skin grafts, muscle flaps, wet-to-dry dressings, Unna boots, hydroxyurea, recombinant human erythropoietin, and arginine butyrate. Ultimately, all patients were treated with topical hydrocolloid dressing (DuoDerm CGF by ConvaTec). The eight patients who had not received surgical treatment healed completely within 2–16 months, with only one recurrence at 4 months. Of the ten patients who had previous surgical treatment, six healed without recurrence at 30 months, two experienced recurrence with resolution upon the reapplication of DuoDerm, and two did not heal though did not experience worsening of their ulcers [2, 54].

7.1.5. Growth factors

Several case reports have used topical growth factors as an approach to treating leg ulcers.

Granulocyte-macrophage colony-stimulating factor (GM-CSF) has been used topically and via intracutaneous injection [55, 56]. The cytokine activates macrophages and induces the proliferation of keratinocytes and differentiation of myofibroblasts. While it was shown to be beneficial in wound healing [55–58], high cost, severe vasoocclusive, and even fatal events have discouraged its use [58].

7.1.6. Use of skin substitutes

There are several skin substitutes that are available commercially. One of them, Apligraf® (Organogenesis, Canton, MA), is a bi-layered bioengineered skin substitute that has been approved by the Food and Drug Administration (FDA) since 2000 for the treatment of diabetic foot ulcers and venous leg ulcers (VLUs) that have not responded within 4 weeks to standard of care (SOC) therapy [7]. Apligraf provides both cells and matrix for the nonhealing wound possibly via production of cytokines and growth factors similar to healthy human skin [59]. Several studies confirm the efficacy of Apligraf in treatment of VLUs, and the Society of Vascular Surgery approves the use of Apligraf for the treatment of VLUs [57, 60–62]. The optimal frequency of use is not known, and current clinical practice is for consideration of reapplication after at least 1–3 weeks of observation after initial application [7].

Gordon and Bui examined the efficacy of Apligraf in their study of sickle cell patients with chronic ulcers. Prior to application, they used a 4-week regimen of hydrogel, followed by 1 week of wet-to-dry dressings and 1 week of wet-to-dry dressings plus application of papain-urea debriding ointment (Accuzyme). After 6 weeks, the ulcer was sufficiently optimized for closure. The use of Apligraf resulted in complete healing, and the ulcer remained healed at the last follow-up (33 months) [63].

7.1.7. Allogeneic keratinocytes

Allogeneic keratinocytes have been used to promote the migration of autologous keratinocytes from the peripheral wound bed. Sheets of cells applied twice per month successfully healed a chronic ulcer within 3 months, without recurrence at follow-up at 8 months [64].

7.1.8. Collagen matrix

Two patients with chronic ulcers were treated with Collistat (collagen matrix) every 4 weeks and experienced complete healing by 10 and 12 weeks [65].

7.1.9. Autologous platelet gel

A case series reported the use of an autologous platelet gel to treat leg ulcers in five SCD patients. Autologous platelet-enriched plasma was applied to the wound margins and fibrin matrix clot to the wound bed, before covering with moist saline gauze. A significant local release of platelet-derived growth factors (PDGFs), transforming growth factor-β (TGF-β), and vascular endothelial growth factor (VEGF) was noted. Three of the patients showed a reduction of the leg ulcer area by 85.7–100% within 6–10 weeks. Two patients with ulcers threefold to tenfold larger experienced 20.5% and 35.2% decreases in the leg ulcer area. The authors concluded that the use of autologous platelet gel offers a promising and cost-effective adjuvant treatment for leg ulcers particularly in small ones [66].

7.1.10. Synthetic heparan sulfate

A synthetic, bioengineered heparan sulfate solution, Cacipliq20, was used to treat a nonhealing leg ulcer. The solution is designed to function as a glycosaminoglycan mimetic, potentially restoring the extracellular matrix scaffold and enhancing growth factor recruitment to aid in collagen production and angiogenesis and to restore tissue homeostasis and protect the wound from further damage. The patient in this case report had failed to respond to several treatments, including moist wound therapy, grafting, and energy-based modalities. The patient experienced complete healing after 8 weeks of twice-weekly applications [67].

7.1.11. Topical nitrite therapy

A phase 1 trial of escalating doses of topical sodium nitrite demonstrated a dose-dependent improvement in ulcer healing and decreasing pain at the ulcer site [68]. Application of topical sodium nitrite twice weekly for 4 weeks was associated with a significant increase in peri-wound cutaneous blood flow measured by laser speckle contrast imaging. It appeared to be well tolerated with no grade 3–4 adverse events. The authors concluded that topical sodium nitrite 2% cream is suitable for additional clinical trials in adults with sickle cell anemia to promote healing of leg ulcers.

7.1.12. Topical honey

Topical honey has been utilized mostly in burns and postoperative wounds as a dressing providing a moist healing environment in addition to its natural anti-inflammatory, healing, and antibacterial properties [69]. Its use has also been described in the sickle cell literature for treatment of leg ulcers [15].

7.1.13. Energy-based modalities

Low-frequency, noncontact ultrasound (e.g., MIST®) has been employed to accelerate healing of sickle cell ulcers. It is believed to act via effective removal of bacteria and biofilm along with reduction of chronic inflammation. It also appears to promote the release of NO and growth factors at the cellular level, thereby stimulating vasodilation, angiogenesis, and collagen deposition. This modality can also be used to optimally prepare the wound for grafting [70].

Low-level laser therapy has been reported to result in 80% reduction in the area of a leg ulcer after just five 10–15-minute sessions, leading to a marked improvement in the patient's quality of life [71]. Low-level laser therapy has previously been reported to modulate wound healing by increasing mitotic activity, fibroblast production, collagen synthesis, and angiogenesis and may have a role in the apoptotic processes of wound healing [72].

7.1.14. Negative-pressure wound therapy

Paggiaro et al. examined the use of negative-pressure wound therapy (NPWT) in leg ulcers. Following surgical debridement and before grafting, three wounds were treated by different methods: a rayon and normal saline solution dressing, calcium alginate and gauze, and negative-pressure therapy. Researchers found that the NPWT-treated wounds had a more homogenous surface with better vascularization in comparison with the other two groups. All three wounds received a split-thickness skin graft. While the other wounds experienced subsequent graft failure, the NPWT-treated wound did not, and the ulcers had not recurred by the time of follow-up (11 months) [73]. However, the painful nature of leg ulcers in SCD may be a limiting factor in the use of NPWT.

7.1.15. Role of leg compression

Bed rest has been shown to promote ulcer healing. Patients who underwent 2–3 weeks of strict bed rest experienced complete closure of their wounds within 2–3 months. In addition to reducing venous back pressure and edema around the ankle, patients developed improvement in RBC deformability, possibly secondary to decreased plasma volume, which also aided healing [74]. However, this approach is not very practical.

The use of compression devices has been shown to be effective in reducing edema and improves healing in other types of ulcers. Although there are no prospective studies evaluating their role in sickle cell-related ulcers specifically, these were universally recommended in a survey of care providers treating these patients [75, 76]. The use of Unna boots is highly recommended by practitioners, as the zinc oxide-impregnated boots are useful in treating lower extremity lesions exacerbated by venous insufficiency. Multicomponent compression systems have been shown to be the most effective in reducing edema and improving venous reflux [20].

As venous insufficiency is often seen in SCD patients, the clinical practice guidelines of the Society for Vascular Surgery and the American Venous Forum are also applicable for treatment of leg ulcers in sickle cell with venous disease. The guidelines recommend compression therapy to increase VLU healing and to decrease the risk of ulcer recurrence. The use of multicomponent compression bandages is encouraged over single-component bandages [62].

7.1.16. Topical analgesics

Topical opioids have been employed by dissolving oxycodone and meperidine tablets in water and applying them locally to provide topical analgesia. Total pain relief was reported likely because of modification of peripheral opioid receptors [77]. While this treatment is not commercially available, these findings warrant further research. Data in mice with SCD show that topical opioids such as morphine and fentanyl not only treat pain but also hasten healing [78]. Inhibition of neurogenic inflammation by topical opioids is advocated as the mechanism of action. A study of nitroglycerin applied above the ulcer demonstrated a significant reduction in ulcer-associated pain, with increased ability to be able to manipulate the ulcer. Pain in fact is often so intense that bedside debridement is not possible, thus ultimately delaying ulcer healing.

7.1.17. Hyperbaric oxygen therapy

Hyperbaric oxygen therapy and its potential benefit in treatment of vasoocclusive crises and leg ulcers have been described in several case reports [76, 79, 80]. However, paucity of research, potential adverse side effects, lack of treatment protocols, limited availability, and economic factors restrict its use [7].

7.1.18. Transdermal continuous oxygen therapy

A case report described the use of transdermal continuous oxygen therapy using a portable device that delivers oxygen directly to the wound site. Two LE wounds received treatment for 15 weeks, and the authors noted that both healed without recurrence in the 42-month follow-up. The authors urge further studies utilizing this form of therapy [81].

7.1.19. Maggot therapy

Maggot therapy has had mixed results when studied in other types of ulcers. One study showed reduced time to debridement, but increased ulcer pain and no improvement in rate of healing [82]. In diabetic ulcers, maggot debridement provided outcomes equal to conventional surgical treatment [83]. At the NIH Clinical Center, Medical Maggots™ (disinfected *Phaenicia sericata* larvae; http://www.monarchlabs.com) has been utilized. Four patients with sickle cell disease received this therapy with mixed results. There was temporary improvement in ulcer appearance, quickly followed by relapse and unclear long-term benefit [7, 16]. Pain has also been a limiting factor for the use of medicinal maggots in this population, and an opioid PCA may be required. This modality is currently reserved only for patients who are poor candidates for surgical debridement [76].

7.2. Systemic treatment

7.2.1. Zinc supplementation

Zinc supplementation has long been believed to promote healing in chronic wounds accompanied by serum zinc deficiency [84]. A placebo-controlled trial reported that 220 mg of zinc sulfate administered orally three times a day significantly improved the healing of leg ulcers in sickle cell patients [43]. However, no further studies have been undertaken to confirm these results, and the results are hard to interpret as neither the length of supplementation with oral zinc or statistical analysis was provided [7].

7.2.2. Pentoxifylline

Pentoxifylline improves RBC and leukocyte deformability potentially decreasing blood viscosity, platelet aggregation, thrombus formation, and plasma fibrinogen levels [7]. This increases microcirculatory flow and tissue oxygenation making it a good modality for treatment of leg ulcers in sickle cell patients. One case report presented that 400 mg of oral pentoxifylline three times a day helped completely heal a leg ulcer in a sickle cell patient within 3 months [85]. In nine RCTs involving 572 patients, pentoxifylline combined with compression bandages improved ulcer healing [86, 87]. The 2014 clinical practice guidelines of the Society for Vascular Surgery and the American Venous Forum recommend the use of pentoxifylline for treatment of long-standing or large VLUs [62]. As venous insufficiency is often present in SCD patients, pentoxifylline may be a good treatment option for them.

7.2.3. L-Carnitine

Systemic therapy of leg ulcers in SCD with L-carnitine has been reported in only one randomized controlled trial and one case study. Data suggests that oral carnitine alters cellular chemistry to favor more efficient oxidative metabolism despite reduced levels of available tissue oxygen. The studies were limited by the fact that transfusion therapy was given concomitantly making it difficult to draw conclusions on the effect of L-carnitine alone [88, 89].

7.2.4. Arginine butyrate

Arginine stimulates collagen production, improves immune function, and prevents vascular restenosis. Butyrate can stimulate PDGF production and downregulate inflammatory cytokines and enzymes that slow wound healing like TGF-β, tumor necrosis factor-alpha (TNF-α), and matrix metalloproteinases [90]. A phase II controlled trial showed significant improvement in ulcer healing in the treatment arm after 3 months (78% vs. 24% in controls, $P < 0.001$). A limitation to this approach is the requirement of an IV catheter. Larger studies are needed to validate this potentially effective treatment modality.

7.2.5. Bosentan

A case report described complete healing of a leg ulcer in a patient with concomitant pulmonary hypertension. The ulcer had previously failed multiple therapies. The researchers attributed the healing to the blockade of the endothelin-1 receptor and vasodilation in the patient with likely decreased NO availability [91]. However, concomitant transfusion therapy might have confounded the observations.

7.2.6. Hydroxyurea

The role of hydroxyurea (HU) in the development or in the treatment of leg ulcers in sickle cell patients is not clear with conflicting data to date [92–97]. HU increases fetal hemoglobin levels, decreasing the intracellular polymerization of HbS, the incidence of painful crises, and the need for transfusions in SCD patients [98]. Moreover, HU is a known NO donor and decreases WBC counts [99]. These effects should theoretically decrease the incidence of leg ulcers. However, leg ulcers observed in patients with chronic myeloproliferative disorders on HU often resolved several months after the discontinuation of this medication [100–103]. A case report suggested that HU causes an acquired blood dyscrasia that increases the risk of ulceration [104]. Other multicenter studies have seen no evidence of an association between hydroxyurea and leg ulceration [76]. There are no prospective trials that specifically address the effects of HU use on leg ulcer healing in the sickle cell population, and therefore, we discourage reflexively stopping HU in patients with leg ulcers who may be benefiting from it for other SCD complications like frequent pain crisis and acute chest syndrome.

7.2.7. Blood transfusions

There are no prospective RCTs addressing the role of blood transfusions for treatment of leg ulcers in sickle cell patients. Transfusions increase the oxygen delivery to tissues by increasing total hemoglobin and decreasing the HbS concentration [76]. Some authors suggest target hemoglobin of 10 g/dl for successful surgical treatment, although a level between 8 and 9 g/dl may be more realistic and adequate for wound healing [20]. However, transfusions come with their own risks including iron overload, alloimmunization, and risk of transfusion reactions and infections. In recent clinical trials and in our clinical practice, we note that there are patients with chronic wounds who are treated with chronic transfusions, either for other indications or because of the ulcer, with no apparent benefit in decreasing the length of ulceration. The author recommends supporting skin grafts with transfusions for a limited time period, 4–6 months, in order to maximize graft success and decrease SCD-related complications.

7.2.8. Antibiotics

As discussed above, bacterial colonization of leg ulcers appears to be common but of uncertain clinical significance. However, colonization may lead to infection or a chronic inflammation, and systemic antimicrobials with anti-inflammatory properties like doxycycline, clindamycin, and metronidazole may improve ulcer healing along with adequate debridement [20].

7.3. Surgical treatment

Surgical treatments for leg ulcers often have high rates of failure and recurrence [7]. Scar tissue becomes denser and less vascular with each subsequent graft, shortening the ulcer-free interval between recurrences [7, 105]. Microsurgical free flap transfers are popular since they include their own blood supply, which is a favorable attribute in these poorly vascular regions [106]. However, they are often limited by complications like thrombi, microemboli, and infection ultimately requiring debridement and split-thickness skin grafts [7].

Aiming to reduce the incidence of graft failure, some experts recommend perioperative and even chronic lifelong transfusions to decrease HbS levels to <30% [106, 107]. Some surgeons support the use of anticoagulation with heparin and/or aspirin, antibiotics, and the rinsing of flaps with heparinized solution prior to attachment [106]. Larger RCTs are required to address these important issues.

8. Nutrition

Nutrition is known to be important in the management of ulcers, and patients should be assessed for nutritional deficiencies and treated appropriately. Zinc deficiency has been shown to be prevalent in SCD patients. The current recommendation is 220 mg of zinc sulfate thrice a day. Serum zinc levels should be remeasured 2 and 4 weeks after initiation of supplementation and therapy discontinued if levels normalize [7, 108]. Others and we have noted that the BMI of SCD patients with recurrent ulcers is lower than patients without leg ulcers [12, Ballas, unpublished data]. We have also noted that several of the most affected patients seem to be almost anorexic, and we speculate that the high state of inflammation that their ulcer causes could be responsible for the presence of TNF-alpha, similar to cancer patients.

9. Thrombosis

Assessment and treatment of occult deep venous thrombosis are essential. Anticoagulation may be necessary to treat known hypercoagulable disorder.

10. Pain control

The pain from leg ulcers in patients with sickle cell disease can be very severe and debilitating leading many patients to require therapy with chronic opioids. Moreover, severe pain may interfere with local therapies and further hinder healing. Nonsteroidal anti-inflammatory agents are often inadequate for optimal pain control. Currently, there are no guidelines recommending topical analgesics in this patient population, but provocative data in sickle cell mice suggest that the application of topical opioids can treat both the pain and increase healing rates [78] although they should be explored in future studies. Some experts recommend regional nerve blocks with good results in pain control and also for secondary vasodilation via reduction of stress-related catecholamine release. This approach is limited by the need for an indwelling catheter, the need for frequent clinic visit for pump refills, and the antecedent risks of infection [7].

11. Wound care

Leg ulcers in SCD are often resistant to treatment and have a high rate of recurrence, making optimizing the wound bed a cornerstone of therapy. The ulcer must be adequately debrided to remove biofilm and necrotic, nonviable tissue from the base and edge of the wound in order to begin the healing process [109]. Various types of debridement techniques may be used including autolytic, enzymatic, biological, mechanical, and sharp, depending on its suitability to the patient, the type of wound, its location, and the extent of debridement required [110]. Regular weekly chronic debridements may be needed for improved healing although the optimal frequency is not established [111]. Sharp debridement can be very painful and may only be possible with some form of analgesia, topical, injectable, or general anesthesia.

Although a multitude of dressings exist, the most important principle of wound care remains maintenance of a moist healing environment. Energy-based modalities like low-frequency, noncontact ultrasound, electrical stimulation, and ultraviolet-C light are good adjuvant treatment options for wounds that fail to respond positively to standard of care methods [7].

The use of RGD peptide matrix, allogeneic keratinocytes, and autologous platelet gel are promising treatments for resistant ulcers, although more research is needed. These are not widely available as yet.

12. Venous insufficiency

Compression therapy is encouraged for the management and prevention of edema, especially if venous insufficiency is present. Compression stockings are useful for prevention, while multilayer compression bandaging is recommended for treatment. An alternative is using a self-applicable and adjustable short-stretch Velcro band [62].

The Society for Vascular Surgery and the American Venous Forum strongly advocate pentoxifylline for treatment of long-standing or large VLUs since venous insufficiency is frequently found in these patients. Apligraf is recommended for ulcers not responding to standard of care therapies within 4–6 weeks.

Minimally, invasive ablation of superficial axial and perforator vein reflux in patients with active venous insufficiency and patent deep venous system is a relatively safe procedure and leads to faster healing and decreased ulcer recurrence when combined with compression therapy [112]. This also underscores prompt referral to a vascular specialist for evaluation and management of leg ulcers in SCD.

13. Antibiotic therapy

The IDSA guidelines do not recommend treating an uninfected wound with antimicrobials since there is no evidence that this prevents infection or improves ulcer healing [113]. When there are clinical signs of infection, post-debridement deep soft tissue or bone biopsy should be sent for culture. Superficial wound cultures are less reliable than tissue biopsies and should be avoided [114]. Hospitalized patients with more severe infections and signs of cellulitis and/or osteomyelitis typically receive intravenous antibiotic therapy at least initially. Finally, topical antibiotics do not significantly affect leg ulcers healing [7]. Further studies are needed to explore the immunomodulatory and anti-inflammatory actions of tetracyclines on ulcer healing.

14. Prevention

A previous history of leg ulcer is the greatest predictor of developing another leg ulcer in patients with sickle cell disease, increasing the risk up to 23-fold in one study [84]. While spontaneous ulcers are unpredictable, traumatic ulcers may be preventable. Encouraging patients to regularly check their skin for signs of early ulcers and preventing local trauma by wearing properly fitting shoes and protecting themselves from insect bites may decrease the risk of developing leg ulcers. Wearing appropriately sized above-the-knee compression stockings can reduce edema and prevent new and recurrent ulcers [16].

15. Complications

15.1. Association of leg ulcers to pulmonary hypertension in adults with SCD

Evidence suggests that SCD patients with hyper-hemolysis phenotype (characterized by severe anemia and markers of hemolysis like high LDH) are at risk for leg ulcers as well as pulmonary hypertension, priapism, and renal disease [115]. Studies have shown that leg ulcers are more common in SCD patients with pulmonary hypertension [12, 116, 117]. Experts recommend that patients with HbS with leg ulcers should be screened for pulmonary hypertension.

This epidemiological relationship between leg ulcers and pulmonary hypertension supports a common pathophysiologic mechanism. Sickle cell patients with leg ulcers have been shown to have higher rates of mortality that those without leg ulcers and are regarded as a marker of disease severity in sickle cell patients [9].

15.2. Local effects

Subcutaneous fibrosis impairing venous and lymphatic drainage may occur and can be severe enough to cause an equinus deformity [4] (**Figure 4**). Osteomyelitis is exceedingly rare but has

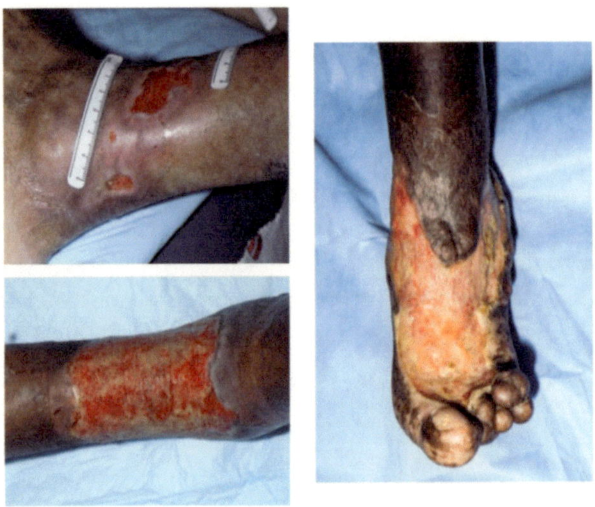

Figure 4. Leg ulcers of varying sizes (from author's personal collection).

http://dx.doi.org/10.5772/64234

been observed on occasion. Acute ankle arthritis complicates some cases of spontaneous leg ulceration, possibly as a result of associated ischemic synovial damage [118]. It resolves spontaneously with improvement of the leg ulcer.

15.3. Social and psychological effects

Leg ulcers can have a profound impact on patients' psychological well-being. Patients often have social withdrawal at school and work places. They often suffer from depression, which may impair their ability to take care of their ulcers adequately and seek medical attention [4].

16. Summary

In summary, sickle cell leg ulcers are a disabling complication of sickle cell disease, and despite being widely described in the medical literature, there remains a paucity of large randomized controlled data pertaining to their treatment. Current recommendations include a multifaceted approach utilizing a combination of topical, systemic, and surgical techniques. We describe a simplified algorithm to aid management of these complex patients (**Figure 5**). While a multidisciplinary team is essential, it is important to retain primary responsibility of the patient as hematologists, optimizing the health of the patient and facilitating plans of care made by various specialties. As we begin to understand more about the complex pathophysiology of these chronic wounds, more research is needed targeting these identified pathways to improve ulcer healing and prevent recurrence.

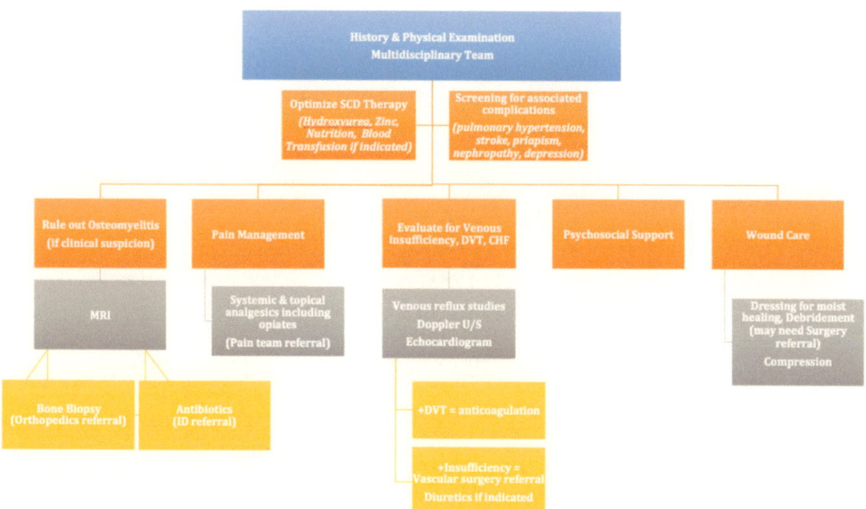

Figure 5. Approach to the management of patients with SCD and wounds.

Author details

Aditi P. Singh and Caterina P. Minniti*

*Address all correspondence to: cminniti@montefiore.org

Department of Hematology-Oncology, Montefiore Medical Center, Bronx, New York, USA

References

[1] Herrick, J. Peculiar elongated and sickle-shaped red blood corpuscles in a case of severe anemia. Arch Intern Med. 1910;6:517–21.

[2] Minniti CP, Kato GJ. Critical reviews: how we treat sickle cell patients with leg ulcers. Am J Hematol. 2016;91(1):22–30. doi: 10.1002/ajh.24134.

[3] Cummer CL, LaRocco CG. Ulcers on the legs in sickle cell anemia. Arch Dermatol Syphilol. 1939;40:459–60.

[4] Serjeant GR, Serjeant BE, Mohan JS, Clare A. Leg ulceration in sickle cell disease: medieval medicine in a modern world. Hematol Oncol Clin North Am. 2005;19:943–9ix.

[5] Perrine RP, Pembrey ME, John P, et al. Natural history of sickle cell anemia in Saudi Arabs. A study of 270 subjects. Ann Intern Med. 1978;88:1–6.

[6] Koshy M, Entsuah R, Koranda A, et al. Leg ulcers in patients with sickle cell disease. Blood. 1989;74:1403–8.

[7] Altman IA, Kleinfelder RE, Quigley JG, Ennis WJ, Minniti CP. A treatment algorithm to identify therapeutic approaches for leg ulcers in patients with sickle cell disease. Int Wound J. 2015. doi: 10.1111/iwj.12522.

[8] Serjeant GR, Higgs DR, Hambleton IR. Elderly survivors with homozygous sickle cell disease. N Engl J Med. 2007;356(6):642–3.

[9] Minniti CP, Taylor JGt, Hildesheim M, et al. Laboratory and echocardiography markers in sickle cell patients with leg ulcers. Am J Hematol. 2011;86:705–8.

[10] Abbade LP, Lastoria S. Venous ulcer: epidemiology, physiopathology, diagnosis and treatment. Int J Dermatol. 2005;44:449–56.

[11] Gabriel A, Przybylski J. Sickle-cell anemia: a look at global haplotype distribution. Nat Educ. 2010;3(3):2.

[12] Minniti CP, Eckman J, Sebastiani P, et al. Leg ulcers in sickle cell disease. Am J Hematol. 2010;85:831–3.

[13] Padmos MA, Roberts GT, Sackey K, et al. Two different forms of homozygous sickle cell disease occur in Saudi Arabia. Br J Haematol. 1991;79:93–8.

[14] Kar BC, Satapathy RK, Kulozik AE, et al. Sickle cell disease in Orissa State, India. Lancet 1986;ii:1198–201.

[15] Ankra-Badu GA. Sickle cell leg ulcers in Ghana. East Afr Med J. 1992;69:366–9.

[16] Minniti CP, Delaney KM, Gorbach AM, et al. Vasculopathy, inflammation, and blood flow in leg ulcers of patients with sickle cell anemia. Am J Hematol. 2014;89:1–6. doi: 10.1002/ajh.23571.

[17] Connes P, Lamarre Y, Hardy-Dessources M-D, et al. Decreased hematocrit-to-viscosity ratio and increased lactate dehydrogenase level in patients with sickle cell anemia and recurrent leg ulcers. PLoS One 2013;8(11):e79680. doi: 10.1371/journal.pone.0079680.

[18] Bartolucci P, Brugnara C, Teixeira-Pinto A, et al. Erythrocyte density in sickle cell syndromes is associated with specific clinical manifestations and hemolysis. Blood 2012;120(15):3136–41. doi: 10.1182/blood-2012-04-424184. Epub 2012 Aug 23.

[19] Reiter CD, Wang X, Tanus-Santos JE, et al. Cell-free hemoglobin limits nitric oxide bioavailability in sickle-cell disease. Nat Med. 2002;8:1383–9.

[20] Ladizinski B, Bazakas A, Mistry N, et al. Sickle cell disease and leg ulcers. Adv Skin Wound Care. 2012;25:420–8. doi: 10.1097/01.ASW.0000419408.37323.0c.

[21] Billett HH, Patel Y, Rivers SP. Venous insufficiency is not the cause of leg ulcers in sickle cell disease. Am J Hematol. 1991;37:133–4.

[22] Saad STO, Zago MA. Leg ulceration and abnormalities of calf blood flow in sickle-cell anemia. Eur J Haematol. 1992;46:188–90.

[23] Norris SL, Gober JR, Haywood J, et al. Altered muscle metabolism shown by magnetic resonance spectroscopy in sickle cell disease with leg ulcers. Magn Reson Imaging 1993;11:119–23.

[24] Mohan JS, Vigilance JE, Marshall JM, et al. Abnormal venous function in patients with homozygous sickle cell (SS) disease and chronic leg ulcers. Clin Sci (Lond). 2000;98:667–72.

[25] Clare A, FitzHenley M, Harris J, Hambleton I, Serjeant GR. Chronic leg ulceration in homozygous sickle cell disease: the role of venous incompetence. Br J Haematol. 2002;119:567–71.

[26] Cumming V, King L, Fraser R, Serjeant G, Reid M. Venous incompetence, poverty and lactate dehydrogenase in Jamaica are important predictors of leg ulceration in sickle cell anaemia. Br J Haematol. 2008;142:119–25. doi: 10.1111/j.1365-2141.2008.07115.x.

[27] Trent JT, Kirsner RS. Leg ulcers in sickle cell disease. Adv Skin Wound Care 2004;17:410–6.

[28] Nsiri B, Gritli N, Bayoudh F, et al. Abnormalities of coagulation and fibrinolysis in homozygous sickle cell disease. Hematol Cell Ther. 1996;38:279–84.

[29] Cacciola E, Giustolisi R, Musso R, Longo A. Antithrombin III concentrate for treatment of chronic leg ulcers in sickle cell-beta thalassemia: a pilot study [Research Support, Non-U.S. Gov't]. Ann Intern Med. 1989;111:534–6.

[30] Bowers AS, Reid HL, Greenidge A, et al. Blood viscosity and the expression of inflammatory and adhesion markers in homozygous sickle cell disease subjects with chronic leg ulcers. PloS One 2013;8:e68929.

[31] de Oliveira Filho RA, Silva GJ, de Farias Domingos I, et al. Association between the genetic polymorphisms of glutathione S-transferase (GSTM1 and GSTT1) and the clinical manifestations in sickle cell anemia. Blood Cell Mol Dis. 2013;51:76–9.

[32] Gniadecka M, Gniadecka R, Serup J, et al. Microvascular reactions to postural changes in patients with sickle cell anaemia. Acta Derm Venereol. 1994;74:191–3.

[33] Mohan JS, Marshall JM, Reid HL, et al. Postural vasoconstriction and leg ulceration in homozygous sickle cell disease. Clin Sci (Lond). 1997;92:153–8.

[34] Grice EA, Kong HH, Conlan S, et al. Topographical and temporal diversity of the human skin microbiome. Science 2009;324(5931):1190–2. doi: 10.1126/science.1171700.

[35] Grice EA, Segre JA. Interaction of microbiome and the innate immune response in chronic wounds. Adv Exp Med Biol. 2012;946:55–68. doi:10.1007/978-1-4614-0106-3_4.

[36] Gardner SE, Hillis SL, Heilmann K, Segre JA, Grice EA. The Neuropathic diabetic foot ulcer microbiome is associated with clinical factors. Diabetes 2013;62(3):923–30. doi: 10.2337/db12-0771.

[37] Ofosu MD, Castro O, Alarif L. Sickle cell leg ulcers are associated with HLA- B35 and Cw4. Arch Dermatol. 1987;123:482–4.

[38] Nolan VG, Adewoye A, Baldwin C, et al. Sickle cell leg ulcers: associations with haemolysis and SNPs in Klotho, TEK and genes of the TGF-beta/BMP pathway. Br J Haematol. 2006;133:570–8.

[39] Vicari P, Adegoke SA, Mazzotti DR, et al. Interleukin-1β and interleukin-6 gene polymorphisms are associated with manifestations of sickle cell anemia. Blood Cells Mol Dis. 2015;54(3):244–9. doi: 10.1016/j.bcmd.2014.12.004. Epub 2014 Dec 26.

[40] Kato GJ, McGowan V, Machado RF, et al. Lactate dehydrogenase as a biomarker of hemolysis-associated nitric oxide resistance, priapism, leg ulceration, pulmonary hypertension, and death in patients with sickle cell disease. Blood 2006;107:2279–85.

[41] Serjeant GR. Leg ulceration in sickle cell anemia. Arch Intern Med. 1974;133:690–4.

[42] Sawhney H, Weedon J, Gillette P, et al. Predilection of haemolytic anemia-associated leg ulcers for the medial malleolus. Vasa. 2002;31:191–3.

[43] Serjeant GR, Galloway RE, Gueri M. Oral zinc sulphate in sickle-cell ulcers. Lancet 1970;2:891–3.

[44] Margraf HW, Covey TH. A trial of silver-zinc-allantoinate in the treatment of leg ulcers. Arch Surg. 1977;112:699–704.

[45] Halabi-Tawil M, Lionnet F, Girot R, et al. Sickle cell leg ulcers: a frequently disabling complication and a marker of severity. Br J Dermatol. 2008;158:339–44.

[46] Queiroz AM, Campos J, Lobo C, et al. Leg amputation for an extensive, severe and intrac-table sickle cell anemia ulcer in a Brazilian patient. Hemoglobin 2014;38:95–8.

[47] Bilgin M, Gunes UY. A comparison of 3 wound measurement techniques: effects of pressure ulcer size and shape. J Wound Ostomy Continence Nurs. 2013;40:590–3.

[48] Mikobi TM, Lukusa Tshilobo P, Aloni MN, et al. Correlation between the lactate dehydrogenase levels with laboratory variables in the clinical severity of sickle cell anemia in congolese patients. PLoS One. 2015;10(5):e0123568. doi: 10.1371/journal.pone.0123568. eCollection 2015.

[49] Alavi A, Kirsner RS. Hemoglobinopathies and leg ulcers. Int J Low Extrem Wounds. 2015;14(3):213–6. doi: 10.1177/1534734615600069.

[50] Baum KF, MacFarlane DE, Maude GH, Serjeant GR. Topical antibiotics in chronic sickle cell leg ulcers. Trans R Soc Trop Med Hyg. 1987;81:847–9.

[51] Martí-Carvajal AJ, Knight-Madden JM, Martinez-Zapata MJ. Interventions for treating leg ulcers in people with sickle cell disease [Research Support, Non-U.S. Gov't Review]. Cochrane Database Syst Rev. 2014;12:CD008394. doi: 10.1002/14651858.CD008394.pub3.

[52] La Grenade L, Thomas PW, Serjeant GR. A randomized controlled trial of solcoseryl and duoderm in chronic sickle-cell ulcers. West Indian Med J. 1993;42:121–3.

[53] Wethers DL, Ramirez GM, Koshy M, et al. Accelerated healing of chronic sickle-cell leg ulcers treated with RGD peptide matrix. RGD Study Group. Blood. 1994;84:1775–9.

[54] Cackovic M, Chung C, Bolton LL, Kerstein MD. Leg ulceration in the sickle cell patient. J Am Coll Surg. 1998;187:307–9.

[55] Alikhan MA, Carter G, Mehta P. Topical GM-CSF hastens healing of leg ulcers in sickle cell disease. Am J Hematol. 2004;76:192. doi: 10.1002/ajh.20063.

[56] Pieters RC, Rojer RA, Saleh AW, Saleh AE, Duits AJ. Molgramostim to treat SS-sickle cell leg ulcers. Lancet. 1995;345:528.

[57] Falanga V, Margolis D, Alvarez O, et al. Rapid healing of venous ulcers and lack of clinical rejection with an allogeneic cultured human skin equivalent. Human Skin Equivalent Investigators Group. [Clinical Trial Multicenter Study Randomized Controlled Trial Research Support, Non-U.S. Gov't]. Arch Dermatol. 1998;134:293–300.

[58] Fitzhugh CD, Hsieh MM, Bolan CD, Saenz C, Tisdale JF. Granulocyte colony-stimulating factor (G-CSF) administration in individuals with sickle cell disease: time for a moratorium? Cytotherapy 2009;11:464–71.

[59] Zaulyanov L, Kirsner RS. A review of a bi-layered living cell treatment (Apligraf) in the treatment of venous leg ulcers and diabetic foot ulcers. Clin Interv Aging 2007;2(1): 93–8.

[60] Falanga V, Sabolinski M. A bilayered living skin construct (APLIGRAF) accelerates complete closure of hard-to-heal venous ulcers [Clinical Trial Multicenter Study Randomized Controlled Trial Research Support, Non-U.S. Gov't Research Support, U.S. Gov't, P.H.S.]. Wound Repair Reg. 1999;7:201–7.

[61] Hankin CS, Knispel J, Lopes M, Bronstone A, Maus E. Clinical and cost efficacy of advanced wound care matrices for venous ulcers [Review]. J Manag Care Pharm. 2012;18:375–84.

[62] O'Donnell TF Jr, Passman MA, Marston WA, et al. Management of venous leg ulcers: clinical practice guidelines of the Society for vascular surgery (R) and the American Venous Forum [Practice Guideline Review]. J Vasc Surg. 2014;60(2 Suppl.):3S–59. doi: 10.1016/j.jvs.2014.04.049.

[63] Gordon S, Bui A. Human skin equivalent in the treatment of chronic leg ulcers in sickle cell disease patients. J Am Podiatr Med Assoc. 2003;93:240–1.

[64] Amini-Adle M, Auxenfants C, Allombert-Blaise C, et al. Rapid healing of long-lasting sickle cell leg ulcer treated with allogeneic keratinocytes. J Eur Acad Dermatol Venereol. 2007;21:707–8. doi: 10.1111/j.1468-3083.2006.02003.x.

[65] Reindorf CA, Walker-Jones D, Adekile AD, Lawal O, Oluwole SF. Rapid healing of sickle cell leg ulcers treated with collagen dressing. J Natl Med Assoc. 1989;81:866–8.

[66] Gilli SC, doValleOliveira SA, Saad ST. Autologous platelet gel: five cases illustrating use on sickle cell disease ulcers. Int J Low Extrem Wounds. 2014;13:120–6. doi: 10.1177/1534734614534979.

[67] Hayek S, Dibo S, Baroud J, Ibrahim A, Barritault D. Refractory sickle cell leg ulcer: is heparan sulphate a new hope? Int Wound J. 2014;13: 35-8 doi: 10.1111/iwj.12217.

[68] Minniti CP, Gorbach AM, Xu D, et al. Topical sodium nitrite for chronic leg ulcers in patients with sickle cell anaemia: a phase 1 dose-finding safety and tolerability trial. Lancet Haematol. 2014;1:e95–103.

[69] Jull AB, Cullum N, Dumville JC, et al. Honey as a topical treatment for wounds. Cochrane Database Syst Rev. 2015;3:CD005083. doi: 10.1002/14651858.CD005083.pub4.

[70] Breuing KH, Bayer L, Neuwalder J, Orgill DP. Early experience using low-frequency ultrasound in chronic wounds. Ann Plast Surg. 2005;55:183–7.

[71] Bonini-Domingos CR, Valente FM. Low-level laser therapy of leg ulcer in sickle cell anemia. Rev Bras Hematol Hemoter. 2012;34:65–6. doi: 10.5581/1516-8484.20120018.

[72] Rocha Junior AM, Vieira BJ, de Andrade LC, Aarestrup FM. Low-level laser therapy increases transforming growth factor-beta2 expression and induces apoptosis of epithelial cells during the tis- sue repair process. Photomed Laser Surg. 2009;27:303–7. doi: 10.1089/pho.2008.2277.

[73] Oliveira Paggiaro A, Fernandes de Carvalho V, Hencklain Fonseca GH, Doi A, Castro Ferreira M. Negative pressure therapy for complex wounds in patients with sickle-cell disease: a case study. Ostomy Wound Manage. 2010;56:62–7.

[74] Keidan AJ, Stuart J. Rheological effects of bed rest in sickle cell disease. J Clin Pathol. 1987;40:1187–8.

[75] O'Meara S, Cullum NA, Nelson EA. Compression for venous leg ulcers. Cochrane Database Syst Rev. 2009;(1):CD000265. PubMed: 19160178

[76] Delaney KM, Axelrod KC, Buscetta A, et al. Leg ulcers in sickle cell disease: current patterns and practices. Hemoglobin 2013;37:325–32. doi: 10.3109/03630269.2013.789968.

[77] Ballas SK. Treatment of painful sickle cell leg ulcers with topical opioids. Blood 2002;99:1096.

[78] Gupta M, Poonawala T, Farooqui M, Ericson ME, Gupta K. Topical fentanyl stimulates healing of ischemic wounds in diabetic rats. J Diabetes 2015;7(4):573–83. doi: 10.1111/1753-0407.12223.

[79] Stirnemann J, Letellier E, Aras N, et al. Hyperbaric oxygen therapy for vaso-occlusive crises in nine patients with sickle-cell disease [Evaluation Studies]. Diving Hyperb Med. 2012;42:82–4.

[80] Reynolds JD. Painful sickle cell crisis. Successful treatment with hyperbaric oxygen therapy. JAMA 1971;216:1977–8.

[81] Massenburg BB, Himel HN. Healing of chronic sickle cell disease-associated foot and ankle wounds using transdermal continuous oxygen therapy. J Wound Care 2016;25(Suppl. 2):S23–7. doi: 10.12968/jowc.2016.25.Sup2.S23.

[82] Dumville JC, Worthy G, Bland JM, et al. Larval therapy for leg ulcers (VenUS II): randomised controlled trial. BMJ 2009;338:b773. PubMed: 19304577

[83] Paul AG, Ahmad NW, Lee HL, et al. Maggot debridement therapy with Lucilia cuprina: a comparison with conventional debridement in diabetic foot ulcers. Int Wound J. 2009;6(1):39–46. PubMed: 19291114

[84] Eckman JR. Leg ulcers in sickle cell disease. Hematol Oncol Clin North Am. 1996;10:1333–44.

[85] Frost ML, Treadwell P. Treatment of sickle cell leg ulcers with pentoxifylline. Int J Dermatol. 1990;29:375–6.

[86] Jull A, Arroll B, Parag V, Waters J. Pentoxifylline for treating venous leg ulcers. Cochrane Database Syst Rev. 2007; Issue 3 :CD001733. doi: 10.1002/14651858.CD001733.pub2.

[87] Sullivan GW, Carper HT, Novick WJ Jr, Mandell GL. Inhibition of the inflammatory action of interleukin-1 and tumor necrosis factor (alpha) on neutrophil function by pentoxifylline [Research Support, Non-U.S. Gov't Research Support, U.S. Gov't, P.H.S.]. Infect Immun. 1988;56:1722–9.

[88] Harrell HL. l-Carnitine for leg ulcers. Ann Intern Med. 1990;113:412.

[89] Serjeant BE, Harris J, Thomas P, Serjeant GR. Propionyl-l-carnitine in chronic leg ulcers of homozygous sickle cell disease: a pilot study. J Am Acad Dermatol. 1997;37(3 Pt 1): 491–3.

[90] McMahon L, Tamary H, Askin M, et al. A randomized phase II trial of arginine butyrate with standard local therapy in refractory sickle cell leg ulcers [Clinical Trial, Phase II Random- ized Controlled Trial Research Support, N.I.H., Extramural Research Support, U.S. Gov't, P.H.S.]. Br J Haematol. 2010;151:516–24. doi: 10.1111/j.1365-2141.2010.08395.x.

[91] Lionnet F, Bachmeyer C, Stankovic K, et al. Efficacy of the endothelin receptor blocker bosentan for refractory sickle cell leg ulcers. Br J Haematol. 2008;142:991–2. doi: 10.1111/j.1365-2141.2008.07206.x.

[92] Chaine B, Neonato MG, Girot R, Aractingi S. Cutaneous adverse reactions to hydroxyurea in patients with sickle cell disease. Arch Dermatol. 2001;137:467–70.

[93] Loukopoulos D, Voskaridou E, Kalotychou V, et al. Reduction of the clinical severity of sickle cell/beta-thalassemia with hydroxyurea: the experience of a single center in Greece. Blood Cell Mol Dis. 2000;26:453–66.

[94] Quattrone F, Dini V, Barbanera S, et al. Cutaneous ulcers associated with hydroxyurea therapy. J Tissue Viability 2013;22:112–21.

[95] Nzouakou R, Bachir D, Lavaud A, et al. Clinical follow-up of hydroxyurea-treated adults with sickle cell disease. Acta Haematol. 2011;125:145–52.

[96] Mendpara S, Clair B, Raza M, et al. Leg ulcers among patients with sickle cell disease on hydroxyurea therapy. ASH Annual Meeting Abstracts 2004;104:1676.

[97] Ferster A, Tahriri P, Vermylen C, et al. Five years of experience with hydroxyurea in children and young adults with sickle cell disease. Blood 2001;97:3628–32.

[98] Kersgard C, Osswald MB. Hydroxyurea and sickle cell leg ulcers. Am J Hematol. 2001;68:215–6.

[99] Almeida CB, Souza LE, Leonardo FC, et al. Acute hemolytic vascular inflammatory processes are prevented by nitric oxide replacement or a single dose of hydroxyurea. Blood 2015;126:711–20.

[100] Sirieix ME, Debure C, Baudot N, et al. Leg ulcers and hydroxyurea: forty-one cases. Arch Dermatol. 1999;135:818–20.

[101] Ravandi-Kashani F, Cortes J, Cohen P, et al. Cutaneous ulcers associated with hydroxyurea therapy in myeloproliferative disorders. Leuk Lymphoma. 1999;35:109–18.

[102] Bader U, Banyai M, Boni R, et al. Leg ulcers in patients with myeloproliferative disorders: disease or treatment-related? Dermatology 2000;200:45–8.

[103] Antonioli E, Guglielmelli P, Pieri L, et al. Hydroxyurea-related toxicity in 3,411 patients with Ph'-negative MPN. Am J Hematol. 2012;87:552–4.

[104] Vélez A, García-Aranda JM, Moreno JC. Hydroxyurea-induced leg ulcers: is macroerythrocytosis a pathogenic factor? J Eur Acad Dermatol Venereol. 1999;12:243–4.

[105] Khouri RK, Upton J. Bilateral lower limb salvage with free flaps in a patient with sickle cell ulcers. Ann Plast Surg. 1991;27:574–6.

[106] Weinzweig N, Schuler J, Marschall M, Koshy M. Lower limb salvage by microvascular free-tissue transfer in patients with homozygous sickle cell disease. Plast Reconstr Surg. 1995;96:1154–61.

[107] Richards RS, Bowen CV, Glynn MF. Microsurgical free flap transfer in sickle cell disease. Ann Plast Surg. 1992;29:278–81.

[108] Kavalukas SL, Barbul A. Nutrition and wound healing: an update. Plast Reconstr Surg. 2011;127(Suppl. 1):38S–43S.

[109] Hoppe IC, Granick MS. Debridement of chronic wounds: a qualitative systematic review of randomized controlled trials [Review]. Clin Plast Surg. 2012;39:221–8. doi: 10.1016/j.cps.2012.04.001.

[110] Madhok BM, Vowden K, Vowden P. New techniques for wound debridement [Meta-Analysis Review]. Int Wound J. 2013;10:247–51. doi: 10.1111/iwj.12045.

[111] Wolcott RD, Kennedy JP, Dowd SE. Regular debridement is the main tool for maintaining a healthy wound bed in most chronic wounds [Review]. J Wound Care 2009;18:54–6. doi: 10.12968/jowc.2009.18. 2.38743.

[112] Alden PB, Lips EM, Zimmerman KP, et al. Chronic venous ulcer: minimally invasive treatment of superficial axial and perforator vein reflux speeds healing and reduces recurrence [Comparative Study]. Ann Vasc Surg. 2013;27:75–83. doi: 10.1016/j.avsg. 2012.06.002.

[113] Lipsky BA, Berendt AR, Cornia PB, et al. 2012 infectious diseases society of america clinical practice guideline for the diagnosis and treatment of diabetic foot infections. J Am Podiatr Med Assoc. 2013;103:2–7.

[114] Lipsky BA, Peters EJ, Senneville E, et al. Expert opinion on the management of infections in the diabetic foot [Review]. Diabetes Metab Res Rev. 2012;28(Suppl 1):163–78. doi: 10.1002/dmrr.2248.

[115] Taylor JG, Nolan VG, Mendelsohn L, et al. Chronic hyper-hemolysis in sickle cell anemia: association of vascular complications and mortality with less frequent vaso-occlusive pain. PLoS One 2008;3:e2095.

[116] De Castro LM, Jonassaint JC, Graham FL, Ashley-Koch A, Telen MJ. Pulmonary hypertension associated with sickle cell disease: clinical and laboratory endpoints and disease outcomes. Am J Hematol. 2008;83:19–25.

[117] Serarslan G, Akgül F, Babayigit C. High prevalence of pulmonary hypertension in homozygous sickle cell patients with leg ulceration. Clin Exp Hypertens. 2009;31(1):44–8.

[118] De Ceulaer K, Forbes M, Roper D, et al. Non-gouty arthritis in sickle cell disease: report of 37 consecutive cases. Ann Rheum Dis. 1984;43:599–603.

Section 5

Precision Medicine and Stem Cell Transplantation

Chapter 11

Stem Cell Transplantation in Patients with Sickle Cell Disease

Murtadha Al-Khabori, Mohammed Al-Huneini and Abdulhakim Al-Rawas

Additional information is available at the end of the chapter

http://dx.doi.org/10.5772/64917

Abstract

Hematopoietic stem cell transplantation (HSCT) is currently the only established cure for sickle cell disease (SCD). Replacement of the stem cell that has the defective beta globin allele with the normal gene decreases hemoglobin S and the risk of complications of SCD. The first case reported was a girl with acute myeloid leukemia and SCD who received HSCT and achieved long-term SCD and leukemia-free survival. Given the favorable outcomes of HSCT with thalassemia major using myeloablative preparative regimens, this approach became widely used in the initial studies of HSCT in SCD. The current standard of care is to use a myeloablative stem cell transplantation in patients with severe disease who have human leukocyte antigen–identical sibling. HSCT improves organ function, quality of life, and overall and disease-free survival. However, this is associated with high risk of gonadal dysfunction and graft versus host disease in addition to the mortality associated with the myeloablative HSCT. Reduced-intensity HSCT has also been reported with high rates of engraftment and favorable outcomes. This has been introduced to lower the gonadal dysfunction, mortality, and graft versus host disease associated with myeloablative approaches. Other approaches include HSCT using matched unrelated donors, cord blood units, and human leukocyte antigen haploidentical donors. Unfortunately, graft rejection is a common complication with these approaches. In this chapter, we review the indications of HSCT for SCD and outcomes of different transplant strategies including alternative donor transplant, graft rejection, and infertility after transplantation.

Keywords: sickle cell disease, hemoglobinopathy, stem cell transplantation, myeloablative, reduced intensity, graft rejection

1. Introduction

Replacement of the stem cell that has the defective beta globin allele with the normal gene decreases Hemoglobin S and the risk of complications of sickle cell disease (SCD). This could be achieved through gene therapy or allogeneic Hematopoietic stem cell transplantation (HSCT). The proof of principle case was an 8-year-old girl with acute myeloid leukemia (AML) and SCD who received HSCT for AML. Her AML was in remission 22 months posttransplantation and she was free of SCD.

The utility of HSCT in patients with SCD was shown in multiple studies since over 20 years with disease-free survival (DFS) of 90% [1, 2]. The improved organ function and decreased risk of SCD-related complications are attractive goals of therapy in these patients [3, 4]. Furthermore, SCD cure by HSCT is associated with improved quality of life scores in the physical, social, and emotional domains [5, 6].

Despite the promising results of HSCT in SCD, there are a number of unresolved issues limiting its' widespread application. The number of HSCT for SCD remains less than expected and cost is one of the major factors behind this knowing that the disease is much more prevalent in countries with low income [7, 8]. The course and severity of the disease cannot be accurately predicted with the currently available tools making it difficult to recommend HSCT early before end organ damage [9, 10]. This is especially important in children without end organ damage where one can debate the utility of HSCT for mild disease before damage occurs. In addition, most of the preparative regimens used are myeloablative [11] and these have led to high rates of gonadal dysfunction in patients who have not yet completed their family. This is even more of an issue in cultures where SCD is prevalent. Another issue is the limited number of siblings in families with SCD potentially giving rise to two problems, the low probability of finding a matched sibling donor (MSD) and the risk of mobilization of siblings with sickle cell trait. Unfortunately, for patients with no MSD, the probability of finding a matched unrelated donor (MUD) is low [12]. The theoretical risk of mobilizing donors with sickle cell trait is probably not real and the safety has been shown in multiple small studies [13].

2. Indications of HSCT in SCD

HSCT is the only curative treatment option for patients with SCD. However, it can be associated with significant toxicities making it a good treatment option for patients with severe disease who have a human leukocyte antigen (HLA) MSD [11]. Therefore, its initial use was limited to severe SCD, which is defined by the presence of one or more of SCD complications that include stroke or central nervous system event lasting longer than 24 hours, acute chest syndrome with recurrent hospitalizations or previous exchange transfusions, recurrent vasoocclusive pain (≥2 episodes per year for several years, recurrent priapism), impaired neuropsychological function and abnormal cerebral MRI scan, stage I or II sickle lung disease, sickle nephropathy (moderate or severe proteinuria or a glomerular filtration rate 30–50% of the predicted normal value), bilateral proliferative retinopathy and major visual impairment in at least in one eye, osteonecrosis of multiple joints, and/or red cell alloimmunization (≥2 antibodies) during long-term transfusion therapy [14]. Unfortunately, besides fetal hemoglobin there are no well-established prognostic markers that can indicate which patients are most likely to develop severe disease making it difficult to determine risk benefit ratio of HSCT for patients with less severe disease.

The indications above were adopted from the inclusion criteria of the first major trial of HSCT in patients with SCD involving 22 children [14]. There is no evidence-based medicine guideline to inform practice and all available guidelines are expert and consensus recommendations. A recent evidence-based focused review [15] divided the indications according to the donor source; however, the quality of evidence is not superior to expert and consensus recommendations. The review suggests that as the severity of SCD worsens, more experimental approaches could be utilized. Below, we list the indications of HSCT according to the donor source as recommended in the review [15].

When MSD is available:

- Stroke or high risk of stroke (elevated transcranial Doppler velocity).
- Recurrent acute chest syndrome.
- Recurrent severe acute painful crises.
- Red cell alloimmunization in patients on chronic transfusion protocol.
- Pulmonary hypertension.
- Recurrent priapism.
- Sickle nephropathy.
- Bone and joint involvement.
- Sickle retinopathy.

When MUD is available:

- Stroke or high risk of stroke (elevated transcranial Doppler velocity).
- Recurrent acute chest syndrome.
- Recurrent severe acute painful crises.
- Red cell alloimmunization in patients on chronic transfusion protocol.
- Pulmonary hypertension.
- Recurrent priapism.
- Sickle nephropathy.
- Bone and joint involvement.

When neither MSD nor MUD is available, mismatched marrow, haploidentical, or unrelated cord blood donor transplantation could be considered when:

- Recurrent stroke in patients on chronic transfusion therapy.
- Failure to tolerate the supportive care (e.g., chronic transfusion) in severe SCD.

HSCT for SCD offers a cure, but with variable morbidity especially graft versus host disease (GvHD) and treatment-related mortality. The risk benefit ratio should be considered when offering HSCT for patients and their families. The risks of complications and options should be discussed with the patients and their families for shared decision making. Outcomes and the nature of evidence for the available transplant donor should be balanced with the severity of SCD and the two should be presented to the patients and their families before a decision to undergo the procedure is made. Finally, the new and experimental approaches should only be performed in experienced transplant centers. Comparison of different transplant outcomes between the different transplant strategies is summarized in **Figure 1**.

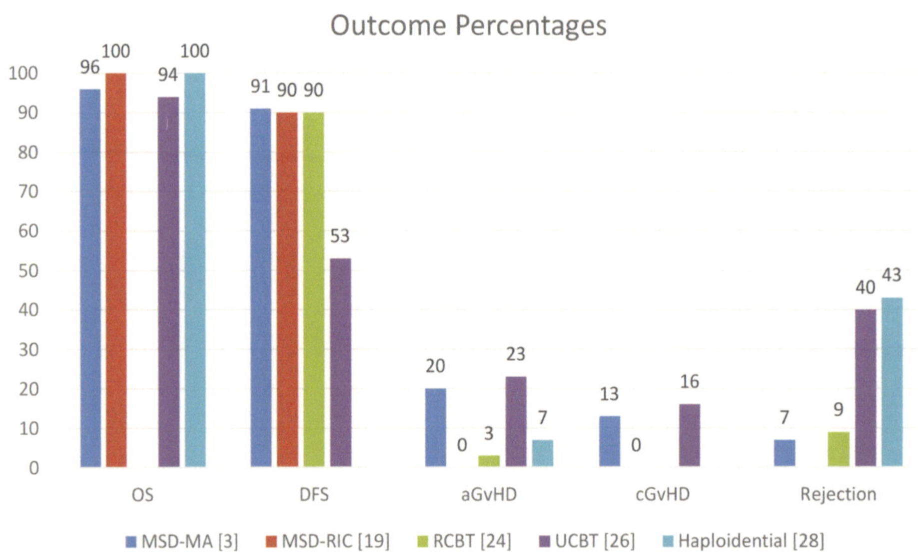

Figure 1. Comparison of transplant outcomes between different transplant strategies. Abbreviations: MSD-MA, matched sibling donor-myeloablative; MSD-RIC, matched sibling donor-reduced intensity conditioning; RCBT, related cord blood transplantation; UCBT, unrelated cord blood transplantation; OS, overall survival; DFS, disease free survival; aGvHD, acute graft versus host disease; cGvHD, chronic graft versus host disease. Note: The numbers in the figure are summarized for representative study of each transplant strategy. In MSD-MA study, the aGvHD rate only represents the high grade.

3. HSCT from MSD using a myeloablative preparative regimen

Preparative regimens and outcomes of HSCT in thalassemia major have influenced the strategies used in HSCT in patients with SCD. Myeloablative, nonradiation-based regimens were commonly used with high rates of engraftment and DFS [11]. The most commonly used was busulfan with cyclophosphamide at myeloablative doses and this became the preferred regimen in many of the future SCD transplant studies [11]. One of the earliest prospective studies was reported by Walters et al. [14]. In this study, a myeloablative regimen using busulfan and cyclophosphamide with antithymocyte globulin (ATG) was used in 22 patients with severe SCD. With a median follow-up of 2 years, overall survival (OS), and DFS were 91 and 73%, respectively. The high grade acute graft versus host disease (aGvHD) and chronic graft versus host disease (cGvHD) rates were 15 and 12%, respectively.

Another study reported by Bernaudin et al. [3] included 87 children with SCD, most of which had cerebrovascular event as the indication of the HSCT. The preparative regimen used was busulfan with cyclophosphamide at myeloablative doses. The ATG was later added to the regimen. The DFS was 91% with OS of 96%. The rates of high grade aGVHD and cGvHD were 20 and 13%, respectively. Two other studies using a similar preparative regimen reported OS of 85–96% [16, 17]. Given the high rates of DFS and OS, myeloablative preparative regimen using MSD is considered the standard of care for patients with SCD undergoing HSCT.

4. HSCT from MSD using reduced intensity preparative regimen

After the encouraging results of myeloablative preparative regimens in children, attempts to include adults using reduced intensity regimens were tried. The rationale was based on the assumption that mixed chimerism may be enough to ameliorate the complications of SCD and unlike in malignant conditions, myeloablation is not needed [18]. The use of reduced intensity regimens has expectedly resulted in less transplant-related organ dysfunction and may have preserved fertility, which is an important limitation of myeloablative transplantation.

Hsieh et al. [19, 20] investigated this approach in 30 adult patients using peripheral stem cell transplants. The preparative regimen constituted of 300 cGy of total body irradiation (TBI) with alemtuzumab and using sirolimus for GvHD prophylaxis. Most patients (26 out of 30) had a successful engraftment and no treatment related mortality, or GvHD was reported. This was attributed to the intensive GvHD prophylaxis using alemtuzumab and sirolimus. The DFS of 90% and OS of 100% were very encouraging. No data are yet available on the gonadal dysfunction of this approach.

Another study by Bhatia et al. [21] using a reduced toxicity, albeit myeloablative, preparative regimen with busulfan, fludarabine, and alemtuzumab in 18 patients with a median age of 8.9 years reported 17% of high grade aGvHD and 11% cGvHD. There was no graft rejection and all patients were alive at the time of the study report.

5. HLA matched unrelated donor transplantation

The probability of finding an HLA MUD is lower than desired in patients with SCD. In a report from the National Marrow Donor Program, the probability of finding a 6/6 MUD for patients with SCD was 60% [12]. The probability is much lower, 20%, when a more strict criteria using

8/8 matching at the allelic level is used [22]. This is likely due to the underrepresentation of the haplotypes of this genetic group in the international stem cell donor registries. Overall, the studies of MUD transplantations in SCD are scarce and include very small number of patients. There is a high risk of graft failure and other transplant-related complications with the MUD approach [23]. A number of prospective studies are currently running and results should be available in the near future. At this time, transplantation for patients with SCD from a MUD donor should only be done in a clinical trial setting.

6. Related cord blood transplantation (RCBT)

Related cord blood transplantation (RCBT) achieves OS and DFS rates similar to that of MSD transplantation, except for a significantly longer engraftment time for neutrophils and platelets. In a comparative study [24] of bone marrow HSCT versus RCBT in patients with hemoglobinopathies, 30 patients received RCBT for SCD. Patients in the RCBT group were mostly children and received a myeloablative preparative regimen. Serotherapy was given in more than half of the patients. The median total nucleated count (TNC) was 3.9×10^7/kg. With a median follow-up of 70 months, the DFS at 6 years for this group was 90% and no patient developed grade IV aGvHD or extensive cGvHD. The cumulative incidence of primary graft failure in the entire RCBT group was 9%. For those who engrafted, the cumulative incidence of day 60 neutrophil and day 180 platelet recovery was 90% (median 23 days) and 83% (median 38 days), respectively. Although the results of RCBT are not markedly different than that of MSD, the delayed recovery of neutrophils and platelets increases the risk of infection and bleeding complications, particularly, the central nervous system. In addition, the probability of finding RCBT unit is limited given the limited number of siblings in families with SCD. Finally, the availability of the RCBT is limited in areas where it is mostly needed, such as Africa.

7. Unrelated cord blood transplantation (UCBT)

The outcomes of unrelated cord blood transplantation (UCBT) are inferior to that of RCBT for patients with SCD. Two of the largest series are the Eurocord study [25] and the SCURT trial [26]. In the Eurocord study [25], 16 patients were transplanted with a mixture of myeloablative (10 received busulfan with cyclophosphamide or fludarabine) and reduced intensity preparative regimens (6 received fludarabine with busulfan, melphalan, or cyclophosphamide). Most patients received serotherapy with either ATG or alemtuzumab. All units were at least 4/6 HLA matched with a median TNC of 6 and 4.9×10^7/kg at the time of collection and infusion, respectively. The engraftment was only 60% with a 2-year OS and DFS of 94 and 53%. The rates of acute and chronic GvHD were 23 and 16%, respectively. In the SCURT trial [26], only eight patients were studied and all received similar nonmyeloablative preparative regimen using melphalan, fludarabine with alemtuzumab. All patients received at least 5/6 HLA matched units with a median TNC of 6.4×10^7/kg. Only three patients engrafted and one died of extensive cGvHD. In a similar small study [27] of eight patients (only five evaluable) using busulfan, fludarabine, and alemtuzumab, only 63 and 50% engrafted neutrophils and platelet, respectively. Twenty-five percent of patients had high grade aGvHD. The overall event-free survival and OS at 2 years were 50 and 63%, respectively.

Given the high rates of graft rejection and the delayed immune reconstitution that is associated with UCBT, this modality should only be used in a study. Possible ways to improve this modality are using higher intensity preparative regimens, using higher TNC, and lower mismatches. Double cord blood or cord blood supplemented with bone marrow are two promising options especially with children.

8. Haploidentical stem cell transplantation

HLA haploidentical HSCT is a promising alternative for patients with SCD with no available MSD. Nevertheless, it is characterized by high rate of graft failure. In a prospective study of 17 patients with SCD [28], 14 patients received a haploidentical transplantation. The preparative regimen was similar to the most widely used T cell-replete haploidentical HSCT with cyclophosphamide, fludarabine, and TBI using bone marrow as the stem cell source. The mycophenolate and the calcineurin inhibitor were used in addition to the posttransplant cyclophosphamide as aGvHD prophylaxis. In this study, ATG was added for 3 days starting Day -9. With a median follow-up 711 days, 10 patients were asymptomatic from SCD and 6 stopped immunosuppression. No deaths were reported and only one patient had GvHD of the skin. Unfortunately, the probability of graft failure was high at 43%. The use of haploidentical transplantation in SCD should be only used in a study setting.

9. Graft rejection

HSCT using myeloablative preparative regimen and HLA MSD has relatively low risk of graft rejection [11]. Bernaudin et al. reported an overall cumulative incidence of rejection of 7.0% at 5 years [3]. The addition of ATG to the preparative regimen resulted in a significant decrease in the 5-year cumulative incidence of rejection from 22.6 to 2.9% in patients who received ATG. A number of other studies using similar myeloablative regimens reported rejection rates of up to 10% [14, 17].

The rejection rate is different outside myeloablative transplantation; graft loss may not be uncommon complication of transplant using nonmyeloablative preparative regimens [11]. Attempts to improve this with higher intensity of nonmyeloablative regimens improved the rejection rate but with high proportion of mixed chimerism [20, 29, 30]. The mixed chimerism, if stable, may be enough to ameliorate the complications SCD [18]. Locatelli et al. reported rejection rate of 9% with RCBT which is similar to the MSD transplantation using myeloablative protocol. The URCB and the HLA haploidentical transplantation are associated with high risk of graft rejection of over 40% [25, 28, 31].

10. Infertility

The risk and fear of infertility is a major limiting factor on the widespread use of HSCT in patients with SCD. This high risk of infertility from HSCT in a benign condition limits the referral of patients. In addition, it also adds to the worries and deferral factors for patients to undergo the procedure.

The assessment of infertility post HSCT in children and young adults is difficult and only surrogate endpoints like gonadal dysfunction are used which limits the interpretation of studies of fertility post HSCT. The use of a standard approach of HSCT in SCD is associated with high risk of gonadal dysfunction. In the prospectively U.S. study [4], the use of a myeloablative preparative regimen lead to hypogonadotropic hypogonadism in most of the pubertal males and primary ovarian failure in the majority of postpubertal females. In another study using a similar preparative myeloablative regimen with ATG or radiation [17], all patients who were transplanted after puberty had gonadal dysfunction. The use of reduced intensity preparative regimens may lower the risk of gonadal dysfunction; however, it is yet to be shown prospectively.

11. Quality of life and long-term complications

Sickle cell disease impacts health related quality of life (HRQL) in children and adults [32–35]. The impact is worse in females and older children [34]. In adults, HRQL scores may be similar to patients receiving hemodialysis [36]. Unfortunately, it is not yet known with confidence that HSCT improves HRQL in patients with SCD. Studies addressing this question are small in number and sample size and predominantly examined reduced intensity HSCT [5, 6, 37]. HRQL scores improved in patients who received reduced intensity chemotherapy-based HSCT. The improvement was more marked with longer follow-up after transplant [5]. The improvement was noticed across all domains of and in parent-reported HRQL. Similar results were observed in patients who received chemotherapy-free (TBI-/alemtuzumab-based) HSCT [37]. The improvement in scores included the bodily pain, general health and vitality.

Long-term complications and reintegration have not been well addressed in literature despite a relatively long history of HSCT in SCD. In a study with a median follow-up of 9 years of 22 children with SCD who received HSCT from MSD [38], the overall survival was 93% and there was no recurrence of graft failure. This study was able to demonstrate that even with long-term follow-up; the engraftment and protection against SCD-related complications were sustained.

12. Conclusions

HSCT for severe SCD offers cure and a chance of amelioration of SCD-related complications. Myeloablative HSCT using HLA MSD remains the standard of care. RCBT offers similar results but longer time to count recovery. Transplantation from MUD, UCBT, or HLA haploidentical donors should only be practiced in a study setting in experienced transplant centers. Reduced intensity transplantations from MSD offer stable mixed chimerism and may decrease the risk of gonadal dysfunction in these young patients. Attempts to expand the pool of donors should continue.

Author details

Murtadha Al-Khabori*, Mohammed Al-Huneini and Abdulhakim Al-Rawas

*Address all correspondence to: khabori@squ.edu.om

Sultan Qaboos University Hospital, Muscat, Oman

References

[1] Bernaudin, F., et al., Bone marrow transplantation (BMT) in 14 children with severe sickle cell disease (SCD): the French experience. GEGMO. Bone Marrow Transplant, 1993. 12(1): 118–121.

[2] Vermylen, C. and G. Cornu, Bone marrow transplantation for sickle cell disease: The European experience. Am J Pediatr Hematol Oncol, 1994. 16(1): 18–21.

[3] Bernaudin, F., et al., Long-term results of related myeloablative stem-cell transplantation to cure sickle cell disease. Blood, 2007. 110(7): 2749–2756.

[4] Walters, M.C., et al., Pulmonary, gonadal, and central nervous system status after bone marrow transplantation for sickle cell disease. Biol Blood Marrow Transplant, 2010. 16(2): 263–272.

[5] Bhatia, M., et al., Health-related quality of life after allogeneic hematopoietic stem cell transplantation for sickle cell disease. Biol Blood Marrow Transplant, 2015. 21(4): 666–672.

[6] Kelly, M.J., et al., Health-related quality of life (HRQL) in children with sickle cell disease and thalassemia following hematopoietic stem cell transplant (HSCT). Pediatr Blood Cancer, 2012. 59(4): 725–731.

[7] Amid, A. and I. Odame, Improving outcomes in children with sickle cell disease: treatment considerations and strategies. Paediatr Drugs, 2014. 16(4): 255–266.

[8] Bhatia, M. and S. Sheth, Hematopoietic stem cell transplantation in sickle cell disease: patient selection and special considerations. J Blood Med, 2015. 6: 229–238.

[9] Galarneau, G., et al., Gene-centric association study of acute chest syndrome and painful crisis in sickle cell disease patients. Blood, 2013. 122(3): 434–442.

[10] Serjeant, G.R., Natural history and determinants of clinical severity of sickle cell disease. Curr Opin Hematol, 1995. 2(2): 103–108.

[11] Gluckman, E., Allogeneic transplantation strategies including haploidentical transplantation in sickle cell disease. Hematol Am Soc Hematol Educ Progr, 2013. 2013: 370–376.

[12] Krishnamurti, L., et al., Availability of unrelated donors for hematopoietic stem cell transplantation for hemoglobinopathies. Bone Marrow Transplant, 2003. 31(7): 547–550.

[13] Al-Khabori, M., et al., Safety of stem cell mobilization in donors with sickle cell trait. Bone Marrow Transplant, 2015. 50(2): 310–311.

[14] Walters, M.C., et al., Bone marrow transplantation for sickle cell disease. N Engl J Med, 1996. 335(6): 369–376.

[15] King, A. and S. Shenoy, Evidence-based focused review of the status of hematopoietic stem cell transplantation as treatment of sickle cell disease and thalassemia. Blood, 2014. 123(20): 3089–3094; quiz 3210.

[16] Panepinto, J.A., et al., Matched-related donor transplantation for sickle cell disease: report from the Center for International Blood and Transplant Research. Br J Haematol, 2007. 137(5): 479–485.

[17] Vermylen, C., et al., Haematopoietic stem cell transplantation for sickle cell anaemia: the first 50 patients transplanted in Belgium. Bone Marrow Transplant, 1998. 22(1): 1–6.

[18] Walters, M.C., et al., Stable mixed hematopoietic chimerism after bone marrow transplantation for sickle cell anemia. Biol Blood Marrow Transplant, 2001. 7(12): 665–673.

[19] Hsieh, M.M., et al., Nonmyeloablative HLA-matched sibling allogeneic hematopoietic stem cell transplantation for severe sickle cell phenotype. JAMA, 2014. 312(1): 48–56.

[20] Hsieh, M.M., et al., Allogeneic hematopoietic stem-cell transplantation for sickle cell disease. N Engl J Med, 2009. 361(24): 2309–2317.

[21] Bhatia, M., et al., Reduced toxicity, myeloablative conditioning with BU, fludarabine, alemtuzumab and SCT from sibling donors in children with sickle cell disease. Bone Marrow Transplant, 2014. 49(7): 913–920.

[22] Justus, D., et al., Allogeneic donor availability for hematopoietic stem cell transplantation in children with sickle cell disease. Pediatr Blood Cancer, 2015. 62(7): 1285–1287.

[23] Fitzhugh, C.D., et al., Hematopoietic stem cell transplantation for patients with sickle cell disease: progress and future directions. Hematol Oncol Clin North Am, 2014. 28(6): 1171–1185.

[24] Locatelli, F., et al., Outcome of patients with hemoglobinopathies given either cord blood or bone marrow transplantation from an HLA-identical sibling. Blood, 2013. 122(6): 1072–1078.

[25] Ruggeri, A., et al., Umbilical cord blood transplantation for children with thalassemia and sickle cell disease. Biol Blood Marrow Transplant, 2011. 17(9): 1375–1382.

[26] Kamani, N.R., et al., Unrelated donor cord blood transplantation for children with severe sickle cell disease: results of one cohort from the phase II study from the Blood and Marrow Transplant Clinical Trials Network (BMT CTN). Biol Blood Marrow Transplant, 2012. 18(8): 1265–1272.

[27] Radhakrishnan, K., et al., Busulfan, fludarabine, and alemtuzumab conditioning and unrelated cord blood transplantation in children with sickle cell disease. Biol Blood Marrow Transplant, 2013. 19(4): 676677.

[28] Bolanos-Meade, J., et al., HLA-haploidentical bone marrow transplantation with posttransplant cyclophosphamide expands the donor pool for patients with sickle cell disease. Blood, 2012. 120(22): 4285–4291.

[29] Krishnamurti, L., B.R. Blazar, and J.E. Wagner, Bone marrow transplantation without myeloablation for sickle cell disease. N Engl J Med, 2001. 344(1): 68.

[30] Krishnamurti, L., et al., Stable long-term donor engraftment following reduced-intensity hematopoietic cell transplantation for sickle cell disease. Biol Blood Marrow Transplant, 2008. 14(11): 1270–1278.

[31] Adamkiewicz, T.V., et al., Transplantation of unrelated placental blood cells in children with high-risk sickle cell disease. Bone Marrow Transplant, 2004. 34(5): 405–411.

[32] Beverung, L.M., et al., Health-related quality of life in children with sickle cell anemia: impact of blood transfusion therapy. Am J Hematol, 2015. 90(2): 139–143.

[33] Beverung, L.M., et al., Health-related quality of life in infants with sickle cell disease. J Pediatr Hematol Oncol, 2015. 37(8): 590–594.

[34] Jackson, J.L., et al., Predictors of health-related quality of life over time among adolescents and young adults with sickle cell disease. J Clin Psychol Med Set, 2014. 21(4): 313–319.

[35] Panepinto, J.A., et al., Health-related quality of life in children with sickle cell disease: child and parent perception. Br J Haematol, 2005. 130(3): 437–444.

[36] McClish, D.K., et al., Health related quality of life in sickle cell patients: the PiSCES project. Health Qual Life Outcomes, 2005. 3: 50.

[37] Saraf, S.L., et al., Nonmyeloablative stem cell transplantation with alemtuzumab/low-dose irradiation to cure and improve the quality of life of adults with sickle cell disease. Biol Blood Marrow Transplant, 2016. 22(3): 441–448.

[38] Dallas, M.H., et al., Long-term outcome and evaluation of organ function in pediatric patients undergoing haploidentical and matched related hematopoietic cell transplantation for sickle cell disease. Biol Blood Marrow Transplant, 2013. 19(5): 820–830.

Chapter 12

Precision Medicine for Sickle Cell Disease: Discovery of Genetic Targets for Drug Development

Betty S. Pace, Nicole H. Lopez, Xingguo Zhu and Biaoru Li

Additional information is available at the end of the chapter

http://dx.doi.org/10.5772/64817

Abstract

Sickle cell disease (SCD) consists of inherited monogenic hemoglobin disorders affecting over three million people worldwide. Efforts to establish precision medicine based on the discovery of genetic polymorphisms associated with disease severity are ongoing to inform strategies for novel drug design. Numerous gene mutations have been associated with the clinical complications of SCD such as frequency of pain episodes, acute chest syndrome, and stroke among others. However, these discoveries have not produced additional treatment options. To date, Hydroxyurea remains the only Food and Drug Administration-approved agent for treating adults with SCD; recently it was demonstrated to be safe and effective in children. The main action of Hydroxyurea is the induction of fetal hemoglobin, a potent modifier of SCD clinical severity. Three inherited gene loci including *XmnI-HBG2, HBS1L-MYB* and *BCL11A* have been linked to *HBG* expression, however the greatest progress has been made to develop *BCL11A* as a therapeutic target. With the expanded availability of next generation sequencing, there exist opportunities to discover additional genetic modifiers of SCD. The progress made over the last two decades to define markers of disease severity and the implications for achieving precision medicine to treat the complications of SCD will be discussed.

Keywords: fetal hemoglobin, single nucleotide polymorphism, drug discovery, genome-wide association studies

1. Introduction

Sickle cell anemia is caused by an A to T point mutation in the sixth codon of the β-globin (*HBB*) gene on chromosome 11 leading to the production of hemoglobin S (HbSS) during adult development. When the sickle mutation is combined with one of over 400 additional mutations reported in the *HBB* locus, different subtypes of sickle cell disease (SCD) are produced. For example, heterozygosity for the sickle *HBB* gene and hemoglobin C produces HbSC disease [1]. A definitive diagnosis of SCD can be made by hemoglobin electrophoresis, isoelectric focusing, or high-performance liquid chromatography. However, DNA testing is required to detect the presence of β-thalassemia mutations, which when inherited with the sickle *HBB* causes HbS-β^0-thalassemia and HbSβ^+-thalassemia.

About one in 500 African-American and one in 36,000 Hispanic-American children are born with SCD disease [2], which is diagnosed at birth by newborn screening in the United States. The carrier state or sickle cell trait is detected in 1:13 African Americans and 1:100 Hispanic Americans [3] with an estimated 2.5 million Americans with sickle cell trait [4]. Worldwide about 3.2 million people have SCD and 43 million have sickle cell trait [5] with 80% occurring in sub-Saharan Africa mainly as a protective mechanism against malaria. Moreover, the *HBB* sickle mutation also occurs in Europe, India, the Arabian Peninsula, and Brazil [6].

Hemoglobin is a tetrameric protein, composed of two α-like and two β-like globin polypeptide chains, which transports oxygen to the body tissues. During human development, two switches in the type of hemoglobin synthesized occur, a process known as hemoglobin switching [1]. The first switch at 6–8 weeks of development involves ε-globin gene silencing and activation of the *HBG2* and *HBG1* genes throughout fetal erythropoiesis, during which $^G\gamma$-globin and $^A\gamma$-globin fetal hemoglobin (HbF; $\alpha_2\gamma_2$) are produced. The second switch occurs shortly after birth when the *HBG1/HBG2* genes are silenced and *HBB* is activated. HbF levels decline to <1% of total hemoglobin by 6–12 months of age [7], and HbF is restricted to a population of erythrocytes called F-cells [8]. During hemoglobin switching, the site of hematopoiesis moves from the yolk sac to the liver/spleen and finally the bone marrow, which becomes the main site of hematopoiesis where adult hemoglobin A (HbA, $\alpha_2\beta_2$) is produced in healthy individuals [1]. As the level of HbF decreases around 5–6 months of age, the clinical symptoms of SCD are observed due to high HbS levels and polymerization under deoxygenated conditions producing sickle-shaped red blood cells (RBCs), vascular occlusion, and tissue ischemia. Therefore, precision medicine based on genetic or pharmacologic approaches to maintain high HbF levels is a proven efficacious strategy to treat SCD.

2. Clinical manifestations of sickle cell disease

Over the last 30 years, survival in people living with SCD has improved significantly due to decreased death rates during infancy. However, morbidity remains high due to central nervous system and pulmonary complications during childhood and end-organ damage in adults [9, 10]. The average life expectancy of people with SCD is 50 years in the United States [11].

Individuals with SCD experience a chronic hemolytic anemia caused by HbS polymerization under deoxygenated conditions, which [12] produces RBC membrane damage and a shortened life span of 14–21 days. As a result, HbSS patients have an average hemoglobin level of 6–8 g/dL with an elevated reticulocyte count and plasma lactate dehydrogenase level [13]. Furthermore, the damaged membrane leads to inflexible and dehydrated sickled RBCs and abnormal adhesion to the vascular endothelium producing the vasculopathy observed in persons with SCD [13].

The most common pathophysiology of SCD is vaso-occlusive (VOC) events produced by tissue ischemia leading to pain and acute or chronic injury to the spleen, brain, lungs, kidneys, and bones [13]. Individuals with a severe SCD sub-phenotype have more frequent VOC events, a higher white blood cell count, a lower HbF level, and increased blood vessel flow resistance under deoxygenation conditions [14–16]. The most common clinical manifestation of SCD is acute painful episodes which occur mainly in the extremities, but can involve the abdomen, back, and chest [17, 18].

As HbF falls below protective levels at around 6–12 months of age, dactylitis involving pain and swelling of the hands and feet is an early manifestation of SCD and is a risk factor for diseased severity [19]. Splenic sequestration occurs in 30% of children between the ages of 6 months to 3 years, which can cause severe life-threatening anemia and death if not treated promptly. Over time, repeated episodes of VOC in the spleen lead to infarction and a markedly increased risk for infection due to encapsulated bacteria such as *Streptococcus pneumonia, Haemophilus influenza, and Staphylococcus aureus* among others [20]. To address this significant cause of early mortality, the Prophylactic Penicillin Study I was conducted which demonstrated the ability of prophylactic penicillin to decrease overwhelming sepsis by 90% and improved survival among infants with SCD [21]. This study provided the rationale for establishing newborn screening for SCD in the late 1980s to facilitate the initiation of penicillin prophylaxis in the first few months of life to protect against infection and prevent early mortality. Penicillin prophylaxis has become the standard of care worldwide.

Other types of VOC events include acute chest syndrome [22, 23], silent and acute cerebral infarcts [24, 25], and osteonecrosis of the femoral head. Episodes of acute chest syndrome can be caused by pulmonary VOC, infection, and/or fat emboli from bone marrow infarcts [22]. Long-term damage in the lungs can precede pulmonary hypertension [26] in older children and adults with SCD causing high morbidity and mortality. By adolescents, 50% of individuals with SCD suffer silent cerebral infarcts [27] and 10% of children over the age of 2 experience overt strokes requiring chronic transfusions [28, 29]. The process of VOC can affect any organ system producing a wide variety of complications in SCD involving the heart, liver, gall bladder, kidney, and skin [30].

3. Treatment of vaso-occlusive complications

Blood transfusions are the mainstay of therapy for individuals suffering from acute and chronic complications of SCD. Red blood cell transfusions improve the oxygen-carrying capacity and prevent sickling by decreasing the HbS level to <30% of total hemoglobin [31–33]. Transfusions are also used for the acute exacerbation of anemia associated with splenic sequestration and aplastic crisis caused by Parvo B19 virus infection [34]. The most common symptom in persons with SCD is acute and chronic pain due to tissue ischemia, which is correlated with long-term survival [35]. Therefore, early aggressive treatment of pain episodes to prevent complications is the standard of care [36]. Recent research has provided insights into mechanisms of pain related to tissue injury (nociceptive), nerve injury (neuropathic), or unknown causes (idiopathic). Effective pain treatment is most often achieved using opioid narcotics combined with nonsteroidal anti-inflammatory drug.

To address the long-term effects of repeated pain episodes, extensive research has been conducted to develop drugs that induce HbF, which inhibits HbS polymerization [37] to improve the clinical symptoms of SCD. Based on findings in the Multicenter Study of Hydroxyurea [38], this agent is the only Food and Drug Administration-approved drug for the treatment of adults with SCD [39]. Subsequent studies in children including BABY HUG demonstrated that hydroxyurea (HU) is an effective HbF inducer and can be used safely in the first year of life [40]. Unfortunately, HU has a 30% nonresponse rate in adults, causes bone marrow suppression, and has detrimental effects on fertility [38, 41]. Therefore, the development of novel therapeutic agents based on inherited mutations that alter the expression of the *HBG1/HBG2* genes to produce high HbF levels is desired to establish precision medicine for SCD.

4. Genetic modifiers of sickle cell disease severity

While homozygosity for the β^S-globin gene mutation (*HBB*; glu6val) causes sickle cell anemia, the clinical diversity of phenotypes and disease severity are similar to the manifestations of multigenic disorders. Intensive studies have been performed to identify genetic risk factors correlated with SCD complications such as stroke, leg ulcers, pulmonary artery hypertension, priapism, and osteonecrosis. To extend the findings of genome-wide association studies of single nucleotide polymorphisms (SNPs) linked with clinical phenotypes, more advanced genomic techniques including next-generation DNA sequencing provide new opportunities to define mechanisms of SCD complications. A comprehensive review of genetic studies conducted in SCD is beyond the scope of this chapter. Therefore, we focus our discussion on efforts to discover SNPs associated with the clinical sub-phenotypes of SCD including pain severity, acute chest syndrome, pulmonary hypertension, osteonecrosis, priapism, leg ulcers, and nephropathy.

4.1. Vaso-occlusive pain

SCD patients experience a wide variety of clinical pain ranging from acute mild/severe to persistent chronic pain. The underlying mechanisms of differences in pain rates are complex and likely involve a number of genetic polymorphisms in several biological systems. Studies have been conducted that provide insights into SNPs associated with the frequency and severity of pain in SCD. Jhun et al. [42] identified mutations in the dopamine D3 receptor (Ser9Gly heterozygotes) associated with a lower acute pain rate. The most commonly used opioid medications including codeine and hydrocodone require cytochrome P450 2D6 (CYP2D6) for drug activation, which can impact the efficacy of these agents. The CYP2D6 gene is highly polymorphic, with variant alleles that result in decreased, absent, or ultra-rapid metabolism [43]. Altered CYP2D6 enzymatic activity in CYP2D6*17 (reduced activity), CYP2D6*5 (gene deletion), and CYP2D6*4 (absent function) is correlated with the analgesic response to codeine and hydrocodone. Therefore, genotyping the CYP2D6 gene is a reasonable approach for developing personalized medicine for the treatment of pain in persons with SCD. Moreover, missense or frame-shift mutations in CYP2C9 decrease or abolish enzymatic activity, respectively, which impairs opioid activation [44, 45]. Likewise, an SNP in the promoter of the gene encoding the enzyme uridine 5′-diphospho (UDP)-glucuronosyltransferase 2B7 (−840G/A) responsible for morphine glucuronidation in the liver is associated with lower morphine metabolites in sickle cell patients suggesting that higher doses of morphine may be required to achieve adequate pain control [46].

4.2. Acute chest syndrome/pulmonary hypertension

Acute chest syndrome continues to contribute to significant morbidity and mortality in children and adults with SCD [47]; therefore, the discovery of genetic modifiers of this complication has the potential for high impact and the design of precision medicine. Redha et al. [48] investigated the association of the vascular endothelial growth factor A (VEGFA) 583C/T mutation with acute chest rates in children with SCD. The presence of the 583T/T genotype was associated with increased serum VEGF levels while the VEGFA 583C/T caused reduced VEGF serum levels.

The rate of RBC hemolysis and release of free heme in the circulation are associated with clinical severity of SCD. Heme oxygenase-1 (*HMOX1*) is the inducible, rate-limiting enzyme in the catabolism of heme which attenuates the severity of VOC and hemolytic events. The (GT)(n) dinucleotide repeat in the promoter of *HMOX1* is highly polymorphic, with long repeats linked to decreased gene activation. Bean et al. [49] examined two *HMOX1* promoter polymorphisms including −413A/T and the (GT)(n) microsatellite (with allele (GT)(n) length from 13 to 45 repeats). The length of the (GT)(n) allele was associated with acute chest syndrome, but not pain rates in children with SCD.

Over the last decade, numerous studies have been conducted to define risk factors associated with pulmonary artery hypertension [50, 51], which defines a severe sub-phenotype of SCD leading to premature death. SNPs in genes involved in the regulation of endothelial function, which alter the synthesis of the endothelium-derived vasodilators nitric oxide and prostacyclin, have been implicated [52]. An extended screen of 297 SNPs in 49 candidate genes [53] identified mutations in the transforming growth factor (TGF) superfamily including the activin A type II-like 1 receptor (ACVRL1), bone morphogenetic protein (BMP) receptor 2, bone morphogenetic protein 6, and the β-1 adrenergic receptor (ADRB1) associated with pulmonary artery hypertension. A multiple regression model using age and hemoglobin as covariates demonstrated that SNPs in ACVRL1, BMP6, and ADRB1 independently contribute to pulmonary hypertension risk. These findings offer promise for identifying patients at risk for this complication and developing novel therapeutic targets for SCD.

A recent study by Al-Habboubi et al. [54] examined the association between VEGF secretion and VOC rates among 210 individuals with SCD. Mutations in VEGFA including rs2010963 heterozygous and rs833068 and rs3025020 homozygous states were associated with increased pain rates. Moreover, Yousry et al. [55] observed that the homozygous mutant eNOS 786T/T was significantly associated with a high risk of acute chest syndrome. By contrast, the wild-type eNOS 4a/4b genotype was protective against VOC and pulmonary hypertension while the homozygous haplotype (C, 4a) was significantly associated with the risk of VOC pain, acute chest syndrome, and pulmonary hypertension. Thus, eNOS SNPs may be useful as a genetic marker of prognostic value in SCD to predict a severe disease sub-phenotype.

4.3. Cerebral vascular disease

SCD is the most common cause of ischemic stroke occurring in 10% of children under 15 years of age; by contrast, hemorrhagic strokes are observed more commonly in adults over 30 years of age [56]. Genetic polymorphisms in multiple genes have been implicated in childhood stroke risk. For example, a mutation in vascular adhesion molecule-1 (*VCAM1*) including the G1238C in the coding region was protective and the intronic T1594C SNP predisposed to small-vessel stroke [57–59]. Mutations in the interleukin (*IL)4R*, tumor necrosis factor (*TNF)*, and *ADRB2* genes were found to be independently associated with stroke susceptibility in the large-vessel stroke subgroup, while SNPs in *VCAM1* and *LDLR NcoI* genes were associated with small-vessel stroke risk [59]. Additional genes have been implicated in stroke risk such as the GT-repeat polymorphism in the angiotensinogen gene including alleles A3 and A4, which conferred a fourfold increase in risk [60]. Hoppe et al. [61] identified SNPs in the cystathionine-β-synthase (278thr) and the *apoE3* genes that were associated with protection and increased risk for stroke, respectively.

Ischemic stroke is common in children with SCD producing high morbidity and mortality. A meta-analysis by Sarecka-Hujar et al. [62] demonstrated the association of SNP 677C/T in the methylenetetrahydrofolate reductase gene with the risk of stroke. Abnormalities in the coagulation pathway have been implicated in the pathogenesis of cerebral bleeding. For example, protein Z, a vitamin K-dependent glycoprotein structurally related to the vitamin K-dependent coagulation factors, is devoid of catalytic activity and inhibits the generation of thrombin. Mahdi et al. [63] identified three SNPs in the protein Z gene promoter (rs3024718, rs3024719, and rs3024731) and one intronic SNP rs3024735 associated with stroke risk suggesting that reduced protein Z levels produced a procoagulant state and increased risk for thrombotic diseases including ischemic stroke. These studies provide evidence for genetic markers that can be used to assess stroke risk in SCD and targeted for therapeutic intervention.

4.4. Osteonecrosis

Repeated episodes of bone infarction caused by vaso-occlusive events precede osteonecrosis of the head of the femur and humerus, a disabling complication of SCD [64, 65]. The discovery of SNPs in genes involved in bone morphogenesis, metabolism, and vascular disease will identify individuals at high risk for osteonecrosis. Previously, 233 SNPs in seven genes including *BMP6, TGFBR2, TGFBR3, EDN1, ERG, KL,* and *ECE1* were shown to be associated with this complication. There were 18 SNPs in the *KL* gene, which encodes the glycosyl hydrolase protein that participates in a negative regulatory network of vitamin D metabolism; moreover, 14 SNPs in *BMP6* and six SNPs in *ANXA2* were significantly associated with osteonecrosis [66]. A second research group [67] demonstrated the association of rs267196 (*BMP6*) and rs7170178 (*ANXA2*) with a higher risk of osteonecrosis. However, additional studies are needed to confirm if these markers are predictive of the clinical risk for this complication.

4.5. Priapism

Thirty percent of males with SCD experience the potentially devastating complication of priapism associated with a clinically severe disease sub-phenotype. Proteins involved in neuro-regulatory and adrenergic pathways, nitric oxide biology, and ion channels have been implicated in the pathophysiology of priapism [68–71]. More recently, clinical studies have identified genetic markers of priapism that produce erectile dysfunction and determine the ability to respond to phosphodiesterase inhibitors. Nolan et al. [72] identified SNPs in the *KLOTHO* gene including rs2249358, rs211239, rs211234, and rs211239 associated with an increased risk for priapism among 148 males with SCD. To support these findings, Elliott et al. [69] examined polymorphisms in a second group of adult male SCD patients with a 42% history of priapism. Mutations in the nitric oxide biology (*NOS2, NOS3,* and *SLC4A1*) and *KLOTHO* genes were associated with priapism risk providing further evidence for modulating nitric oxide levels as a therapy for this complication.

4.6. Nephropathy

Sickle nephropathy is a serious complication of SCD that can lead to renal failure and is rapidly becoming a major cause of death in adults. In view of the high medical burden and poor health outcome of end-stage renal disease, genetic markers of nephropathy risk are desirable. Youssry et al. [73] identified soluble FMS-like tyrosine kinase-1, a member of the vascular endothelial growth factor receptor family, as a biomarker for sickle nephropathy. In addition, Ashley-Koch et al. [53] demonstrated that the myosin, heavy chain 9, non-muscle (*MYH9*), and apolipoprotein L1 (*APOL1*) genes are associated with risk for focal segmental glomerulosclerosis and end-stage renal disease in African Americans. Seven SNPs in *MYH9* and one in *APOL1* remained significantly associated with proteinuria after multiple testing corrections. The causative role of these proteins in the development of sickle nephropathy needs to be tested further.

4.7. Leg ulcers

Cutaneous leg ulcers occur more often in adult sickle cell patients with low baseline hemoglobin levels and increased hemolysis rates indicated by high lactate dehydrogenase, bilirubin, and reticulocyte levels. The V34L G/T SNP (rs5985) in the factor XIII gene (F13A1) has been associated with leg ulcers [74]. Other studies have implicated factor V Leiden [75], the fibroblast growth factor receptor [76], and the HLA-B3525 antigen [77] in the pathogenesis of leg ulcers. A larger study involving 243 sickle cell patients [78] examined SNPS in 60 candidate genes that have a putative role in the pathophysiology of SCD. The association of SNPs in *KLOTHO, TEK,* and the TGF-β/BMP-signaling pathway was implicated in leg ulcer risk. Of these, *KLOTHO* promotes endothelial nitric oxide production and the TEK receptor tyrosine kinase is involved in angiogenesis. The TGF-β/BMP-signaling pathway modulates wound healing and angiogenesis, among other functions. Hemolysis-driven phenotypes such as leg ulcers could be improved by agents that increase nitric oxide bioavailability.

5. Genetic modifiers of fetal hemoglobin

5.1. *HBB* locus haplotypes

Inherited genetic mutations that modulate *HBG1/HBG2* gene expression enable persons with SCD to maintain high HbF levels, which ameliorates their clinical symptoms and long-term survival [17]. Individual SNPs inherited in set patterns define *HBB* haplotypes and determine the ancestral origin of the β^S-globin gene mutation in different ethnic and racial groups. Five common haplotypes including Senegal, Benin, Central African Republic (Bantu), Cameroon, and Asian (Indian/Saudi-Arabian) have been identified [1]. HbF levels vary greatly among individuals with different and the same *HBB* haplotype, which has precluded the establishment of a consistent correlation between the two parameters. However, individuals with the Senegal haplotype generally have higher HbF levels and milder disease [79], whereas individuals with the Benin haplotype tend to have lower HbF levels and more severe disease [80]. To address this limitation, a genomic study by Liu et al. [81] established the complexity of the *HBB* locus providing insights into the challenges of defining distinct *HBB* haplotypes for the prediction of disease severity and the development of therapeutic strategies.

5.2. Genome-wide association studies (GWAS)

The normal switch from HbF to HbA synthesis occurs during the first year of life reaching adult levels of HbF <1% by 12 months of age. A group of disorders known as hereditary persistence of HbF expression is caused by inherited deletions in the *HBB* locus or point mutations in the promoter region of the *HBG* genes. HbF levels range from 10 to 40% depending on whether heterozygous or homogeneous mutations are inherited. To gain insights into loci outside the *HBB* locus that control HbF heritability, GWAS to identify quantitative trait loci were conducted [82]. Three major loci were discovered including the *Xmn1-HBG2* (Gγ-globin) on chromosome 11, *HBS1L-MYB* intergenic region (HMIP) on chromosome 6q23, and *BCL11A* gene on chromosome 2p16 that control up to 40% of HbF variance in different populations [83]. These loci will be discussed subsequently in the context of the development of precision medicine for persons with SCD.

http://dx.doi.org/10.5772/64817

5.3. *Xmn1-HBG2*

In 1985, the C/T SNP at nucleotide −158 of the *HBG2* gene (rs7482144; T/T) was shown to be associated with high HbF levels with an increase in HbF expressing erythrocytes or F-cells (**Figure 1A**), and a milder disease phenotype in persons with SCD and β-thalassemia [84]. The positive association between the rs7482144 minor alleles (C/T) and HbF levels was replicated in European and Native Indian populations. However, this SNP was not associated with HbF levels in the people of African ancestry [85]. By contrast, the rs7482144 (G/A) allele occurred at a higher frequency in sickle cell patients with the Senegal and Arab-Indian haplotypes suggesting that the A allele is associated with the geographical origin of the study population. The ancestry for African Americans with SCD showed a high degree of European, African, and Native American admixture at 39.6, 29.6, and 30.8%, respectively.

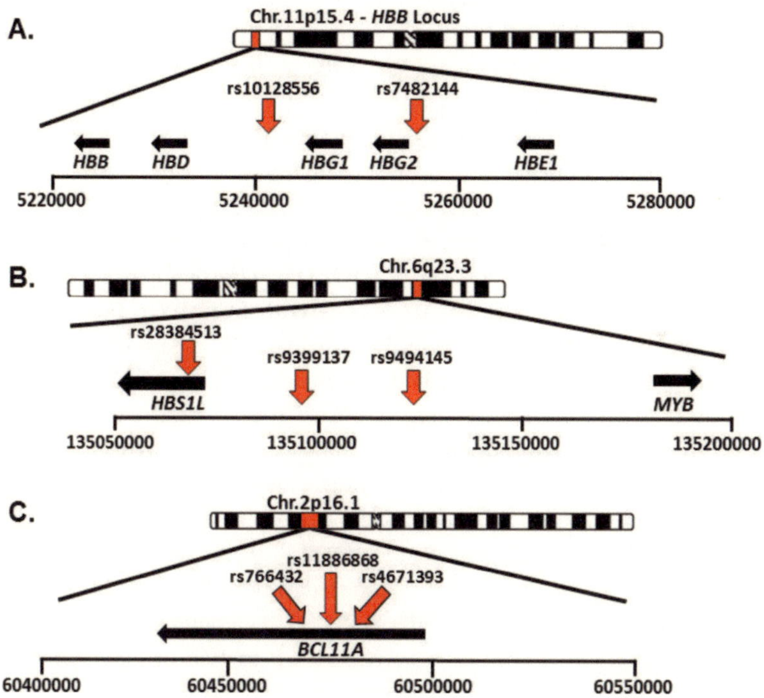

Figure 1. Summary of major single nucleotide polymorphisms (SNPs) associated with inherited genetic modifiers of HbF variance. Genome-wide genetic studies and GWAS identified SNPs associated with inherited levels of HbF in various ethnic and racial groups. Shown are SNPs in the *HBB* locus (A), the *HBS1L-MYB* intergenic region (B), and intron 2 of the *BCL11A* gene (C) associated with *HBG* regulation.

5.4. *HBS1L-MYB* (HMIP) region

Early studies conducted in a family of Asian Indian origin using segregation analysis demonstrated a modifier of *HBG* gene expression independent of the *HBB* locus [86]. Using a regressive model, a major locus was discovered on chromosome 6q23–q24 in the HMIP region.

Of the three SNPs identified, only rs4895441 was significantly associated with HbF levels, explaining 9.2% of variance. Later studies showed an association of the other two SNPs, rs28384513 and rs9399137, with HbF levels in the Northern European population (**Figure 1B**). Subsequently, these SNPs were also demonstrated to control HbF expression in African American, Brazilian, African British, and Tanzanian sickle cell patients [87]. The minor allele frequency of rs9399137 (C) is most significantly associated with HbF expression, but is less common in African populations, with a frequency of 1–2% in African sickle cell patients without European admixture. Similarly, a 3-bp (TAC) deletion on chromosome 6q23 is common in non-African populations, whereas the minor allele of rs9399137 occurs at a higher frequency in African Americans with SCD and elevated HbF levels [88].

5.5. *BCL11A*

After the completion of the Human Genome Project and the development of genome-wide techniques, GWAS became the preferred approach to identify inherited genetic modifiers of disease phenotypes. The first GWAS to identify HbF modifiers utilized a selected genotyping study design, targeting 179 individuals with contrasting extremes of F-cell numbers [89]. The *Xmn1-HBG2* and HMIP regions were identified along with a novel locus in the second intron of the oncogene *BCL11A* located at chromosome 2p16; the A allele of rs4671393 was associated with increased HbF levels. Subsequently, Uda et al. [90] confirmed SNPs in the *BCL11A* gene associated with high HbF in Sardinian thalassemia patients, establishing the first major repressor of *HBG1/HBG2* gene expression (**Figure 1C**). The majority of GWAS to identify inherited HbF determinants in African Americans with SCD have been conducted using samples collected during the Cooperative Study of Sickle Cell Disease [91–94]. The first GWAS conducted by Solovieff et al. [93] confirmed the *BCL11A* SNP (rs766432) and identified a polymorphism in the *ORB1B5/OR51B6* locus (rs4910755) associated with HbF levels in sickle cell patients (**Figure 1A**). A subsequent meta-analysis was conducted using GWAS data generated in seven African-American SCD cohorts totaling 2040 patients [95]. The most significant SNPs were identified in *BCL11A* (rs766432) and the HMIP region (rs9494145), which represented 11.1 and 3.2% of the phenotypic variability in HbF expression, respectively. Recently, the first GWAS was conducted in a Tanzanian population of 1213 individuals with SCD [96]. Similar to African Americans, SNPs in the *BCL11A* gene and the HMIP region were replicated in Tanzanians. Other studies have shown up to 10% of HbF variance associated with the *BCL11A* SNP rs4671393 in sickle cell patients from Northern Brazil (**Figure 1C**).

5.6. Mechanism of regulating *HBG* expression

Many decades of research have revealed that two types of mechanisms play a major role in modifying HbF levels: (1) direct transactivation of the *HBG1/HBG2* genes through the *Xmn1-HBG2* site or (2) an indirect effect on *HBG1/HBG2* through the repression of silencers such as *BCL11A* or *MYB*. The *Xmn1-HBG2* variant rs7482144 mediates a direct effect on Gγ-globin gene expression by functioning as a promoter [1]. By contrast, SNPs in the 14-kb second intron of *BCL11A* produces a strong enhancement of HbF expression. High levels of the short BCL11A isoform are associated with enhanced HbF expression in primitive erythroblasts, whereas full-length BCL11A isoforms are present in adult-stage erythroblasts when the *HBG* genes are silenced. BCL11A interacts with several DNA-binding proteins such as the corepressors LSD1/CoREST [97], DNMT1 [98], GATA1/FOG1/NuRD complex [99], and Sox6 [100] to facilitate γ-globin gene silencing through binding in the HbF-silencing region located upstream of the δ-globin gene [101]. Other studies have shown direct binding of BCL11A to a core motif 5′-GGCCGG-3″ in the *HBG* promoters to form a repressor complex in K562 cells [102]. Recently, an erythroid-specific enhancer was discovered in the second intron of BCL11A [103], which can be targeted to achieve lineage-specific gene silencing to achieve gene therapy for SCD directed at inhibiting *BCL11A* in erythroid progenitors.

SNP	Gene	Phenotype	Reference
rs1186868	*BCL11A*	Baseline HbF	Uda et al. [90]
rs766432	*BCL11A*	Baseline HbF	Sedgewick et al. [92]
rs4671393	*BCL11A*	Baseline HbF	Lettre et al. [94]
rs7557939	*BCL11A*	Baseline HbF	Lettre et al. [94]
rs7482144	*HBB*	Baseline HbF	Lettre et al. [94]
rs10128556	*HBB*	Baseline HbF	Galarneau et al. [110]
rs3759070	*HBE1*	Baseline HbF	Sebastiani et al. [91]
rs5024042	*OR51B5/OR51B6*	Baseline HbF	Solovieff et al. [93]
rs4895441	*HBS1L-MYB*	Baseline HbF	Lettre et al. [94]
rs9494145	*HBS1L-MYB*	Baseline HbF	Bae et al. [95]
rs9399137	*HBS1L-MYB*	Baseline HbF	Creary et al. [107]
rs28384513	*HBS1L-MYB*	Baseline HbF	Galarneau et al. [110]
rs12103880	*GLP2R*	Baseline F-cells	Bhatnagar et al. [109]
rs4769058	ALOX5AP	HbF induced by HU	Sebastiani et al. [91]
rs1867380	*AQP9*	HbF induced by HU	Sebastiani et al. [91]
rs17599586	*ARGI*	HbF induced by HU	Ware et al. [108]
rs2295644	*ARG2*	HbF induced by HU	Ware et al. [108]
rs10483802	*ARG2*	HbF induced by HU	Ma et al. [105]
rs2182008	*FTL I*	HbF induced by HU	Ma et al. [105]
rs10494225	*HAO2*	HbF induced by HU	Ma et al. [105]
rs7130110	*HBE1*	HbF induced by HU	Sebastiani et al. [91]
rs7977109	*NOSI*	HbF induced by HU	Ma et al. [105]
rs944725	*NOS2A*	HbF induced by HU	Ma et al. [105]
rs4282891	*SAR1A*	HbF induced by HU	Kumkhaek et al. [111]
rs2310991	*SAR1A*	HbF induced by HU	Kumkhaek et al. [111]

HbF, fetal hemoglobin; HU, hydroxyurea.

Table 1. SNPs known to modulate HbF levels and response to hydroxyurea therapy.

The mechanism by which the HMIP region silences *HBG* expression is less clear. It is known that a 24-kb nonprotein-coding region exists between the *HBS1L* and *MYB* oncogenes. A recent study identified a distal regulatory locus HMIP 2, which contains a regulatory element composed of several GATA-1 motifs that coincided with DNaseI-hypersensitive sites associated with intergenic transcripts in erythroid precursor cells [104]. It was suggested that the HMIP 2 element might regulate *MYB*, which is a repressor of the *HGB* genes.

5.7. Genetic modifiers of response to hydroxyurea therapy

Data from the Multicenter Hydroxyurea Study [38] suggest that not all persons with SCD respond to HU treatment with increased HbF expression. Therefore, genetic markers to predict response to HU would support the development of precision medicine by limiting unnecessary exposure to a chemotherapy drug that causes bone marrow suppression and decreased fertility [41]. Although limited, studies have identified genetic modifiers of HbF response to HU. For example, SNPs in the *ARG2, FLT1, HAO2,* and *NOS1* genes were associated with increased HbF expression based on HapMap data [105]. Interestingly, 29 genes involved in HU metabolism were located in loci previously reported to be linked to HbF levels including 6q22.3–q23.2, 8q11–q12, and Xp22.2–p22.3 [105, 106]. A novel bioinformatics method Random Forest was used to investigate the association between SNPs and the change in HbF after stable long-term HU therapy. SNPs in the *ARG2, FLT1, HAO2,* and *NOS1* genes and 6q22.3–23.2 and 8q11–q12 regions were associated with the HbF response to HU [105]. A summary of the SNP-associated *HBG* expression at baseline or in response to HU treatment in sickle cell patients is shown in **Table 1** [90-92, 94, 95, 107–111].

5.8. MicroRNA-mediated control of *HBG* gene expression

Recent studies have focused on posttranscriptional mechanisms of *HBG* regulation via microRNA (miRNA) gene expression. For example, Miller and colleagues [112] demonstrated the ability of LIN28 to silence miRNA let-7 to activate HbF in human primary erythroid progenitors. Likewise, miR-15a and miR-16-1 [113] enhance *HBG* expression through the inhibition of *MYB* expression. Studies by Walker et al. correlated miR-26b with baseline HbF levels and miR-151-3p expression with the maximal tolerated dose of HU in children with SCD [114].

Other miRNAs have been implicated in *HBG* regulation including miR-96 [115], miR-486-3p, miR-210 [116], and miR-34a [117]. Recent studies demonstrated the preferential expression of miR-96 in adult erythroid cells and its ability to directly target the open-reading frame of γ-globin mRNA; the inhibition of miR-96 resulted in a 20% increase in γ-globin expression in erythroid progenitors [115]. BCL11A is directly targeted by miR-486-3p, and its overexpression reduces BCL11A levels followed by an increase in γ-globin expression [118]. The role of MYB as a repressor of γ-globin was demonstrated in children with trisomy 13 where increased miR-15a and miR-16 expression targets MYB expression directly to mediate high HbF levels [113]. By contrast, a subset of miRNAs has been shown to be associated with enhanced γ-globin expression. For example, miR-210 was elevated in a β-thalassemia patient with high HbF expression [116]. Similarly, the Pace group recently demonstrated the ability of miR-34a to exert a positive regulatory effect on the *HBG1/HBG2* genes when stably expressed in K562 cells [117] suggesting that these miRNAs target repressor proteins. These studies demonstrate the potential of developing miRNAs as targets for precision medicine and the development of therapeutic options for individuals with SCD.

6. Precision medicine for sickle cell disease

Completion of the Human Genome Project greatly improved efforts to develop gene-based treatment strategies for β-hemoglobinopathies. Early efforts to identify genetic modifiers of clinical severity and sub-phenotypes of disease severity in SCD consisted of candidate gene studies. Insights were gleamed into risk factors for acute VOC pain events such as SNPs in the dopamine D3 receptor [42]. Expanded investigations to understand the wide range of opioid dose required by individual sickle cell patients led to the characterization of mutations in the CYP2D6 gene required for opioid activation and classification of slow, intermediate, and rapid metabolizers [43]. However, additional studies with larger sample sizes and/or direct DNA sequencing are required to develop gene markers of disease severity for the development of precision medicine to inform clinical decision making.

A great urgency exists to identify genetic factors associated with risk for acute chest syndrome, the leading cause of morbidity and mortality in children and adults with SCD. Mutations in *VEGF* [48] and the *HMOX1* [49] genes hold promise since they serve as markers of endothelial damage and hemolysis associated with the release of free heme in the vascular space, respectively. Long-term repeated episodes of acute chest syndrome can lead to pulmonary hypertension and early death. With a paucity of effective therapies for this complication, genetic markers that identify subgroups of sickle cell patients at risk will support efforts to develop precision medicine. For example, SNPs in the TGF superfamily of proteins and the ADRB1gene can be targeted for drug development to improve clinical outcomes. Likewise, SNPs in the *eNOS* genes [55] required for maintaining normal nitric oxide levels might serve as excellent targets for pharmacologic modulation. Interestingly, SNPs in the *KLOTHO* [72] and *NOS2/NOS3* [69] genes have been associated with the occurrence of priapism in SCD. These observations suggest that developing drug therapy-targeting genes involved in nitric oxide regulation might treat multiple complications of SCD. Genome-wide studies involving next-generation DNA sequencing technology will move the field closer to achieving precision medicine in SCD.

Based on the absence of clinical symptoms in infants and the amelioration of symptoms in persons with hereditary persistence of HbF, the most effective strategy to modulate disease severity in persons with SCD is *HBG* activation. Therefore, understanding molecular mechanisms of *HBG1/HBG1* gene silencing during hemoglobin switching is an attractive but challenging strategy adopted by many investigators over the last three decades. Early genome-wide family genetic studies [82] and subsequent GWAS identified the *XmnI-HBG2, HBS1-MYB*, and *BCL11A* loci that account for ~40% of inherited HbF variance [83]. Orkin and colleagues advanced the field significantly by defining mechanisms of BCL11A-mediated γ-globin gene repression during murine development and correction of the SCD phenotype [119]. Genetic studies in an extended family identified mutations in *KLF1* that produce hereditary persistence of HbF [120, 121] suggesting this transcription factor is a viable target for gene therapy. However, the efficacy of targeting transcription factors for therapeutic development remains to be demonstrated.

Additional genetic studies that utilize high-throughput DNA (whole genome and exome) and RNA/miRNA (RNA-seq) sequencing will increase our knowledge of mechanisms involved in *HBG* regulation. With the expanded availability of genome-wide approaches, novel technologies for gene editing, and preclinical mouse models, the translation of bench research findings to clinical trials will be accelerated to improve treatment options for SCD and β-thalassemia.

Funding source

National Heart Lung and Blood Institute, National Institutes of Health to BSP (R01HL069234).

Author details

Betty S. Pace*, Nicole H. Lopez, Xingguo Zhu and Biaoru Li

*Address all correspondence to: bpace@augusta.edu

Department of Pediatrics, Augusta University, Augusta, GA, USA

References

[1] Stamatoyannopoulos G, Grosveld F. Hemoglobin switching. In: Stamatoyannopoulos G, Majerus PW, Perlmutter RM, Varmus H, editors. The Molecular Basis of Blood Disease. Vol. 3. Philadelphia: Saunders. 2001.

[2] September is Sickle Cell Awareness Month. CDC. February 2011.

[3] Sickle Cell Disease and Your Baby. March of Dimes. February 2008.

[4] Vichinsky EP, Mahoney DH, Landlaw SA. Uptodate: Sickle Cell Trait, November 2011.

[5] Global Burden of Disease Study 2013 Collaborators. Global, regional, and national incidence, prevalence, and years lived with disability for 301 acute and chronic diseases and injuries in 188 countries, 1990–2013: a systematic analysis for the global burden of disease study 2013. *Lancet* 386:743–800, 2015.

[6] Silva WS, de Oliveira RF, Ribeiro SB, da Silva IB, de Araújo EM, Baptista AF. Screening for structural hemoglobin variants in Bahia, Brazil. *Int J Environ Res Public Health* 13:pii(E225), 2016.

[7] Maier-Redelsperger M, Noguchi CT, de Montalembert M, Rodgers GP, Schechter AN, Gourbil A, Blanchard D, Jais JP, Ducrocq R, Peltier JY. Variation in fetal hemoglobin parameters and predicted hemoglobin S polymerization in sickle cell children in the first two years of life: Parisian Prospective Study on Sickle Cell Disease. *Blood* 84:3182–8, 1984.

[8] Boyer SH, Belding TK, Margolet L, Noyes AN. Fetal hemoglobin restriction to a few erythrocytes (F cells) in normal human adults. Science 188:361–3, 1975.

[9] Hassell KL. Population estimates of sickle cell disease in the U.S. *Am J Prev Med* 38:S512–21, 2010.

[10] Manci EA, Culberson DE, Yang YM, Gardner TM, Powell R, Haynes J Jr, Shah AK, Mankad VN. Investigators of the Cooperative Study of Sickle Cell Disease. Causes of death in sickle cell disease: an autopsy study. *Br J Haematol* 123:359–65, 2003.

[11] Werner EM. NHLBI Activities in Hemoglobinopathies. National Heart Blood and Lung Institute/National Institute of Health. NICHD Newborn Screening Translational Research Network Meeting. pp. 1–38, 2013.

[12] Quinn CT. Clinical severity in sickle cell disease: the challenges of definition and prognostication. *Exp Biol Med* 241:679–88, 2016.

[13] Bender MA, Seibel GD. Sickle Cell Disease. 2003 Sep 15 [Updated 2014 Oct 23]. In: Pagon RA, Adam MP, Ardinger HH, et al., editors. GeneReviews® [Internet]. Seattle (WA): University of Washington, Seattle; 1993–2016. Available from: http://www.ncbi.nlm.nih.gov/books/NBK1377/

[14] Charache S, Barton FB, Moore RD, Terrin ML, Steinberg MH, Dover GJ, Ballas SK, McMahon RP, Castro O, Orringer EP. Hydroxyurea and sickle cell anemia. Clinical utility of a myelosuppressive "switching" agent. The multicenter study of hydroxyurea in sickle cell anemia. *Medicine* 75:300–26, 1996.

[15] Darbari DS, Onyekwere O, Nouraie M, Minniti CP, Luchtman-Jones L, Rana S, Sable C, Ensing G, Dham N, Campbell A, Arteta M, Gladwin MT, Castro O, Taylor JG 6th, Kato GJ, Gordeuk V. Markers of severe vaso-occlusive painful episode frequency in children and adolescents with sickle cell anemia. *J Pediatr* 160:286–90, 2012.

[16] Wood DK, Soriano A, Mahadevan L, Higgins JM, Bhatia SN. A biophysical indicator of vaso-occlusive risk in sickle cell disease. *Sci Transl Med* 4:123ra26, 2014.

[17] Platt OS, Thorington BD, Brambilla DJ, Milner PF, Rose WF, Vichinsky E, Kinney TR. Pain in sickle cell disease. Rates and risk factors. *N Eng J Med* 325:11–6, 1991.

[18] Gill FM, Sleeper LA, Weiner SJ, Brown AK, Bellevue R, Grover R, Pegelow CH, Vichinsky E. Clinical events in the first decade in a cohort of infants with sickle cell disease. Cooperative study of sickle cell disease. *Blood* 86:776–83, 1995.

[19] Miller ST, Sleeper LA, Pegelow CH, Enos LE, Wang WC, Weiner SJ, Wethers DL, Smith J, Kinney TR. Prediction of adverse outcomes in children with sickle cell disease. *N Engl J Med* 342:83–9, 2000.

[20] Powars D, Overturf G, Weiss J, Lee S, Chan L. Pneumococcal septicemia in children with sickle cell anemia. Changing trend of survival. *JAMA* 245:1839–42, 1981.

[21] Cober MP, Phelps SJ. Penicillin prophylaxis in children with sickle cell disease. *J Pediatr Pharmacol Ther* 15:152–159, 2010.

[22] Vichinsky EP, Neumayr LD, Earles AN, Williams R, Lennette ET, Dean D, Nickerson B, Orringer E, McKie V, Bellevue R, Daeschner C, Manci EA. Causes and outcomes of the acute chest syndrome in sickle cell disease. National Acute Chest Syndrome Study Group. *N Engl J Med* 342:1855–65, 2000.

[23] Vichinsky EP, Styles LA, Colangelo LH, Wright EC, Castro O, Nickerson B. Acute chest syndrome in sickle cell disease. Clinical presentation and course. Cooperative Study of Sickle Cell Disease. *Blood* 89:1787–92, 1997.

[24] DeBaun MR, Gordon M, McKinstry RC, Noetzel MJ, White DA, Sarnaik SA, Meier ER, Howard TH, Majumdar S, Inusa BPD, Telfer PT, Kirby-Allen M, McCavit TL, Kamdem A, Airewele G, Woods GM, Berman B, Panepinto JA, Fuh, BR, Kwiatkowski JL, King AA, Fixler JM, Rhodes MM, Thompson AA, Heiny ME, Redding-lallinger RC, Kirkham FJ, Dixon N, Gonzalez CE, Kalinyak KA, Quinn CT, Strouse JJ, Miler JP, Lehmann H, Kraut MA, Ball Jr. WS, Hirtz D, Casella JF. Controlled trial of transfusion for silent cerebral infarcts in sickle cell anemia. *N Engl Med* 371:699–710, 2014.

[25] Meier ER, Wright EC, Miller JL. Reticulocytosis and anemia are associated with an increased risk of death and stoke in the newborn cohort of the Cooperative Study of Sickle Cell Disease. *Am J Hematol* 89:904–6, 2014.

[26] Ataga KI, Moore CG, Jones S, Olajide O, Strayhorn D, Hinderliter A, Orringer EP. Pulmonary hypertension in patients with sickle cell disease: a longitudinal study. *Br J Haematol* 134:109–15, 2006.

[27] Bernaudin F, Verlhac S, Arnaud C, Kamdem A, Chevret S, Hau I, Coïc L, Leveillé E, Lemarchand E, Lesprit E, Abadie I, Medejel N, Madhi F, Lemerle S, Biscardi S, Bardakdjian J, Galactéros F, Torres M, Kuentz M, Ferry C, Socié G, Reinert P, Delacourt C. Impact of early transcranial Doppler screening and intensive therapy on cerebral vasculopathy outcome in newborn sickle cell anemia cohort. *Blood* 117:1130–40, 2011.

[28] Schatz J, Brown RT, Pascual JM, Hsu L, DeBaun MR. Poor school and cognitive functioning with silent cerebral infarcts and sickle cell disease. *Neurology* 56:1109–11, 2001.

[29] Pegelow CH, Macklin EA, Moser FG, Wang WC, Bello JA, Miller ST, Vichinsky EP, DeBaun MR, Guarini L, Zimmerman RA, Younkin DP, Gallagher DM, Kinney TR. Longitudinal changes in brain magnetic resonance imaging findings in children with sickle cell disease. *Blood* 99:3014–8, 2002.

[30] Bonds DR. Three decades of innovation in the management of sickle cell disease: the road to understanding the sickle cell disease clinical phenotype. *Blood Rev* 19:99–110, 2005.

[31] Reed W, Vichinsky E. New considerations in the treatment of sickle cell disease. *Annu Rev Med* 49:461–74, 1998.

[32] Nifong T, Domen R. Oxygen saturation and hemoglobin a content in patients with sickle cell disease undergoing erythrocytapheresis. *Ther Apher* 6:390–3, 2002.

[33] Thurston G, Henderson N, Jeng M. Effects of erythrocytapheresis transfusion on the viscoelasticity of sickle cell blood. *Clin Hemorheol Microcirc* 30:83–97, 2004.

[34] Josephson CD, Su LL, Hillyer KL, Hillyer CD. Transfusions in the patient with sickle cell disease: a critical review of the literature and transfusion guidelines. *Transfusion Med Rev* 21:118–33, 2007.

[35] Platt OS. Easing the suffering caused by sickle cell disease. *N Engl J Med* 330:783–4, 1994.

[36] Benjamin L. Pain management in sickle cell disease: palliative care begins at birth? *Am Soc Hematol* 1:466–74, 2008.

[37] Fard AD, Hosseini SA, Shahjahani M, Salari F, Jaseb K. Evaluation of novel fetal hemoglobin inducer drugs in treatment of β-hemoglobinopathy disorder. *Int J Hematol Oncol Stem Cell Res* 7:47–54, 2013.

[38] Charache S, Terrin ML, Moore RD, Dover GJ, Barton FB, Eckert SV, McMahon RP, Bonds DR. Effect of hydroxyurea on the frequency of painful crises in sickle cell anemia. Investigators of the Multicenter Study of Hydroxyurea in Sickle Cell Anemia. *N Engl J Med* 332:1317–22, 1995.

[39] Wong TE, Brandow AM, Lim W, Lottenberg R. Update on the use of hydroxyurea therapy in sickle cell disease. *Blood* 124:3850–7, 2014.

[40] Wang WC, Ware RE, Miller ST, Iyer RV, Casella JF, Minniti CP, Rana S, Thornburg CD, Rogers ZR, Kalpatthi RV, Barredo JC, Brown RC, Sarnaik SA, Howard TH, Wynn LW, Kutlar A, Armstrong FD, Files BA, Goldsmith JC, Waclawiw MA, Huang X, Thompson BW; BABY HUG investigators. Hydroxycarbamide in very young children with sickle-cell anaemia: a multicentre, randomised, controlled trial (BABY HUG). *Lancet* 377:1663–72, 2011.

[41] Steinberg MH, Lu ZH, Barton FB, Terrin ML, Charache S, Dover GJ. Fetal hemoglobin in sickle cell anemia: determinants of response to hydroxyurea. Multicenter Study of Hydroxyurea. *Blood* 89:1078–88, 1997.

[42] Jhun E, He Y, Yao Y, Molokie RE, Wilkie DJ, Wang ZJ. Dopamine D3 receptor Ser9Gly and catechol-o-methyltransferase Val158Met polymorphisms and acute pain in sickle cell disease. *Anesth Analg* 119:1201–7, 2014.

[43] Yee MM, Josephson C, Hill CE, Harrington R, Castillejo MI, Ramjit R, Osunkwo I. Cytochrome P450 2D6 polymorphisms and predicted opioid metabolism in African American children with sickle cell disease. *J Pediatr Hematol Oncol* 35:e301–5, 2013.

[44] Jaja C, Bowman L, Wells L, Patel N, Xu H, Lyon M, Kutlar A. Preemptive genotyping of CYP2C8 and CYP2C9 allelic variants involved in NSAIDs metabolism for sickle cell disease pain management. *Clin Transl Sci* 8:272–80, 2015.

[45] Jaja C, Patel N, Scott SA, Gibson R, Kutlar A. CYP2C9 allelic variants and frequencies in a pediatric sickle cell disease cohort: implications for NSAIDs pharmacotherapy. *Clin Transl Sci* 7:396–401, 2014.

[46] Darbari DS, van Schaik RH, Capparelli EV, Rana S, McCarter R, van den Anker J. UGT2B7 promoter variant -840G>A contributes to the variability in hepatic clearance of morphine in patients with sickle cell disease. *Am J Hematol* 83:200–2, 2008.

[47] Vichinsky EP, Neumayr LD, Earles AN, et al. Causes and outcomes of the acute chest syndrome in sickle cell disease. *N Engl J Med* 342:1855–65, 2000.

[48] Redha NA, Mahdi N, Al-Habboubi HH, Almawi WY. Impact of VEGFA -583C>T polymorphism on serum VEGF levels and the susceptibility to acute chest syndrome in pediatric patients with sickle cell disease. *Pediatr Blood Cancer* 61:2310–2, 2014.

[49] Bean CJ, Boulet SL, Ellingsen D, Pyle ME, Barron-Casella EA, Casella JF, Payne AB, Driggers J, Trau HA, Yang G, Jones K, Ofori-Acquah SF, Hooper WC, DeBaun MR. Heme oxygenase-1 gene promoter polymorphism is associated with reduced incidence of acute chest syndrome among children with sickle cell disease. *Blood* 120:3822–8, 2012.

[50] Kato GJ, Onyekwere OC, Gladwin MT. Pulmonary hypertension in sickle cell disease: relevance to children. *Pediatr Hematol Oncol* 24:159–70, 2007.

[51] Potoka KP, Gladwin MT. Vasculopathy and pulmonary hypertension in sickle cell disease. *Am J Physiol Lung Cell Mol Physiol* 308:L314–24, 2015.

[52] Bunn HF, Nathan DG, Dover GJ, Hebbel RP, Platt OS, Rosse WF, Ware RE. Pulmonary hypertension and nitric oxide depletion in sickle cell disease. *Blood* 116:687–92, 2010.

[53] Ashley-Koch AE, Elliott L, Kail ME, De Castro LM, Jonassaint J, Jackson TL, Price J, Ataga KI, Levesque MC, Weinberg JB, Orringer EP, Collins A, Vance JM, Telen MJ. Identification of genetic polymorphisms associated with risk for pulmonary hypertension in sickle cell disease. *Blood* 111:5721–6, 2008.

[54] Al-Habboubi HH, Mahdi N, Abu-Hijleh TM, Abu-Hijleh FM, Sater MS, Almawi WY. The relation of vascular endothelial growth factor (VEGF) gene polymorphisms on

VEGF levels and the risk of vasoocclusive crisis in sickle cell disease. *Eur J Haematol* 89:403–9, 2012.

[55] Yousry SM, Ellithy HN, Shahin GH. Endothelial nitric oxide synthase gene polymorphisms and the risk of vasculopathy in sickle cell disease. *Hematology* 4:1–9, 2016.

[56] Ohene-Frempong K, Weiner SJ, Sleeper LA, Miller ST, Embury S, Moohr JW, Wethers DL, Pegelow CH, Gill FM. Cerebrovascular accidents in sickle cell disease: rates and risk factors. *Blood* 91:288–94, 1998.

[57] Belisário AR, Nogueira FL, Rodrigues RS, Toledo NE, Cattabriga AL, Velloso-Rodrigues C, Duarte FO, Silva CM, Viana MB. Association of alpha-thalassemia, TNF-alpha (-308G>A) and VCAM-1 (c.1238G>C) gene polymorphisms with cerebrovascular disease in a newborn cohort of 411 children with sickle cell anemia. *Blood Cells Mol Dis* 54:44–50, 2015.

[58] Taylor JG 6th, Tang DC, Savage SA, Leitman SF, Heller SI, Serjeant GR, Rodgers GP, Chanock SJ. Variants in the VCAM1 gene and risk for symptomatic stroke in sickle cell disease. *Blood* 100:4303–9, 2002.

[59] Hoppe C, Klitz W, Cheng S, Apple R, Steiner L, Robles L, Girard T, Vichinsky E, Styles L; CSSCD Investigators. Gene interactions and stroke risk in children with sickle cell anemia. *Blood* 103:2391–6, 2004.

[60] Tang DC, Prauner R, Liu W, Kim KH, Hirsch RP, Driscoll MC, Rodgers GP. Polymorphisms within the angiotensinogen gene (GT-repeat) and the risk of stroke in pediatric patients with sickle cell disease: a case-control study. *Am J Hematol* 68:164–9, 2001.

[61] Hoppe C, Cheng S, Grow M, Silbergleit A, Klitz W, Trachtenberg E, Erlich H, Vichinsky E, Styles L. A novel multilocus genotyping assay to identify genetic predictors of stroke in sickle cell anaemia. *Br J Haematol* 114:718–20, 2001.

[62] Sarecka-Hujar B, Kopyta I, Pienczk-Reclawowicz K, Reclawowicz D, Emich-Widera E, Pilarska E. The TT genotype of methylenetetrahydrofolate reductase 677C>T polymorphism increases the susceptibility to pediatric ischemic stroke: meta-analysis of the 822 cases and 1,552 controls. *Mol Biol Rep* 39:7957–63, 2012.

[63] Mahdi N, Abu-Hijleh TM, Abu-Hijleh FM, Sater MS, Al-Ola K, Almawi WY. Protein Z polymorphisms associated with vaso-occlusive crisis in young sickle cell disease patients. *Ann Hematol* 91:1215–20, 2012.

[64] Milner PF, Kraus AP, Sebes JI, Sleeper LA, Dukes KA, Embury SH, Bellevue R, Koshy M, Moohr JW, Smith J. Sickle cell disease as a cause of osteonecrosis of the femoral head. *N Engl J Med* 325:1476–81, 1991.

[65] Almeida A, Roberts I. Bone involvement in sickle cell disease. *Br J Haematol* 129:482–90, 2005.

[66] Baldwin C, Nolan VG, Wyszynski DF, Ma QL, Sebastiani P, Embury SH, Bisbee A, Farrell J, Farrer L, Steinberg MH. Association of KLOTHO, bone morphogenic protein 6, and annexin A2 polymorphisms with sickle cell osteonecrosis. *Blood* 106:372–5, 2005.

[67] Chaouch L, Kalai M, Jbara MB, Chaabene AB, Darragi I, Chaouachi D, Mallouli F, Hafsia R, Ghanem A, Abbes S. Association between rs267196 and rs267201 of BMP6 gene and osteonecrosis among sickle cell anaemia patients. *Biomed Pap Med Fac Univ Palacky Olomouc Czech Repub* 159:145–9, 2005.

[68] Chrouser KL, Ajiboye OB, Oyetunji TA, Chang DC. Priapism in the United States: the changing role of sickle cell disease. *Am J Surg* 201:468–74, 2011.

[69] Elliott L, Ashley-Koch AE, De Castro L, Jonassaint J, Price J, Ataga KI, Levesque MC, Brice Weinberg J, Eckman JR, Orringer EP, Vance JM, Telen MJ. Genetic polymorphisms associated with priapism in sickle cell disease. *Br J Haematol* 137:262–7, 2007.

[70] Rogers ZR. Priapism in sickle cell disease. *Hematol Oncol Clin North Am* 19:917–28, 2005.

[71] Broderick GA. Priapism and sickle-cell anemia: diagnosis and nonsurgical therapy. *J Sex Med* 9:88–103, 2012.

[72] Nolan VG, Baldwin C, Ma Q, Wyszynski DF, Amirault Y, Farrell JJ, Bisbee A, Embury SH, Farrer LA, Steinberg MH. Association of single nucleotide polymorphisms in KLOTHO with priapism in sickle cell anaemia. *Br J Haematol* 128:266–72, 2005.

[73] Youssry I, Makar S, Fawzy R, Wilson M, AbdAllah G, Fathy E, Sawires H. Novel marker for the detection of sickle cell nephropathy: soluble FMS-like tyrosine kinase-1 (sFLT-1). *Pediatr Nephrol* 30:2163–8, 2015.

[74] Gemmati D, Tognazzo S, Serino ML, Fogato L, Carandina S, De Palma M, Izzo M, De Mattei M, Ongaro A, Scapoli GL, Caruso A, Liboni A, Zamboni P. Factor XIII V34L polymorphism modulates the risk of chronic venous leg ulcer progression and extension. *Wound Repair Regen* 12:512–7, 2004.

[75] Brandt HRC, Messina MCD, Belda W, Martins JEC, Criado PR. Leg ulcers associated with factor V Leiden and prothrombin G20210A and methyltetrahydrofolate reductase mutations: successful treatment with warfarin. *Int J Dermatol* 46:1319–20, 2007.

[76] Nagy N, Németh IB, Szabad G, Szolnoky G, Belsõ N, Bata-Csörgõ Z, Dobozy A, Kemény L, Széll M. The altered expression of syndecan 4 in the uninvolved skin of venous leg ulcer patients may predispose to venous leg ulcer. *Wound Repair Regen* 16:495–502, 2008.

[77] Ofosu MD, Castro O, Alarif L. Sickle cell leg ulcers are associated with HLA-B35 and Cw4. *Arch Dermatol* 123:482–4, 1987.

[78] Nolan VG, Adewoye A, Baldwin C, Wang L, Ma Q, Wyszynski DF, Farrell JJ, Sebastiani P, Farrer LA, Steinberg MH. Sickle cell leg ulcers: associations with haemolysis and SNPs in KLOTHO, TEK and genes of the TGF-beta/BMP pathway. *Br J Haematol* 133:570–8, 2006.

[79] Nagel RL, Erlingsson S, Fabry ME, Fabry ME, Croizat H, Susuka SM, Lachman H, Sutton M, Driscoll C, Bouhassira E, Billett, HH. The Senegal DNA haplotype is associated with the amelioration of anemia in African-American sickle cell anemia patients. *Blood* 77:1371–5, 1991.

[80] Powars DR. 1990. Sickle cell anemia and major organ failure. *Hemoglobin* 14:573–98.

[81] Liu Li, Onykwere O, Quinn, C Sylvan C, Kalra I, Muralidar S, Amekar S, Pace BS. High density SNP-chip genotyping and haploview analysis to define γ-globin locus haplotypes. *Blood Cell Mol Dis* 42:16–24, 2009.

[82] Menzel S, Garner C, Gut I, Matsuda F, Yamaguchi M, Heath S, Foglio M, Zelenika D, Boland A, Rooks H. et al. A QTL influencing F cell production maps to a gene encoding a zinc-finger protein on chromosome 2p15. *Nat Genet* 39:1197–9, 2007.

[83] Thein SL, Menzel S, Lathrop M, Garner C. Control of fetal hemoglobin: new insights merging from genomics and clinical implications. *Hum Mol Genet* 18:216–23. 2009.

[84] Labie D, Dunda-Belkhodja O, Rouabhi F, Pagnier J, Ragusa A, Nagel RL. The -158 site 50 to the Gg gene and Gg expression. *Blood* 66:1463–5, 1985.

[85] Efremov GD, Gjorgovski I, Stojanovski N, Diaz-Chico JC, Harano T, Kutlar F, Huisman THJ. One haplotype is associated with the Swiss type of hereditary persistence of fetal hemoglobin in the Yugoslavian population. *Hum Genet* 77:132–6, 1987.

[86] Thein SL, Weatherall DJ. A non-deletion hereditary persistence of fetal hemoglobin (HPFH) determinant not linked to the beta-globin gene complex. *Prog Clin Biol Res* 316B: 97–111, 1989.

[87] Pissard S, Beuzard Y. A potential regulatory region for the expression of fetal hemoglobin in sickle cell disease. *Blood* 84:331–8, 1994.

[88] Old JM, Ayyub H, Wood WG, Clegg JB, Weatherall DJ. Linkage analysis of nondeletion hereditary persistence of fetal hemoglobin. *Science* 215:981–2, 1982.

[89] Thein SL, Menzel S, Peng X, Best S, Jiang J, Close J, Silver N, Gerovasilli A, Ping C, Yamaguchi M, Wahlberg K, Ulug P, Spector TD, Garner C, Matsuda F, Farrall M, Lathrop M. Intergenic variants of HBS1L-MYB are responsible for a major quantitative trait locus on chromosome 6q23 influencing fetal hemoglobin levels in adults. *Proc Natl Acad Sci* 104:11346–51, 2007.

[90] Uda M, Galanello R, Sanna S, Lettre G, Sankaran VG, Chen W, Usala G, Busonero F, Maschio A, Albai G, Piras MG, Sestu N, Lai S, Dei M, Mulas A, Crisponi L, Naitza S, Asunis I, Deiana M, Nagaraja R, Perseu L, Satta S, Cipollina MD, Sollaino C, Moi P, Hirschhorn JN, Orkin SH, Abecasis GR, Schlessinger D, Cao A. Genome-wide association study shows BCL11A associated with persistent fetal hemoglobin and amelioration of the phenotype of beta-thalassemia. *Proc Natl Acad Sci USA* 105:1620–5, 2008.

[91] Sebastiani P, Wang L, Nolan VG, Melista E, Ma Q, Baldwin CT, Steinberg MH. Fetal hemoglobin in sickle cell anemia: Bayesian modeling of genetic associations. *Am J Hematol* 83:189–95, 2008.

[92] Sedgewick AE, Timofeev N, Sebastiani P, So JC, Ma ES, Chan LC, Fucharoen G, Fucharoen S, Barbosa CG, Vardarajan BN, Farrer LA, Baldwin CT, Steinberg MH, Chui DH. BCL11A is a major HbF quantitative trait locus in three different populations with beta-hemoglobinopathies. *Blood Cells Mol Dis* 41:255–8, 2008.

[93] Solovieff N, Milton JN, Hartley SW, Sherva R, Sebastiani P, Dworkis DA, Klings ES, Farrer LA, Garrett ME, Ashley-Koch A, Telen MJ, Fucharoen S, Ha SY, Li CK, Chui DH, Baldwin CT, Steinberg MH. Fetal hemoglobin in sickle cell anemia: genome-wide association studies suggest a regulatory region in the 5' olfactory receptor gene cluster. *Blood* 115:1815–22, 2010.

[94] Lettre G, Sankaran VG, Bezerra MA, Araujo AS, Uda M, Sanna S, Cao A, Schlessinger D, Costa FF, Hirschhorn JN, Orkin SH. DNA polymorphisms at the BCL11A, HBS1L-MYB, and beta-globin loci associate with fetal hemoglobin levels and pain crises in sickle cell disease. *Proc Natl Acad Sci* 105:11869–74, 2008.

[95] Bae HT, Baldwin CT, Sebastiani P, Telen MJ, Ashley-Koch A, Garrett M, Hooper WC, Bean CJ, Debaun MR, Arking DE, Bhatnagar P, Casella JF, Keefer JR, Barron-Casella E, Gordeuk V, Kato GJ, Minniti C, Taylor J, Campbell A, Luchtman-Jones L, Hoppe C, Gladwin MT, Zhang Y, Steinberg MH. Meta-analysis of 2040 sickle cell anemia patients: BCL11A and HBS1L-MYB are the major modifiers of HbF in African Americans. *Blood* 120:1961–2, 2012.

[96] Mtatiro SN, Singh T, Rooks H, Mgaya J, Mariki H, Soka D, Mmbando B, Msaki E, Kolder I, Thein SL, Menzel S, Cox SE, Makani J, Barrett JC. Genome wide association study of fetal hemoglobin in sickle cell anemia in Tanzania. *PLoS One* 9:e111464, 2014.

[97] Xu J, Bauer DE, Kerenyi MA, Vo TD, Hou S, Hsu YJ, Yao H, Trowbridge JJ, Mandel G, Orkin SH. Corepressor-dependent silencing of fetal hemoglobin expression by BCL11A. *Proc Natl Acad Sci* 110:6518–23, 2013.

[98] Roosjen M, McColl B, Kao B, Gearing LJ, Blewitt ME, Vadolas J. Transcriptional regulators Myb and BCL11A interplay with DNA methyltransferase 1 in developmental silencing of embryonic and fetal β-like globin genes. *FASEB J* 28:1610–20, 2014.

[99] Amaya M, Desai M, Gnanapragasam MN, Wang SZ, Zu Zhu S, Williams DC Jr, Ginder GD. Mi2β-mediated silencing of the fetal γ-globin gene in adult erythroid cells. *Blood* 121:3493–501, 2013.

[100] Xu J, Sankaran VG, Ni M, Menne TF, Puram RV, Kim W, Orkin SH. Transcriptional silencing of γ-globin by BCL11A involves long-range interactions and cooperation with SOX6. *Genes Dev* 24:783–98, 2010.

[101] Sankaran VG, Xu J, Byron R, Greisman HA, Fisher C, Weatherall DJ, Sabath DE, Groudine M, Orkin SH, Premawardhena A, Bender MA. A functional element necessary for fetal hemoglobin silencing. *N Engl J Med* 365:807–14, 2011.

[102] Chen Z, Luo HY, Steinberg MH, Chui DH. BCL11A represses HBG transcription in K562 cells. *Blood Cells Mol Dis* 42:144–9, 2009.

[103] Bauer DE, Kamran SC, Lessard S, Xu J, Fujiwara Y, Lin C, Shao Z, Canver MC, Smith EC, Pinello L, Sabo PJ, Vierstra J, Voit RA, Yuan GC, Porteus MH, Stamatoyannopoulos JA, Lettre G, Orkin SH. An erythroid enhancer of BCL11A subject to genetic variation determines fetal hemoglobin level. *Science* 342:253–7, 2013.

[104] Menzel S, Rooks H, Zelenika D, Mtatiro SN, Gnanakulasekaran A, Drasar E, Cox S, Liu L, Masood M, Silver N, Garner C, Vasavda N, Howard J, Makani J, Adekile A, Pace B, Spector T, Farrall M, Lathrop M, Thein SL. Global genetic architecture of an erythroid quantitative trait locus, HMIP-2. *Ann Hum Genet* 78:434–51, 2014.

[105] Ma Q, Wyszynski DF, Farrell JJ, Kutlar A, Farrer LA, Baldwin CT, Steinberg MH. Fetal hemoglobin in sickle cell anemia: genetic determinants of response to hydroxyurea. *Pharmacogenomics J* 7:386–94, 2007.

[106] Chang YP, Maier-Redelsperger M, Smith KD, Contu L, Ducroco R, de Montalembert M, Belloy M, Elion J, Dover GJ, Girot R. The relative importance of the X-linked FCP locus and beta-globin haplotypes in determining haemoglobin F levels: a study of SS patients homozygous for beta S haplotypes. *Br J Haematol* 96:806–14, 1997.

[107] Creary LE, Ulug P, Menzel S, McKenzie CA, Hanchard NA, Taylor V, Farall M, Forrester TE, Thein SL. Genetic variation on chromosome 6 influences F cell levels in healthy individuals of African descent and HbF levels in sickle cell patients. PLoS One 4:e4218, 2009.

[108] Ware RE, Despotovic JM, Mortier NA, Flanagan JM, He J, Smeltzer MP, Kinble AC, Aygun B, Wu S, Joward T, Sparrebom A. Pharmacokinetics, pharmacodynamics, and pharmacogenetics of hydroxyurea treatment for children with sickle cell anemia. *Blood* 118:4985–91, 2011.

[109] Bhatnagar P, Purvis S, Barron-Casella E, et al. Genome-wide association study identifies genetic variants influencing F-cell levels in sickle-cell patients. *J Hum Genet* 56:316–23, 2011.

[110] Galarneau G, Palmer CD, Sankaran VG, Orkin SH, Hirschhorn JN, Lettre G. Fine-mapping at three loci known to affect fetal hemoglobin levels explains additional genetic variation. *Nat Genet* 42:1049–51, 2010.

[111] Kumkhaek C, Taylor JG 6th, Zhu J, Hoppe C, Kato GJ, Rodgers GP. Fetal haemoglobin response to hydroxycarbamide treatment and sar1a promoter polymorphisms in sickle cell anaemia. *Br J Haematol* 141:254–9, 2008.

[112] Lee YT, de Vasconcellos JF, Yuan J, Byrnes C, Noh SJ, Meier ER, Kim KS, Rabel A, Kaushal M, Muljo SA, Miller JL. LIN28B-mediated expression of fetal hemoglobin and

production of fetal-like erythrocytes from adult human erythroblasts ex vivo. *Blood* 122:1034–41, 2013.

[113] Sankaran VG, Menne TF, Scepanovic D, Vergilio JA, Ji P, Kim J, Thiru P, Orkin SH, Lander ES, Lodish HF. MicroRNA-15a and -16-1 act via MYB to elevate fetal hemoglobin expression in human trisomy 13. *Proc Natl Acad Sci* 108:1519–24, 2011.

[114] Walker AL, Steward S, Howard TA, Mortier N, Smeltzer M, Wang YD, Ware RE. Epigenetic and molecular profiles of erythroid cells after HU treatment in sickle cell anemia. *Blood* 118:5664–70, 2011.

[115] Azzouzi I, Moest H, Winkler J, Fauchere JC, Gerber AP, Wollscheid B, Stoffel M, Schmugge M, Speer O. MicroRNA-96 directly inhibits gamma-globin expression in human erythropoiesis. *PLoS One* 6:28, 2011.

[116] Bianchi N, Zuccato C, Lampronti I, Borgatti M, Gambari R. Expression of miR-210 during erythroid differentiation and induction of gamma-globin gene expression. *BMB Rep* 42:493–9, 2009.

[117] Ward CM, Li B, Pace BS. Stable expression of miR-34a mediates fetal hemoglobin induction in K562 cells. *Exp Biol Med (Maywood)* 241:719–29, 2016.

[118] Lulli V, Romania P, Morsilli O, Cianciulli P, Gabbianelli M, Testa U, Giuliani A, Marziali G. MicroRNA-486-3p regulates gamma-globin expression in human erythroid cells by directly modulating BCL11A. *PLoS One* 8, 2013.

[119] Xu J, Peng C, Sankaran VG, Shao Z, Esrick EB, Chong BG, Ippolito GC, Fujiwara Y, Ebert BL, Tucker PW, Orkin SH. Correction of sickle cell disease in adult mice by interference with fetal hemoglobin silencing. *Science* 334:993–6, 2011.

[120] Borg J, Papadopoulos P, Georgitsi M, Gutiérrez L, Grech G, Fanis P, Phylactides M, Verkerk AJ, van der Spek PJ, Scerri CA, Cassar W, Galdies R, van Ijcken W, Ozgür Z, Gillemans N, Hou J, Bugeja M, Grosveld FG, von Lindern M, Felice AE, Patrinos GP, Philipsen S. Haploinsufficiency for the erythroid transcription factor KLF1 causes hereditary persistence of fetal hemoglobin. *Nat Genet* 42:801–5, 2010.

[121] Zhou D, Liu K, Sun CW, Pawlik KM, Townes TM. KLF1 regulates BCL11A expression and gamma- to beta-globin gene switching. *Nat Genet* 42:742–4, 2010.

Section 6

New Dimensions in the Management of Chronic Complication

Chapter 13

Phytotherapy and the Relevance of Some Endogenous Antioxidant Enzymes in Management of Sickle Cell Diseases

Israel Sunmola Afolabi, Iyanuoluwa O. Osikoya and Adaobi Mary-Joy Okafor

Additional information is available at the end of the chapter

http://dx.doi.org/10.5772/64273

Abstract

Introduction: Sickle cell disease (SCD) is one of the most devastating diseases ravaging most populations.

Methodology, results, and discussion: The numerous plants earlier reported to be used for treating SCD were compiled along with their geographical locations (using relevant online databases when not provided in cited articles for each plant) and relative antisickling strength. The process of hemolysis in sickle cell diseases, a brief overview of the current treatments, and management of sickle cell diseases is considered in the chapter. The activities of endogenous antioxidants and some biochemical enzyme markers coupled to these plants' ability to maintain the integrity of red blood cell membrane are discussed in line with their antisickling health benefits and are also used to proffer more reliable molecular therapeutic strategies for managing sickle cell diseases. Furthermore, the operational principles of some enzymes, as well as their contributions to advancement of knowledge for management of the disease, were examined.

Conclusion: Geographical spread of these identified antisickling plants contributes to low levels of sickle cell patients where the potentials are known. More efforts should therefore be channeled toward increasing awareness about the plants, as well as harnessing their active principles to obtain a more lasting solution to sickle cell disease at the molecular level.

Keywords: plants, sickle cell diseases, enzymes, antisickling, antioxidants

1. Introduction

Sickle cell disease (SCD) is an autosomal recessive genetic disorder that is caused by a mutation in the β-globin gene on chromosome 11q [1]. This mutation involves glutamic acid being substituted with valine at the 6th position along the β-globin chain. $\alpha_2\beta_2$ is expressed as normal hemoglobin, $\alpha_2\beta^S$ (heterozygote) is expressed as sickle trait, while α_2S_2 (homozygote recessive) is expressed as sickle cell anemia. Most of the time as a result of repeated series of sickling and unsickling, the erythrocytes become permanently damaged and consequently lyse. Some acute and chronic tissue injuries result when these abnormally shaped red cells impede blood flow through the vessels [2].

Sickle cell disease is one of the most devastating diseases ravaging most populations. It is a disease that affects numerous nations and ethnic groups. It is associated with painful symptoms and is a genetic disease in which an individual inherits the allele for sickle cell hemoglobin from both parents. Patients with this disease possess lower level of erythrocytes than the normal healthy human. In addition to an unusually large number of immature cells such as transferrin receptor-positive, reticulocytes, erythroblasts that sometimes manifest in the form of granular bodies in the cytoplasm of red blood cells, the blood contains many long, thin, crescent-shaped erythrocytes that look like the blade of a sickle [3]. The hemoglobin (hemoglobin S) in blood of patients with sickle cell disease becomes insoluble and forms polymers that aggregate into tubular fibers when deoxygenated. The altered properties of hemoglobin S result from a single amino acid substitution, which leads to the presence of a valine (Val) with no electric charge instead of a glutamate (Glu) residue with a negative charge when pH is 7.4 at position 6 in the two chains, resulting in two fewer negative charges than normal hemoglobin A [3]. Glutamine residue replaces the valine residue at position 6 of β-chain of hemoglobin in the normal blood to form a "sticky" hydrophobic interaction outside the surface of the sickle cell blood. It is the resultant sticky points on the surface of sickle cell blood that makes deoxyhemoglobin S molecules to interact abnormally with each other to form the long, fibrous aggregates peculiar to this disorder that eventually cause the deformation of the normal disc biconcave red blood cell 'RBC' [4].

Polymerization of the sickled cells thereby alters the integrity of the red cell membrane, leading to loss of K^+, water, and a corresponding gain of Na^+. Increased intracellular free Ca^{2+} occurs during sickling, resulting in a loss of K^+ with accompanying movements of Cl^- and water [5]. The clumping of sickled RBCs leads to blockage of small blood vessels, preventing blood supply to various organs. The deoxygenation process in tissue capillaries causes damage to its endothelium, leading to exudation of plasma into the surrounding soft tissue [6]. The integrity of the red blood cell membrane is maintained by hydration and sickling is generated when there is dehydration of the membrane. It is also believed that increase in synthesis of endogenous nitric oxide may be beneficial to SCD patients by preventing the mopping up of the nitric oxide by the hemoglobin released during hemolysis, which may trigger a cascade of events that ultimately inhibit blood flow [7].

There is high incidence of the sickle cell disease in different parts of the world, especially in Africa and Asia. The traditional people in these regions have learnt to manage the problem using plants which are God's gift of nature, especially among the lower socio-economic class who cannot afford the high cost of western medicine, as well as traditionalists who simply believe in their efficacy [6]. There has been increasing insight into gaining understanding about the management approaches of sickle cell disease in several African countries on the efficacy of conventional and traditional medicines. However, no substantial evidence exists to support the efficacy of herbal medications in actually curing the disease. Research into phytotherapy of diseases is a current trend in the management of sickle cell disease, with the hope of finding inexpensive and less toxic alternative medicines that people can easily access [8].

Nutritional evaluation of *S. monostachyus* leaves revealed the presence of carbohydrate, protein, ash, fiber, and fat as well as potassium and vitamin C in higher concentrations; calcium, magnesium, vitamin A, vitamin B_6, vitamin E in lower concentrations; and others in trace quantities. Phytochemical screening revealed the presence of tannins, saponins, alkaloids, flavonoids, cyanogenic glycosides, and phytate [9]. Caffeic acid is one of the bioactive phenolic components of *Solenostemon monostachyus* leaves (unpublished report). It is a potent antioxidant. The study of antioxidants especially in various antisickling agents is of great significance because antisickling agents vary in their degree of efficacy. Antioxidants constitute a major component of these antisickling agents; thus, it is believed that the higher the antioxidant property of an antisickling agent, the higher its possible antisickling and therapeutic effect. Thus, reducing oxidative stress may ameliorate sickle cell crisis [8].

As a reference point, African/Nigerian medicinal plants are applied in the treatment of diseases, such as HIV/AIDS, malaria, tuberculosis, sickle cell diseases, diabetes, mental disorders, and so on. Research on these medicinal plants has shown various results such as antimicrobial (16%), molluscicidal (11%), antimalarial (7%), plant toxicology (7%), antitumor (4%), and many others. The major challenge with these medicinal plants is the lack of scientifically based evidence, quality standards, and regulations [6]. The antisickling activity of *S. monostachyus* on human sickle blood cells resulting in the alleviation of SCD symptoms has been reported [10]. Sickle cell disease and thalassemia are hemoglobinopathies characterized by chronic hemolysis [11].

2. Contribution of phytomedicine in the management of sickle cell diseases

The use of medicinal plants in the control of many diseases such as sickle cell diseases may be useful, especially in developing countries. The cost of treatment provided by orthodox medical practitioners largely contributes to the dependence on the use of traditional medicine in low-income settings. Much of the medicinal use of plants seems to have been developed through observations of wild animals, and by trial and error. It has been estimated by the World Health Organization that 80% of the world's population relies on traditional medicine to meet their daily health needs. Thiocyanate-rich foods, erythropoietin, nutritional supplements, food extracts, phytochemicals, and synthetic compounds have been tested in vitro and in vivo on their possible roles in the management of sickle cell disease [12]. Many medicinal plants with antisickling properties are indicated in **Table 1**. The leaves from most of the above-identified plants have been successfully proven to play a role in the management of sickle cell diseases possibly by antioxidant phytochemicals, proximate nutrients, amino acids, and minerals. Phytochemical testing revealed the presence of folic acid, vitamin B12, alkaloids, spooning, glycosides, tannins, and anthraquinones. Studies also indicated the plant extracts contained flavonoids and the antioxidants vitamins A and C [13, 14].

S.n	Natural antisickling resources	Name of country where identified	Natural habitat and geographical locations	References
1	*Zanthoxylum zanthoxyloides* (Fagara) root	Nigeria	Senegal and other west African countries	[23]
2	*Cajanus cajan* seeds	Nigeria	West/South Africa, southern India, and northern Australia	[24, 25]
3	*Solenostemon monostachyus* (P. Beauv.) Briq.	Nigeria	Anthrogenic habitat and rocky savanna in Cameroon, Gabon, Equatorial Guinea, Ivory Coast, Benin, Nigeria, Liberia, Guinea, Ghana, Togo, Burkina Faso, Republic of the Congo, Sao Tome and Principe, Central African Republic, Mali, and Brazil	[10]
4	*Ipomea involucrata*	Nigeria	Tropical Asia (possibly India); South and South-East Asia, tropical Africa, South and Central America; and Oceania	[10]
5	*Carica papaya* seed oil	Nigeria	Originated in Central America and is now grown in tropical areas worldwide	[10]
6	*Carica papaya* unripe fruit	Nigeria	Originated in Central America and is now grown in tropical areas worldwide	[13, 26]
7	*Parquetina nigrescens* (whole plant extracts) with ability to boost blood volume	Nigeria	A large part of Africa, from Senegal east to Sudan and south through Central and East Africa to Zambia, Angola and eastern Zimbabwe	[27]
8	Nicosan (drug)	Nigeria	Commercially distributed by National Institute for Pharmaceutical Research and Development (NIPRD), Nigeria	[8, 15, 19, 28]
9	Ciklavit (drug)	Nigeria	Commercially distributed by Neimeth International Pharmaceuticals Plc, Lagos, Nigeria	[8, 24, 29, 30]
10	*Walthera indica* (Malvaceae)	Nigeria	Widely distributed across tropical part of the world.	
11	Dried fish (Tilapia) and dried prawn (*Astacus red*)	Nigeria	Globally	[31–33]
12	Fermented *Sorghum bicolor* leaves	Nigeria	Widely cultivated in tropical part of Africa and Asia	[12]
13	*Terminalia catappa* (Tropica Almond)	Nigeria	Well-distributed globally but has abundant presence in regions between Seychelles and India; Southeast Asia; Papua New Guinea and Northern Australia; South Pacific Region; China, Taiwan, Cambodia, and New Caledonia	[12]
14	*Scoparia dulcis* Linnaeus	Nigeria	Tropical America and South-East Asia	[34]

S.n	Natural antisickling resources	Name of country where identified	Natural habitat and geographical locations	References
15	*Zanthoxylum macrophylla* (aqueous extract of roots)	Nigeria	Savannah and dry forest vegetation of Southwestern Nigeria	[35, 36]
16	*Garcinia kola* (aqueous extracts)	Nigeria	Tropical rain forests with moist lowland especially in part of west Africa	[37, 38]
17	*Adansonia digitata* (bark)	Nigeria	Africa, Madagascar, and Australia	[37, 39]
18	*Fagara zanthoxyloides* (root extracts)	Nigeria	West Africa and Cameroon	[40, 41]
19	*Vernonia amygdalina* (extracts)	Nigeria	Tropical Africa and Asia	[42]
20	*Parquetina nigrescens*	Nigeria	Most part of Africa	
21	Grape (*Citrus paradise*)	Nigeria	Tropical and subtropical part of the world	[10]
22	Lemon grass (*Citrus lemon*)	Nigeria	Widely distributed globally particularly in Mediterranean region	
23	Pumpkin, *Telfeira occidentalis* (fresh leaves)	Nigeria	Forest zone of West and Central Africa, particularly in Benin (Nigeria) and Cameroon	[8]
24	*Pterocarpus santolinoides* DC	Nigeria	Africa and South America	[43]
25	*Aloe vera*	Nigeria	Indigenous to most parts of Africa, widely distributed in the tropical and subtropical regions of the world	[43]
26	*Alchornea cordifolia*	Democratic Republic of Congo	West and Central Africa	[44–47]
27	*Afromomum albo violaceum*	Democratic Republic of Congo	West and Central Africa	[48]
28	*Annona senegalensis*	Democratic Republic of Congo	West and Central Africa.	[49]
29	*Cymbopogon densiflorus*	Democratic Republic of Congo	Widely distributed across the globe	[50]
30	*Bridelia ferruginea*	Democratic Republic of Congo	West Africa	[50]
31	*Ceiba pentandra*	Democratic Republic of Congo	Tropical regions of America and Africa	[50]
32	*Morinda lucida*	Democratic Republic of Congo	West and Central Africa	[50]
33	*Hymenocardia acida*	Democratic Republic of Congo	Tropical region of Africa	[50]

S.n	Natural antisickling resources	Name of country where identified	Natural habitat and geographical locations	References
34	*Coleus kilimandcharis*	Democratic Republic of Congo	Subtropical and warm temperate region of India, Nepal, Myanmar, Sri Lanka, Thailand, and Africa	[50–52]
35	*Dacryodes edulis*	Democratic Republic of Congo	Rainforests of Central and West Africa, particularly Angola, Benin, Cameroon, Central African Republic, Congo, Cote d'Ivoire, Democratic Republic of Congo, Equatorial Guinea, Gabon, Ghana, Liberia, Nigeria, Sierra Leone, Togo, and Uganda	[50]
36	*Caloncoba welwithsii*	Democratic Republic of Congo	Tropical forest of Africa, particularly in West Africa	[50]
37	*Vigna unguiculata*	Democratic Republic of Congo	Originated in Africa. Present across the globe particularly in savanna regions of West and Central Africa	[50]

Table 1. Geographical locations of some identified antisickling plants.

The use of phytomaterials such as *Piper guineense, Pterocarpus osun, Eugenia caryophyllata,* and *Sorghum bicolor* extracts in the drug Nicosan, previously NIPRISAN (Nix-0699), for the treatment of sickle cell disease was reported to possess antisickling properties. Nicosan was developed by a research team led by Prof. Charles O. Wambebe at the National Institute for Pharmaceutical Research and Development, Abuja, Nigeria. The efficacy of the drug had been reported with minor fear of toxicity since the constituents are largely from commonly consumed food items such as *Piper guineense, Eugenia caryophyllata,* and *Pterocarpus osun* [15–19]. A major constituent of a herbal formula (Ajawaron HF) consists of the extracts of the roots of *Cssus populnea* L. CPK had also been effectively used to reverse sickling in the management of sickle cell disease in south west of Nigeria. The most prominent and widely used of them all is Ciklavit developed by Prof G. Ekeke after 18 years of intensive research in collaboration with Neimeth Pharmaceuticals, Lagos, Nigeria. These efforts led to the development of WHO-approved drugs such as Niprisan and Ciklavit from some of these plants traditionally identified for treating sickle cell diseases [8, 20, 21].

The role of other components in Ciklavit (apart from *Cajanus cajan*) is essentially nutritional. A study on children with sickle cell disease suggests that nutritional supplements can help improve growth and weight gain. It can also boost the immune system and thus help in protecting against bacterial infections. Zinc deficiency is a major nutritional problem seen in sickle cell disease [8, 22]. Also reported are amino acids, glycine, phenylalanine, and tyrosine, which have been reported to possess antisickling properties. Particularly, extracts from underutilized plants such as *S. monostachyus, Carica papaya* seed oil, and *Ipomoea involucrata* were proven to reverse human sickle cell blood almost completely coupled with the ability to also reduce stress in sickle cell disease patients. Hence, each plant individually or in combination can be used in the management of sickle cell disease [10].

http://dx.doi.org/10.5772/64273

Local mixtures of herbivores, pollinators, and micro-organisms generated from the application of plants usually upregulate or downregulate certain biochemical pathways. These actions are often a result of their secondary metabolites as well as pigments, which can be refined to produce drugs [53]. Many drugs originally derived from plants, such as salicylic acid (a precursor of aspirin) originally derived from white willow bark and the meadowsweet plant, have been developed using this approach. Quinine—antimalarial drug, Vincristine—an anticancer drug, and drugs (morphine, codine, and paregoric) for treating diarrhea were developed from Cinchona bark, periwinkle, and the opium poppy, respectively [54].

3. Plants as sources of antioxidants in the management of sickle cell diseases

In addition to depletion in iron level, the generation of reactive oxygen species (ROS) in the erythrocytes is a major factor contributing to the occurrence of anemia in sickle cell diseases. ROS are defined as substances generated by one electron reduction of molecular oxygen, including oxygen radicals and reactive nitrogen species (RNS) [55]. Common radical species include peroxide, superoxide, and the hydroxyl radical that contain an unpaired electron and as such are extremely reactive, allowing them to react immediately with any biological molecule to produce cellular damage. ROS contributes to the pathogenesis of several hereditary disorders of erythrocytes, including sickle cell disease, thalassemia, and glucose-6-phosphate dehydrogenase (G6PD) deficiency. Oxidative stress is defined as the imbalance between pro-oxidants and antioxidants, which is a result of the formation of reactive oxygen species (ROS) in excess of the capacity of antioxidants to remove them [56].

3.1. Antioxidants

Antioxidants are the first line of defense against free radical damage and are critically needed for the maintenance and optimization of human health and well-being. Defence mechanisms against free radical-induced oxidative stress involve: (i) preventative mechanisms, (ii) repair mechanisms, (iii) physical defenses, and (iv) antioxidant defences. The body is also equipped with natural enzymatic antioxidant defences that include superoxide dismutase (SOD), glutathione peroxidase (GPx), and catalase (CAT). Antioxidants terminate these chain reactions by removing free radical intermediates and inhibit other oxidation reactions (**Figure 1**). They do this by being oxidized themselves, so antioxidants are often reducing agents such as thiols, ascorbic acid, or polyphenols [57].

In order to protect the cells and organ systems of the body against reactive oxygen species, a highly sophisticated and complex antioxidant protection system has been evolved by humans. This involves a variety of components such as nutrient-derived antioxidants, antioxidant enzymes, metal-binding proteins, and numerous other antioxidant phytonutrients, which are both endogenous and exogenous in origin, that function interactively and synergistically to neutralize free radicals [59]. The natural antioxidants are naturally occurring antioxidants having high or low molecular weights and can differ in their physical and chemical properties.

The mechanisms by which these antioxidants act at molecular and cellular levels include role in gene expression and regulation, apoptosis, and signal transduction. Thus, antioxidants are involved in fundamental metabolic and homeostatic processes [58]. General patterns of behavior of some endogenous antioxidant enzymes and other relevant enzymes associated with sickle cell disease patients are subsequently described to provide more insight into how to solve the numerous challenges of the disease. Furthermore, introduction to a few selected enzymes that uniquely interact with constituents in these medicinal plants and are more relevant to the advancement of sickle cell diseases are provided subsequently.

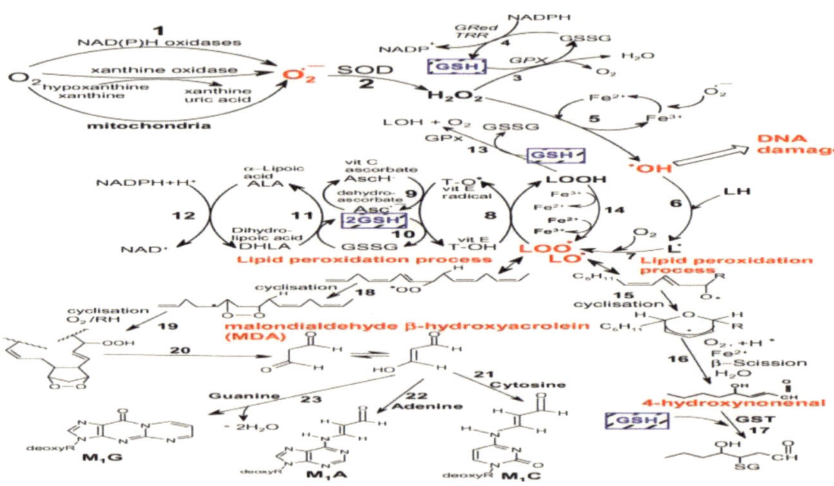

Figure 1. Pathways of ROS formation, the lipid peroxidation process, and the role of glutathione (GSH) and other antioxidants (vitamin E, vitamin C, lipoic acid) in the management of oxidative stress (equations are not balanced) [58].

3.2. Glucose-6-Phosphate Dehydrogenase (G6PD)

Glucose-6-phosphate dehydrogenase (G6PD) is the limiting enzyme that catalyzes the first reaction in the pentose phosphate pathway (**Figure 2**) in which glucose is converted into the pentose sugars required for glycolysis and various biosynthetic reactions. The pentose phosphate pathway (also known as the HMP shunt pathway) has a major biochemical role of providing reducing power to all cells in the form of NADPH (reduced form of nicotinamide adenine dinucleotide phosphate). This is possible in the presence of enzyme G6PD and 6-phosphogluconate dehydrogenase. NADPH enables cells to neutralize oxidative stress often induced by several oxidant agents and to preserve the reduced form of glutathione [57]. The hemoglobin in the blood, enzymes, and other proteins are damaged by the oxidants after all the leftover reduced glutathione is consumed. This leads to the generation of cross-bonding, protein deposition, and electrolyte imbalance in the red cell membranes. The hemoglobin from damaged red blood cells is metabolized to bilirubin that causes jaundice after attaining high concentrations [60]. High incidence of G6PD has been associated with areas of high prevalence of sickle cell disease. G6PD deficiency screening among SCD patients has provided the opportunity to administer appropriate preventive and therapeutic measures. The enzyme is

http://dx.doi.org/10.5772/64273

becoming an increasingly strong confirmatory indicator of blood associated with sickle cell diseases and other closely associated ailments like malaria [10, 61]. The enzyme provides information on the link between malaria and sickle cell diseases so as to understand strategies for the adoption of resistance of SCD patients to malaria to improve human health.

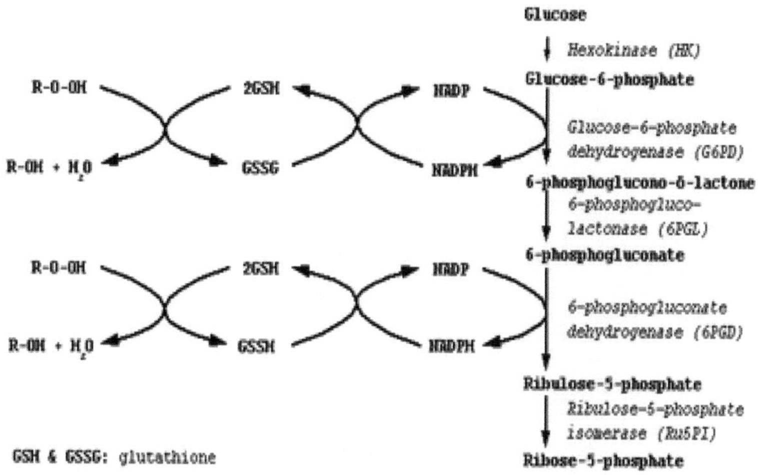

Figure 2. The pentose phosphate pathway. Source: [60].

3.3. Heme oxygenase

Heme oxygenases (HO) consists of a family of evolutionarily conserved endoplasmic reticulum (ER) enzymes [62]. Heme oxygenase (HO) plays a central role in regulating the levels of intracellular heme by catalyzing the oxidative degradation of heme into equimolar amounts of biliverdin, carbon monoxide, and iron as shown in **Figure 3a** and **b** [63]. They are central in determining what happens with regard to the central components of mammalian stress response and defense against oxidative stress [64]. Heme oxygenase activity is a key determinant of the health status of sickle cell anemia patients. Human sickle blood enhances endothelial heme oxygenase (HO) activity and the positive effects of HO-1 induction, biliverdin, and CO in reducing sickle blood adherence and in promoting vasodilation, indicating the need to further explore the therapeutic potentials of the HO pathway in the treatment of SCD [64]. The human HO-1 is comprised of a protein fold that primarily contains α-helices. The heme is held between two of these helices (**Figure 3b**). HO-1 acts as a cytoprotective stress protein and provides defense against oxidative stress associated with sickle cell disease by accelerating the degradation of pro-oxidant heme and hemo proteins to the radical scavenging bile pigments, biliverdin, and bilirubin [65]. HO-1 helps the body's defense in response to physical stress. The levels of heme are strictly controlled by the balance between heme biosynthesis and catabolism as indicated in **Figure 4** [65]. The key factor in the transcriptional activation of HO-1 is transcription factor Nrf2 (**Figure 4**). It interacts with many other genes that encode phase II drug-metabolizing enzymes so as to respond to oxidative stress [68].

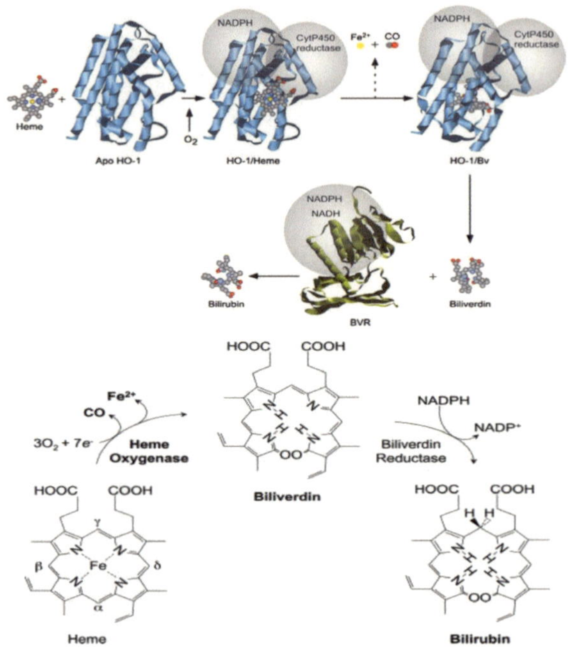

Figure 3. (a) The Heme oxygenase system. Source: [66]. (b) The Heme oxygenase system. Source: [67].

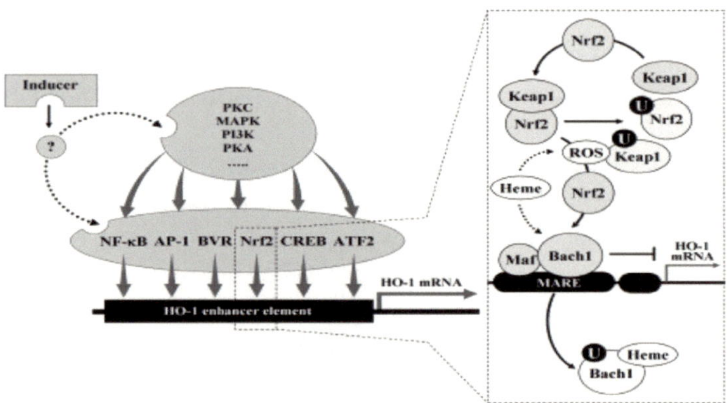

Figure 4. Regulation of HO-1 induction by transcription factors and kinases. Source: [69].

Sickle hemoglobin induces the expression of heme oxygenase-1 (HO-1) in hematopoietic cells through a mechanism that involves the ubiquitination-degradation of Kelch-like ECH-associated protein 1 (Keap1), a cytoplasmic repressor of the transcription factor NF-E2-related factor-2 (Nrf2). Upon nuclear translocation, Nrf2 binds to the stress-responsive elements in the Hmox1 promoter, a regulatory mechanism that plays a central role in the control of Hmox1 expression in response to heme [70]. Moreover, the higher rate of free heme released from sickle versus normal human subjects, in the absence of inflammation, induces HO-1 expression

http://dx.doi.org/10.5772/64273

without causing cytotoxicity and this explains how sickle human Hb may also cause the expression of HO-1 in human and mouse peripheral blood mononuclear cells and in human endothelial cells as well [54]. Although a link between sickle cell disease and resistance to severe malaria is well established, the biochemical relationship between the two is unknown.

3.4. Inducible nitric oxide synthase

Nitric oxide (NO) also influences the outcome of sickle cell disease. This outcome may sometimes be beneficial to SCD patients, provided there is increase in the production of endogenous NO so as to prevent the release of hemoglobin during hemolysis [7]. Inducible nitric oxide synthase (iNOS) is not normally expressed in the cells, but can be induced by the action of bacterial endotoxins (lipopolysaccharide), cytokines, and other agents. Though it is mainly identified in macrophages, iNOS expression may be stimulated in virtually any cell or tissue type, provided the appropriate inducing agents have been identified [71]. Upon its expression, iNOS remains constantly active and independent of intracellular Ca^{2+} concentrations. Cell and tissue damage can be linked to the NO radical itself or NO interaction with $O_2^{-\bullet}$ resulting in the formation of peroxynitrite ($ONOO^-$). Most of the inflammatory and autoimmune lesions are characterized by large amounts of activated macrophages and neutrophils. NO can be secreted in large quantities by the cells, causing damage to the surrounding tissues [72].

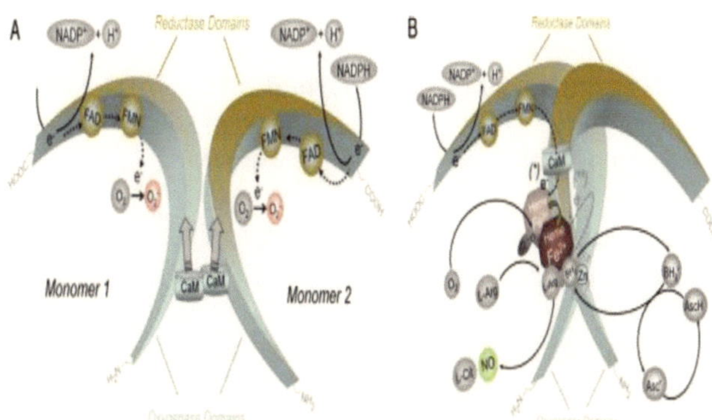

Figure 5. Structure of NOS monomers (A) and the functional dimer (B) Source: [71].

Finally, the excessive production of NO by iNOS plays a critical role in septic shock. This condition is characterized by massive microvascular lesions, arteriolar vasodilatation, and hypotension. Symptoms are usually initiated by bacterial endotoxins. Nonetheless, decrease in blood pressure can occur as a result of excessive production of NO by iNOS induced in the vascular wall [73]. In mammals, nitrous oxide (NO) is produced by the calcium-calmodulin-regulated constitutive isoenzymes eNOS (endothelial NOS) and nNOS (neuronal NOS), while the inducible isoform, iNOS, binds to calmodulin at physiologically significant concentrations producing NO free radicals as an immune defense mechanism (this is the direct cause of septic shock), and it may also play a role in autoimmune diseases. NOS-derived NO represents most of the NO produced in the vasculature and is associated with plasma membranes around cells including the membranes of red blood cells [71]. The structure and catalytic mechanisms of functional NOS are shown in **Figure 5**.

4. Conclusion

In conclusion, it is worthwhile to increase the search for potential plants that could supply bioactive compounds useful for the treatment of sickle cell disease. More so, concerted efforts are needed to further generate drugs to complement the already few drugs in existence, while taking into account the synergistic effect on these bioactives. This will help to standardize the administration of the bioactives to avoid any impediment to health due to overdose. Furthermore, it is necessary to exploit understanding of the interaction of these bioactives with the genes of sickle cell disease patient to increase our chances of getting a permanent solution to the disease. Geographical spread of these identified antisickling plants contributes to low levels of sickle cell patients where the potentials are known. More efforts should therefore be channeled toward increasing awareness about the plants.

Author details

Israel Sunmola Afolabi[1*], Iyanuoluwa O. Osikoya[1] and Adaobi Mary-Joy Okafor[2]

*Address all correspondence to: afolabisunmola@yahoo.com

1 Molecular Biology Research Laboratory, Biochemistry Unit, Biological Sciences Department, College of Science and Technology, Covenant University, Ota, Ogun State, Nigeria

2 Department of Computer and Information System, Covenant University Bioinformatics Research (CUBRe), Ota, Ogun State, Nigeria

References

[1] Pauling L, Itano HA, Singer SJ, Wells IC. Sickle cell anaemia, a molecular disease. Science 1949; 110: 543–548. doi:10.1126/science.110.2865.543

[2] Steinberg MH. SNPing away at sickle cell pathophysiology. Blood 2008; 111: 5420–5421. doi:10.1182/blood-2008-01-135392

[3] Voet D, Voet JG, Pratt CW. Protein function. In: Voet JG ed, Fundamentals of Biochemistry. Second ed. New York: John Wiley; 2002

[4] Iyamu EW, Ernest A, Toshio A. Niprisan (Nix-0699) improves the survival rates of transgenic sickle cell mice under acute severe hypoxic conditions. British Journal of Haematology 2003; 122: 1001–1008

[5] Brugnara C, De Franceshi L, Alper SL. Inhibition of Ca^{2+} dependent K^{+} transport and cell dehydration in sickle erythrocytes by CLT and other imidazole derivatives. Journal of Clinical Investigation 1993; 92: 520–526

[6] Okpuzor J, Adebesin O, Ogbunugafor H, Amadi I. The potential of medicinal plants in sickle cell disease control: a review. International Journal of Biomedical and Health Sciences 2008; 4: 47–55

[7] Mack AK, Kato GJ. Sickle cell disease and nitric oxide: a paradigm shift? International Journal of Biochemistry & Cell Biology 2006; 38: 1237–1243. doi:10.1016/j.biocel. 2006.01.010

[8] Imaga NA. Phytomedicines and nutraceuticals: alternative therapeutics for sickle cell anemia. The Scientific World Journal 2013; 2013: 269659. doi: http://dx.doi.org/ 10.1155/2013/269659

[9] Obichi EA, Monago CC, Belonwu DC. Nutritional qualities and phytochemical compositions of *Solenostemon monostachyus* (Family Lamiaceae). Journal of Environment and Earth Science 2015; 5: 105–112

[10] Afolabi IS, Osikoya IO, Fajimi OD, Usoro PI, Ogunleye DO, Bisi-Adeniyi T, O.Adeyemi A, Adekeye BT. *Solenostemon monostachyus, Ipomoea involucrata* and *Carica papaya* seed oil versus Glutathione, or *Vernonia amygdalina*: methanolic extracts of novel plants for the management of sickle cell anemia disease. BMC Complementary and Alternative Medicine 2012; 12: 262. doi:10.1186/1472-6882-12-262

[11] Platt OS, Brambilla DJ, Rosse WF, Milner PF, Castro O, Steinberg MH, Klug PP. Mortality in sickle cell disease. Life expectancy and risk factors for early death. The New England Journal of Medicine 1994; 330: 1639–1644. doi:10.1056/ NEJM199406093302303

[12] Nwaoguikpe RN, Uwakwe AA. The antisickling effects of dried fish (tilapia) and dried prawn (*Astacus red*). Journal of Applied Science and Environment Management 2005; 9: 115–119

[13] Imaga NOA, Gbenle GO, Okochi VI, Akanbi SO, Edeoghon SO, Oigbochie V, Kehinde MO, Bamiro SB. Antisickling property of Carica papaya leaf extract. African Journal of Biochemistry Research 2009; 3: 102–106

[14] Imaga NOA. The use of phytomedicines as effective therapeutic agents in sickle cell anemia. Scientific Research and Assays 2010; 5: 3803–3807

[15] Wambebe C, Khamofu H, Momoh JA, Ekpeyong M, Audu BS, Njoku OS, Bamgboye EA, Nasipuri RN, Kunle OO, Okogun JI, Enwerem MN, Audam JG, Gamaniel KS, Obodozie OO, Samuel B, Fojule G, Ogunyale O. Double-blind, placebo-controlled,

randomised cross-over clinical trial of NIPRISAN in patients with Sickle Cell Disorder. Phytomedicine 2001; 8: 252–261. doi:10.1078/0944-7113-00040

[16] Wambebe CO, Bamgboye EA, Badru BO, Khamofu H, Momoh JA, Ekpeyong M, Audu BS, Njoku SO, Nasipuri NR, Kunle OO, Okogun JI, Enwerem NM, Gamaniel SK, Obodozie OO, Samuel B, Fojule G, Ogunyale PO. Efficacy of niprisan in the prophylactic management of patients with sickle cell disease. Current Therapeutic Research 2001; 62: 26–34. 10.1016/s0011-393x(01)80039-4

[17] Ameh SJ, Obodozie OO, Afolabi EK, Oyedele EO, Ache TA, Onanuga CE, Ibe MC, Inyang US. Some basic requirements for preparing an antisickling herbal medicine - NIPRISAN® African Journal of Pharmacy and Pharmacology 2009; 3: 259–264

[18] Perampaladas K, Masum H, Kapoor A, Shah R, Daar AS, Singer PA. The road to commercialization in Africa: lessons from developing the sickle-cell drug Niprisan. BMC International Health and Human Rights 2010; 10(Suppl 1): S11. 10.1186/1472-698X-10-S1-S11

[19] Obodozie OO, Ameh SJ, Afolabi EK, Oyedele EO, Ache TA, Onanuga CE, Ibe MC, Inyang US. A normative study of the components of niprisan--an herbal medicine for sickle cell anemia. Journal of Dietary Supplements 2010; 7: 21–30. doi: 10.3109/19390210903534988

[20] Iweala EEJ, Uhegbu FO, Ogu GN. Preliminary in vitro antisickilng properties of crude juice extracts of *Persia americana, Citrus sinensis, Carica papaya* and Ciklavit®. African Journal of Traditional, Complementary and Alternative Medicines 2010; 7: 113–117

[21] Iwu MM, Igboko AO, Onwubiko H, Ndu UE. Effect of cajaminose from *Cajanus cajan* on gelation and oxygen affinity of sickle cell haemoglobin. Journal of Ethnopharmacology 1988; 23: 99–104. doi:10.1016/0378-8741(88)90118-3

[22] Nagalla S, Ballas SK. Drugs for preventing red blood cell dehydration in people with sickle cell disease. The Cochrane Database of Systematic Reviews 2010; 4: CD003426. doi:10.1002/14651858.CD003426.pub3

[23] Sofowora EA, Isaac Sodeye WA, Ogunkoya LO. Isolation and characterisation of an antisickling agent from *Fagara zanthoxyloides* root. Lloydia 1975; 38: 169–171

[24] Ekeke GI, Shode FO. The reversion of sickled cells by *Cajanus cajan*. Planta Medica 1985; 51: 504–507. doi:10.1055/s-2007-969576

[25] Khoury CK, Castañeda-Alvarez NP, Achicanoy HA, Sosa CC, Bernau V, Kassa MT, Norton SL, van der Maesen LJG, Upadhyaya HD, Ramírez-Villegas J, Jarvis A, Struik PC. Crop wild relatives of pigeonpea [*Cajanus cajan* (L.) Millsp.]: distributions, ex situ conservation status, and potential genetic resources for abiotic stress tolerance. Biological Conservation 2015; 184: 259–270. doi:10.1016/j.biocon.2015.01.032

[26] Mojisola OC, Adebolu EA, Alani DM. Antisickling Properties of Carica papaya Linn. Journal of Natural Products 2008; 1: 56–58

[27] Kade IJ, Kotila OO, Ayeleso AO, Olaleye AA, Olawoye TL. Antisickling properties of Parquetina nigrescens. Biomedical Research 2003; 14: 185–188

[28] Hankins J, Aygun B. Pharmacotherapy in sickle cell disease--state of the art and future prospects. British Journal of Haematology 2009; 145: 296–308. doi:10.1111/j.1365-2141.2009.07602.x

[29] Ekeke GI, Uwakwe AA, Nwaoguikpe R. Edible legumes as nutritionally beneficial antisickling agents. Nigerian Journal of Biochemistry and Molecular Biology 2000; 15: 200–203

[30] Imaga NA, Chukwu CE, Blankson A, Gbenle GO. Biochemical assessment of Ciklavit®, a nutraceutical used in sickle cell anaemia management. Journal of Herbal Medicine 2013; 3: 137–148. doi:10.1016/j.hermed.2013.05.003

[31] Abubakar MS, Musa AM, Ahmed A, Hussaini IM. The perception and practice of traditional medicine in the treatment of cancers and inflammations by the Hausa and Fulani tribes of Northern Nigeria. Journal of Ethnopharmacology 2007; 111: 625–629. doi:10.1016/j.jep.2007.01.011

[32] Gbadamosi IT. An Inventory of ethnobotanicals used in the management of sickle cell disease in Oyo State, Nigeria. Botany Research International 2015; 8: 65–72. doi:10.5829/idosi.bri.2015.8.4.523

[33] Vaishnava S, Rangari VD. A review on phytochemical and pharmacological research – Remedy for sickle cell disease. International Journal of Pharmaceutical Sciences and Research 2016; 7: 472–481. doi:10.13040/ijpsr.0975-8232.7

[34] Mgbemene CN, Ohiri FC. Anti-sickling potential of *Terminalia catappa* leaf extract. Pharmaceutical Biology 2008; 37: 152–154. doi:10.1076/phbi.37.2.152.6090

[35] Orhue NEJ, Nwanze EAC, Okafor A. Serum total protein, albumin and globulin levels in *Trypanosoma brucei* infected rabbits: effects of orally administered *Scoparia dulcis*. African Journal of Biotechnology 2005; 4: 1152–1155

[36] Aguilar NO, Schmelzer GH. Scoparia dulcis L.[Internet] record from Proseabase. In: van Valkenburg JLCH, Bunyapraphatsara N, eds, PROSEA (Plant Resources of South-East Asia) Foundation, Bogor, Indonesia; 2001

[37] Elekwa I, Monanu MO, Anosike EO. In vitro effects of aqueous extracts of *Zanthoxylum macrophylla* roots on adenosine triphosphatases from human erythrocytes of different genotypes. Biokemistri 2005; 17: 19–25

[38] Adesina SK. The Nigerian Zanthoxylum; chemical and biological values. African Journal Traditional, Complementary and Alternative Medicines 2005; 2: 282–301

[39] Farombi EO, Owoeye O. Antioxidative and chemopreventive properties of *Vernonia amygdalina* and Garcinia bioflavonoid. International Journal of Environmental Research and Public Health 2011; 8: 2533–2555

[40] Bell KL, Rangan H, Kull CA, Murphy DJ. The history of introduction of the African baobab (*Adansonia digitata*, Malvaceae: Bombacoideae) in the Indian subcontinent. Royal Society Open Science 2015; 2: 150370. doi:10.1098/rsos.150370

[41] Egunyomi A, Moody JO, Eletu OM. Antisickling activities of two ethnomedicinal plant recipes used for the management of sickle cell anaemia in Ibadan, Nigeria. African Journal of Biotechnology 2009; 8: 20–25

[42] Isaacs-Sodeye WA, Sofowora EA, Williams AO, Marquis VO, Adekunle AA, Anderson CO. Extract of *Fagara zanthoxyloides* root in sickle cell anaemia. Acta Haematology 1975; 53: 158–164. doi:10.1159/000208177

[43] Ekeke GI, Uwakwe AA, Nwaoguikpe R. The action of ripe fruit juices on hemoglobin polymerization, Fe^{2+}/Fe^{3+} ratio and lactate dehydrogenase activity of sickle cell (HbSS) blood. Nigerian Journal of Biochemistry and Molecular Biology 2001; 16: 31–35

[44] Alada ARA. The hematological effect of *Telfelria occidentalis* diet preparation. African Journal of Biomedical Resources 2000; 3: 185–186

[45] Dina OA, Adedapo AA, Oyinloye OP, Saba AB. Effect of *Telfairia occidentalis* extract on experimentally induced anaemia in domestic rabbits. African Journal of Biomedical Resources 2006; 3: 181–183

[46] Aderibigbe AO, Lawal BAS, Oluwagbemi JO. The anti-hyperglycaemic effect of *Telfairia occidentalis* in mice. African Journal of Medical Sciences 1999; 28: 171–175

[47] Alegbejo JO. Production, marketing, nutritional value and uses of fluted pumpkin (*Telfairia occidentalis* Hook. F.) in Africa. Journal of Biological Science and Bioconservation 2012; 4: 20–27

[48] Ameh SJ, Tarfa FD, Ebeshi BU. Traditional herbal management of sickle cell anemia: lessons from Nigeria. Anemia 2012; 2012: 607436. doi:10.1155/2012/607436

[49] Nwaoguikpe RN, Braide W, Ezejiofor TIN. The effect of aloe vera plant (*Aloe barbadensis*) extracts on sickle cell blood (hbss). African Journal of Food Science and Technology 2010; 1: 58–63

[50] Mpiana PT, Tshibangu DS, Shetonde OM, Ngbolua KN. In vitro antidrepanocytary actvity (anti-sickle cell anemia) of some congolese plants. Phytomedicine 2007; 14: 192–195. doi:10.1016/j.phymed.2006.05.008

[51] FAO. Non-wood forest products 9: Domestication and commercialization of non-timber forest products in agroforestry systems. In: Leakey RRB, Temu AB, Melnyk M, Vantomme P ed, Development of *Coleus forskohlii* as a medicinal crop. Rome (Italy): Food and Agricultural Organisation of the United Nations; 1996: 212–217

[52] Khatun S, Chatterjee NC, Cakilcioglu U. The strategies for production of forskolin vis-a-vis protection against soil borne diseases of the potential herb *Coleus forskohlii* Briq. European Journal of Medicinal Plants 2011; 1: 1–9

[53] Santos JLd, Lanaro C, Lima LM, Gambero S, Franco-Penteado CF, Alexandre-Moreira MS, Wade M, Yerigenahally S, Kutlar A, Meiler SE, Costa FF, Chung M. Design, synthesis, and pharmacological evaluation of novel hybrid compounds to treat sickle cell disease symptoms. Journal of Medicinal Chemistry 2011; 54: 5811–5819. doi: 10.1021/jm200531f

[54] Todou G. Climatic niche of *Dacryodes edulis* (G. Don) H.J. Lam (Burseraceae), a semi-domesticated fruit tree native to Central Africa. Journal of Ecology and The Natural Environment 2013; 5: 231–240. doi:10.5897/jene12.075

[55] Sabri A, Hughie HH, Lucchesi PA. Regulation of hypertrophic and apoptotic signaling pathways by reactive oxygen species in cardiac myocytes. Antioxidants and Redox Signalling 2003; 5: 731–740

[56] Halliwell B. Oxidative stress and cancer: have we moved forward? Biochem J 2007; 401: 1–11. doi:10.1042/BJ20061131

[57] Tenore GC, Campiglia P, Ritieni A, Novellino E. In vitro bioaccessibility, bioavailability and plasma protein interaction of polyphenols from Annurca apple (M. pumila Miller cv Annurca). Food Chemistry 2013; 141: 3519–3524. doi:10.1016/j.foodchem.2013.06.051

[58] Finco FDBA, Kammerer DR, Carle R, Tseng W-H, Böser S, Graeve L. Antioxidant activity and characterization of phenolic compounds from bacaba (*Oenocarpus bacaba* Mart.) fruit by HPLC-DAD-MSn. Journal of Agricultural and Food Chemistry 2012; 50: 7665–7673. doi:10.1021/jf3007689

[59] Jacob RA. The integrated antioxidant system. Nutrition Research 1995; 15: 755–766. doi: 10.1016/0271-5317(95)00041-g

[60] Capellini MD, Fiorelli G. Glucose-6-phosphate dehydrogenase deficiency. Lancet 2008; 371: 64–65

[61] Benkerrou M, Alberti C, Couque N, Haouari Z, Ba A, Missud F, Boizeau P, Holvoet L, Ithier G, Elion J, Baruchel A, Ducrocq R. Impact of glucose-6-phosphate dehydrogenase deficiency on sickle cell anaemia expression in infancy and early childhood: a prospective study. British Journal of Haematology 2013; 163: 646–654. 10.1111/bjh.12590

[62] Bansal S, Biswas G, Avadhani NG. Mitochondria-targeted heme oxygenase-1 induces oxidative stress and mitochondrial dysfunction in macrophages, kidney fibroblasts and in chronic alcohol hepatotoxicity. Redox Biology 2014; 2: 273–283. doi:10.1016/j.redox.2013.07.004

[63] Xia ZW, Zhou WP, Cui WJ, Zhang XH, Shen QX, Li YZ, Yu SH. Structure prediction and activity analysis of human heme oxygenase-1 and its mutant. World Journal of Gastroenterology 2004; 10: 2352–2356

[64] Bolisetty S, Traylor A, Zarjou A, Johnson MS, Benavides GA, Ricart K, Boddu R, Moore RD, Landar A, Barnes S, Darley-Usmar V, Agarwal A. Mitochondria-targeted heme

oxygenase-1 decreases oxidative stress in renal epithelial cells. American Journal of Physiology Renal Physiology 2013; 305: F255–F264. doi:10.1152/ajprenal.00160.2013

[65] Morimatsu H, Takahashi T, Shimizu H, Matsumi J, Kosaka J, Morit K. Heme Proteins, Heme Oxygenase-1 and Oxidative Stress. In: Lushchak DV, ed, Oxidative stress – Molecular mechanisms and biological effects. First ed. Rijeka (Croatia): InTech; 2012: 109–124. doi:10.5772/33757

[66] Ferreira A, Marguti I, Bechmann I, Jeney V, Chora A, Palha NR, Rebelo S, Henri A, Beuzard Y, Soares MP. Sickle hemoglobin confers tolerance to plasmodium infection. Cell 2011; 145: 398–409. doi:10.1016/j.cell.2011.03.049

[67] Stocker R, Perrella MA. Heme oxygenase-1: a novel drug target for atherosclerotic diseases? Circulation 2006; 114: 2178–2189. doi:10.1161/CIRCULATIONAHA.105.598698

[68] Liu XM, Peyton KJ, Ensenat D, Wang H, Hannink M, Alam J, Durante W. Nitric oxide stimulates heme oxygenase-1 gene transcription via the Nrf2/ARE complex to promote vascular smooth muscle cell survival. Cardiovascular Research 2007; 75: 381–389. doi:10.1016/j.cardiores.2007.03.004

[69] Kim H, Hwang JS, Woo CH, Kim EY, Kim TH, Cho KJ, Kim JH, Seo JM, Lee SS. TNF-alpha-induced up-regulation of intercellular adhesion molecule-1 is regulated by a Rac-ROS-dependent cascade in human airway epithelial cells. Experimental & Molecular Medicine 2008; 40: 167–175. doi:10.3858/emm.2008.40.2.167

[70] Kwak MK, Wakabayashi N, Greenlaw JL, Yamamoto M, Kensler TW. Antioxidants enhance mammalian proteasome expression through the Keap1-Nrf2 signaling pathway. Molecular & Cellular Biology 2003; 23: 8786–8794. doi:10.1128/mcb.23.23.8786-8794.2003

[71] Forstermann U, Sessa WC. Nitric oxide synthases: regulation and function. Eur Heart J 2012; 33: 829–837, 837a–837d. doi:10.1093/eurheartj/ehr304

[72] Vandelle E, Delledonne M. Peroxynitrite formation and function in plants. Plant Science: An International Journal of Experimental Plant Biology 2011; 181: 534–539. doi:10.1016/j.plantsci.2011.05.002

[73] Li Z, Zhao ZJ, Zhu XQ, Ren QS, Nie FF, Gao JM, Gao XJ, Yang TB, Zhou WL, Shen JL, Wang Y, Lu FL, Chen XG, Hide G, Ayala FJ, Lun ZR. Differences in iNOS and arginase expression and activity in the macrophages of rats are responsible for the resistance against *T. gondii* infection. PLoS One 2012; 7: e35834. doi:10.1371/journal.pone.0035834

Chapter 14

Digital Health Interventions (DHIs) to Support the Management of Children and Adolescents with Sickle-Cell Disease

Stephan Lobitz, Kristina Curtis and Kai Sostmann

Additional information is available at the end of the chapter

http://dx.doi.org/10.5772/64315

Abstract

Sickle-cell disease (SCD) is a very complex disorder alluding to all areas of medicine. Nevertheless, basic preventive and therapeutic interventions in patients suffering from SCD are extremely simple. However, in everyday life it is sometimes virtually impossible to motivate children and young adolescents to effectively self-manage their disorder at an early stage. Digital health interventions (DHIs) provide new opportunities to support self-management behaviours. DHIs may facilitate daily and recurrent routines such as drug intake or appointments along with helping the patients to better cope with their disease. This may be realized through mobile-training programmes, disease-specific social networks using secure communication channels, diaries, blogs and even games. Indeed, there are fascinating opportunities for modern disease-training programmes to take advantage of several media that can be combined and didactically optimized to meet the individual needs and intellectual abilities of different patients. The technological progress is rapid, extremely dynamic and highly creative. Our chapter gives an overview of the multifarious world of DHIs with a focus on smartphone applications known as mobile health apps (mHealth apps). We elucidate the potential reasons why we think that numerous apps for SCD patients have not been successful and which app features developers should consider if they want to create a popular patient app.

Keywords: mHealth, smartphone application, app, DHI, sickle-cell disease

1. Introduction

The rapid technological progress of the last two decades has had a deep impact on medical practice and research. In particular, searching for health information has become significantly easier today compared to the last few decades, where it was necessary to visit a library or a bookstore to access a certain publication. Today, health information is just a mouse-click away. You can download it to your computer, tablet or smartphone at any place in the world provided you are connected to the Internet. The latest scientific health evidence, therapies and guidelines to name but a few can be spread at lightning speed.

Health communication itself has been profoundly revolutionized in many ways. Undeniably, previous forms of communication such as letters and faxes have been largely replaced by mobile phones in the form of text, photo and video messaging. In particular, the smartphone plays a crucial role. Smartphones are a combination of a mobile phone and a personal digital assistant (PDA), often combined with inbuilt sensors such as accelerometers, cameras and GPS. They are generally categorized by their manufacturer or operating system (OS) with the most prevalent systems running on Android, iOS, Windows phone and Blackberry OS platforms [1, 2]. Smartphones enable people to exchange information around the world in a matter of seconds. This offers considerable advantages to both patients and health-care staff, and hence health-care providers should be open-minded towards this rapid and continuous stream of information. Ultimately, these new technologies have the potential capability to improve patient care significantly. However, any concrete application requires a very critical assessment, in particular in terms of usefulness and data security, since many applications may not keep their promises and potentially cause more harm than good [3–7]. Although it should be noted that no digital application in the world replaces the personal contact between the patient and the doctor, some may support this sensitive relationship in a reasonable and timely manner. This may help to make daily routines easier and save considerable resources in a time of underfinanced health-care systems.

This chapter provides an introduction to the multifarious and versatile world of digital health interventions with a focus on smartphone applications ('apps') for patients with sickle-cell disease (SCD).

2. Digital health interventions (DHIs)

DHIs are composed of software solutions on personal computers, mobile phones or tablets and, finally, web-based resources. DHIs are synonymously used with the term 'eHealth' and comprise a wide range of technologies and health conditions. The World Health Organization (WHO) classifies DHIs into the following categories [8]:

- The delivery of health information, for health professionals and health consumers, through the Internet and telecommunications.
- Using the power of IT and e-commerce to improve public health services, for example, through the education and training of health workers.
- The use of e-commerce and e-business practices in health system management.

http://dx.doi.org/10.5772/64315

Digital health technologies may involve tools that help to support the management of particular health conditions. For example, the miniaturization of sensor technology for use in mobile devices allows for the recognition and recording of motion patterns with increasing accuracy and permitting non-invasive synchronization with a multitude of bodily functions such as heart rate, blood pressure, perspiration, facial expression or haemoglobin levels. Invasively measured data can be entered manually for the purpose of documentation (e.g. blood glucose) [9–16]. Automated interpretation of the data entered by the software allows for an immediate feedback to the user. The technological progress is rapid, extremely dynamic and highly creative.

Along with simple tasks such as the documentation of pharmacotherapy or reminders of appointments, modern devices may also monitor correct drug intake, for example, by reading barcodes on the drug package with the smartphone's inbuilt camera. Motion sensors help to achieve predefined daily activity goals or detect patterns typical of certain disease states or complications such as pain. The presence and immediate availability of mobile devices enable their user to keep records at any time and place—an exciting feature in terms of documenting the natural history of a disease in a patient and of particular interest in clinical research.

DHI providers and users are able to interact by means of diverse forms of text, picture and video messaging. There are also fascinating opportunities for modern disease-training programmes to combine several media that can be didactically optimized for the individual needs and intellectual abilities of a range of patients. Video conferences between patients and doctors may help to facilitate real-time exchange of information and medical findings, even between individuals who live thousands of miles away from each other. This is a highly beneficial feature monitoring injuries and symptoms such as wounds or skin rashes.

Currently, there is a trend in developing DHIs to help modify behaviour [17]. In the majority of cases, these DHIs are smartphone applications that can be easily adapted to the individual needs. Many of them are health promoting and preventive in character and aim to support users to start or reinforce one of more health behaviours (e.g. health eating) and/or reduce risk behaviours (e.g. smoking cessation) [18]. The majority of these apps are aimed at healthy people, but not for patients—developing a huge market.

2.1. Mobile health apps

One of the most important sub-disciplines of DHIs is mobile health (mHealth), outlined by the Global Observatory of eHealth (GOe) as mobile devices such as mobile phones, personal digital assistants (PDA), and other wireless devices supporting medical or public health routines [19]. mHealth interventions can be structured into eight categories [2]:

- point-of-care diagnostics
- wellness
- education and reference
- efficiency and productivity

- patient monitoring
- compliance
- behaviour modification
- environmental mentoring

Within mHealth, it is the arrival of the smartphone, complemented by an eruption of commercial mobile health and medical apps (mHealth apps), that is revolutionizing approaches to personal health management [20]. A mobile app is a small programme or application downloaded from a website (e.g. Apple's App Store) which operates on a smartphone or a tablet computer [1, 2]. Originally, apps have served to improve productivity (e.g. a simple calendar app) or handle small data sets and information (e.g. phone book). However, as a result of a tremendous demand, mobile apps for smartphones and tablets have been developed for use in all areas of life. Inevitably, the app market has grown exponentially within the last years. By 2016, it is expected that over 44 billion apps will have been downloaded which equates to six apps downloaded for every person across the globe [21].

Currently, the two big app stores, the Apple App Store and the Google Play Store, host more than 150,000 health apps, ready to be downloaded and claiming to provide a health-promoting benefit for the user or an entrusted person. Approximately 20,000 apps are medical apps in a strict sense, that is, they are directed to patients, doctors and other medical service providers with the ultimate goals of supporting medical care [7].

The global sales volume of mobile health technologies is expected to reach 31 billion Euros by 2020 [22], creating a highly competitive market. The wide choice of products generates a trade rivalry of formerly unknown enormity resulting in many apps being discarded after first use. Indeed, the consumer decides whether an app will survive or not, although it is important to recognize that even well-liked apps are thought to have a life expectancy of less than 6 months. Many factors are important when considering what makes a 'good' app. Many of which are intangible, that is, factors that affect the decision, but that cannot be expressed in monetary or rational terms. Is an app useful? Is it easy to handle? Is it self-explanatory? Is it visually appealing? The decision on success or failure depends on nuances. Ultimately, it is difficult to predict how certain population groups will respond to a health app. However, a range of sub-disciplines from the design, psychology, engineering and computer science fields seeks to understand the nature of app usage. Among these fields, there is strong consensus that app development requires drawing on theory, evidence and formative research with the target audience. Mobile health interventions should have a high degree of social validity and acceptability among its users, helping to establish the trend towards the adoption of a user-centred approach [23]. User-Centred Design (USD) places the users' needs and desires at the core of the development process. It represents a participatory design approach focusing on the user and on 'incorporating the user's perspective in all stages of the design process' [24].

http://dx.doi.org/10.5772/64315

3. Wearables

Further developments in the field of mobile interactive devices comprise the introduction of so-called wearable electronic devices ('wearables'). Most of these microelectronic items are at the size of a wrist watch or so small that they can be delivered on the size of a credit card or as a piece of jewellery. They are developed mainly to measure and deliver data in real time or to record long-term data. Sensors of these items can track the activity, velocity and the location of their users (GPS, accelerometers, speedometers). Other sensor technology measures physical functions such as heart frequency rates, oxygen saturation in the blood, blood pressure or skin humidity. They are applied at two levels to the health-care market. On the consumer side of the market, the distribution of these items exploded and founded a market on its own, where there has been a drive towards people measuring every aspect of their physical and mental life known as the 'Quantified Self-Movement' [25]. Within the context of the health-care system, data collection is fundamental to the improvement of health-care services for patients with SCD. The collection, analysis and interpretation of data enabled through the application of recently developed new software technologies have led to a new discipline known as 'Big Data'. The sheer volume of patient data represents new opportunities and new challenges for multiple stakeholders regarding data storage and interpretation.

4. Digital health interventions (DHIs) for SCD

Sickle-cell disease is a very complex disorder alluding to virtually all areas of medicine. Nevertheless, basic preventive and therapeutic interventions in patients suffering from SCD are extremely simple. Minor behavioural changes may reduce the incidence of several complications. Wearing warm clothes prevents pain crises. Vaccinations and penicillin prophylaxis virtually eliminate life-threatening bacterial infections. Patients with febrile illnesses require urgent medical care. Parents who are able to palpate spleen size can diagnose splenic sequestration at home at a very early stage and seek medical attention immediately. Most patients who have internalized this simple code of conduct show a great improvement in their condition.

The groundwork is laid in childhood. It is up to the paediatricians to communicate this information and knowledge during childhood and adolescence. Experience has taught us that the transition to adult care is often inadequate and that those patients who get lost at this critical stage of care have not understood the gravity of their individual situation—resulting in serious consequences for their health.

However, in everyday life it is sometimes virtually impossible to support children and adolescents to self-manage their condition. For the first time ever, DHIs provide new opportunities to support self-management behaviours [26, 27]. As a minimum, DHIs may facilitate daily and recurrent routines such as drug intake or appointments through simple reminders. However, at an advanced level, they may also help the patient to cope better with their disease.

This may be realized through a number of modes of delivery such as mobile-training programmes, disease-specific social networks using secure communication channels, diaries and blogs.

It is an absolute prerequisite to awaken a patient's interest and motivation in their own disease to establish understanding and create awareness for disease-specific needs. DHIs, in particular apps, for children and adolescent with SCD aim to create an improved sense of self and disease in the very first instance.

Despite the enormous prevalence of SCD, there are still a limited number of SCD apps available to patients suffering from SCD, their families, peers and caregivers as well as a paucity of publications on SCD apps. Nevertheless, so far research has shown promise for the acceptability and usability of SCD apps aimed at tracking multiple symptoms such as pain and tiredness [28–30], facilitating reminders for medication [31], enhancing communication with health-care providers and general health management [30] and delivering therapeutic interventions such as cognitive behavioural therapy [32, 33]. Indeed, research- and industry-led apps have chosen diverse approaches to address SCD. Consequently, the diverging SCD-related apps on the market pursue a variety of objectives. Most apps have several functions and behavioural targets, but they can be classified on the basis of their primary objective.

There are apps that:

- facilitate the diagnosis of SCD
- help to educate patients about the disease
- record symptoms and complications
- aim to change the behaviour of patients, in particular, their adherence to medication
- support therapeutic approaches to coping with the disease
- improve the communication between patients and between patients and caregivers

A number of SCD apps have been developed by academic institutions or pharmaceutical companies, while other apps are the product of more or less fruitful cooperation between different stakeholders. However, most app developers fail to involve patients in the design, development or evaluation process. Consequently, most apps for SCD patients have one feature in common: they have been rejected by the patient community and disappeared rapidly from the market.

5. Identifying the gaps in SCD apps: the case of Germany

The clinical course of an individual suffering from SCD is highly dependent on where the patient actually lives. For example, there are massive problems in providing state-of-the-art care in most African countries. Many patients have none or limited access to public health care.

In addition, most health-care systems in Africa where many drugs are not widely available are not comparable to the high-resource countries in Europe and North America. In particular, most patients in Africa have no access to penicillin prophylaxis and to hydroxycarbamide despite the fact that the latter is comparatively cheap and on the WHO Model List of Essential Medicines [34]. Additional adverse factors such as malaria and malnutrition also have a high impact on the outcome of SCD in Africa. Consequently, regionally up to 90% of children suffering from SCD die before they are 5 years of age [35]. In the second decade of the twenty-first century, this is horrifying. In stark comparison, during the last four decades, SCD care has improved considerably in Europe and North America. Newborn screening, infection prophylaxis and the wide use of hydroxyurea have probably had the most important impact on the survival rates that are now close to 100% in childhood and adolescence in the large cohort studies from the UK and USA, respectively [36–40].

However, the quality of care for patients suffering from SCD is not only dependent on the unlimited access to an efficient health-care system and medication. It is also dependent on national and local prevalence rates and the comprehensiveness of care centres for the treatment of SCD and other disorders. Globally, SCD is the most common monogenetic disease of all, a fact that is mainly attributed to its high prevalence in Sub-Saharan Western and Central Africa, the Persian Gulf and India. SCD is quite uncommon in the Middle and Northern European countries and actually even fulfils the criteria of a rare disease in most European countries. The European Medicines Agency's (EMEA) definition of a rare disease is 'less than five affected persons in 10,000'. Consequently, many countries with high-performance health-care systems (such as Germany) have problems in offering comprehensive SCD care, simply because they do not have enough patients in most centres. It took the German Society of Paediatric Oncology and Haematology (GPOH) until 2012 to implement a structured disease-management program and to establish a national registry for patients with SCD. A national guideline for the treatment of children and adolescents with SCD was released in 2015. And finally, three pilot studies have shown that the prevalence of SCD in Germany is high enough to justify integrating the highly political SCD-screening procedure into the national newborn screening programme [41–44].

Although the number of SCD in Germany is expected to be in an order of 3000–5000 (estimate based on personal communications and reference [45]), 58 GPOH hospitals, several non-GPOH hospitals and a number of paediatricians in private practice are involved in primary SCD care. Consequently, most doctors look after much less than 30 patients. And unfortunately, there are no prominent patient-support groups.

Another important aspect is that in Germany, SCD only affects people with a personal or a familial history of migration [45]. In the majority of cases, patients are poorly integrated and have a poor educational background. Their influence on the society is low and so is their impact on political decisions. In other words, they have no voice.

Accordingly, it is difficult to acquire funding for clinical research and development for patients suffering from SCD. Not even clinical routine care is financed adequately. For example, the German compulsory health insurance companies do not cover liver iron MRI examinations for polytransfused patients on a reliable legal basis. Decisions are made on a case-by-case basis and require a yearly time-consuming formal application for each individual.

The main problems in Germany are summarized as follows:

- no dedicated treatment centre(s) for haemoglobinopathies
- few specialized contact persons
- poor utilization of present resources
- poor knowledge about the disease among the patient population
- low levels of awareness and virtually no knowledge about the disease among the general population
- poor education levels of most patients and their families
- little willingness towards understanding the 'basics' of the disease in conjunction with a suboptimal support from the health-care providers

Within the context of Germany, a smartphone application for SCD patients requires app features to:

- improve the patient's interest in his/her own illness, hopefully leading to a better understanding of sickle-cell disease,
- support the patient in taking their medication (improve adherence),
- improve appointment adherence,
- improve the documentation of complications and other disease-related symptoms to get a more objective overall picture of the individual clinical course between two consultations,
- improve the communication with the health-care service providers,
- improve the communication between patients,
- educate the surrounding family and community about the condition,
- support the patients whenever and wherever they are looking for a doctor specialized in SCD care, in particular when they are not at home (e.g. on a holiday).

Certainly, these objectives may differ from other countries where there may already be well-working educational programmes in place. However, there is strong consensus among some health-app developers, that the needs defined by doctors differ significantly from the needs defined by patients. It is thus an indispensable prerequisite to develop a successful app to involve patients into the whole development process right from the start [26]. To keep the balance between the patients' and doctors' needs is the 'art of health-app development'.

http://dx.doi.org/10.5772/64315

Author details

Stephan Lobitz[1*], Kristina Curtis[2] and Kai Sostmann[3]

*Address all correspondence to: stephan.lobitz@charite.de

1 Department of Pediatric Oncology, Hematology and BMT, Charité-University Medicine Berlin, Berlin, Germany

2 The Centre for Technology Enabled Health Research (CTEHR), Coventry University, Coventry, United Kingdom

3 Department of eLearning, Vice Deanery for Academic Studies and Teaching, Charité – University Medicine Berlin, Berlin, Germany

References

[1] Curtis, K.E., The development of a theory and evidence based, user-centred family healthy eating app in The University of Warwick. 2016.

[2] Olla, P. and Shimskey, C., mHealth taxonomy: a literature survey of mobile health applications. Health Technol, 2014. 4: p. 299–308.

[3] Wolf, J.A., et al., Diagnostic inaccuracy of smartphone applications for melanoma detection. JAMA Dermatol, 2013. 149(4): p. 422–426.

[4] Wallace, L.S. and Dhingra, L.K., A systematic review of smartphone applications for chronic pain available for download in the United States. J Opioid Manag, 2014. 10(1): p. 63–68.

[5] Baig, M.M., GholamHosseini, H. and Connolly, M.J., Mobile healthcare applications: system design review, critical issues and challenges. Australas Phys Eng Sci Med, 2015. 38(1): p. 23–38.

[6] BinDhim, N.F., Hawkey, A. and Trevena, L., A systematic review of quality assessment methods for smartphone health apps. Telemed J E Health, 2015. 21(2): p. 97–104.

[7] Wiechmann, W., et al., There's an app for that? Highlighting the difficulty in finding clinically relevant smartphone applications. West J Emerg Med, 2016. 17(2): p. 191–194.

[8] WHO Trade foreign policy diplomacy and health E-Health 2016; Available from: http://www.who.int/trade/glossary/story021/en/

[9] Collings, S., et al., Non-invasive detection of anaemia using digital photographs of the conjunctiva. PLoS One, 2016. 11(4): p. e0153286.

[10] Kim, E.K., et al., Feasibility of a patient-centered, smartphone-based, diabetes care system: a pilot study. Diabetes Metab J, 2016.

[11] Franc, S., et al., Telemedicine and type 1 diabetes: is technology per se sufficient to improve glycaemic control? Diabetes Metab, 2014. 40(1): p. 61–66.

[12] McGillicuddy, J.W., et al., Mobile health medication adherence and blood pressure control in renal transplant recipients: a proof-of-concept randomized controlled trial. JMIR Res Protoc, 2013. 2(2): p. e32.

[13] Simon, S.K. and Seldon, H.L., Personal health records: mobile biosensors and smartphones for developing countries. Stud Health Technol Inform, 2012. 182: p. 125–132.

[14] Gregoski, M.J., et al., Development and validation of a smartphone heart rate acquisition application for health promotion and wellness telehealth applications. Int J Telemed Appl, 2012. 2012: p. 696324.

[15] Lowres, N., et al., Atrial fibrillation screening in pharmacies using an iPhone ECG: a qualitative review of implementation. Int J Clin Pharm, 2015. 37(6): p. 1111–1120.

[16] Lowres, N., et al., Self-monitoring for atrial fibrillation recurrence in the discharge period post-cardiac surgery using an iPhone electrocardiogramdagger. Eur J Cardiothorac Surg, 2016.

[17] Neubeck, L., et al., The mobile revolution—using smartphone apps to prevent cardiovascular disease. Nat Rev Cardiol, 2015. 12(6): p. 350–360.

[18] Curtis, K.E. and Karasouli, E., An assessment of the potential of health promotion apps to support health behaviour change. Health Psychol Update, 2014. 23(2): p. 43–49.

[19] WHO, mHealth: new horizons for health through mobile technologies. Global Observatory for eHealth Series, 2011. 3; Available from: http://www.who.int/goe/publications/ehealth_series_vol3/en/.

[20] Bert, F., et al., Smartphones and health promotion: a review of the evidence. J Med Syst, 2014. 38(1): p. 9995.

[21] West, J.H., et al., Health behavior theories in diet apps. J Cons Health Int, 2013. 17(1): p. 10–24.

[22] Vranova, Z., The mHealth app market will grow by 15% to reach $31 billion by 2020. 2016; Available from: http://research2guidance.com/2015/11/11/the-mhealth-app-market-will-grow-by-15-to-reach-31-billion-by-2020/.

[23] Curtis, K.E., Lahiri, S. and Brown, K.E., Targeting parents for childhood weight management: development of a theory-driven and user-centered healthy eating app. JMIR Mhealth Uhealth, 2015. 3(2): p. e69.

[24] Devi, K.R., Sen, A.M. and Hemachandran, K., A working framework for the user-centered design approach and a survey of the available methods. Int J Sci Res Publ, 2012. 2(4): p. 1–8.

[25] Appelboom, G., et al., The quantified patient: a patient participatory culture. Curr Med Res Opin, 2014. 30(12): p. 2585–2587.

[26] Badawy, S.M., Thompson, A.A. and Liem, R.I., Technology access and smartphone app preferences for medication adherence in adolescents and young adults with sickle cell disease. Pediatr Blood Cancer, 2016. 63(5): p. 848–852.

[27] Issom, D.Z., et al., Exploring the challenges and opportunities of ehealth tools for patients with sickle cell disease. Stud Health Technol Inform, 2015. 216: p. 898.

[28] Jacob, E., et al., Remote monitoring of pain and symptoms using wireless technology in children and adolescents with sickle cell disease. J Am Assoc Nurse Pract, 2013. 25(1): p. 42–54.

[29] Jonassaint, C.R., et al., Usability and feasibility of an mhealth intervention for monitoring and managing pain symptoms in sickle cell disease: the sickle cell disease mobile application to record symptoms via technology (SMART). Hemoglobin, 2015. 39(3): p. 162–168.

[30] Shah, N., Jonassaint, J. and De Castro, L., Patients welcome the sickle cell disease mobile application to record symptoms via technology (SMART). Hemoglobin, 2014. 38(2): p. 99–103.

[31] Creary, S.E., et al., A pilot study of electronic directly observed therapy to improve hydroxyurea adherence in pediatric patients with sickle-cell disease. Pediatr Blood Cancer, 2014. 61(6): p. 1068–1073.

[32] Cheng, C., et al., iACT--an interactive mHealth monitoring system to enhance psychotherapy for adolescents with sickle cell disease. Conf Proc IEEE Eng Med Biol Soc, 2013. 2013: p. 2279–2282.

[33] Schatz, J., et al., Changes in coping, pain, and activity after cognitive-behavioral training: a randomized clinical trial for pediatric sickle cell disease using smartphones. Clin J Pain, 2015. 31(6): p. 536–547.

[34] McGann, P.T., et al., Hydroxyurea therapy for children with sickle cell anemia in sub-saharan africa: rationale and design of the REACH trial. Pediatr Blood Cancer, 2016. 63(1): p. 98–104.

[35] Grosse, S.D., et al., Sickle cell disease in Africa: a neglected cause of early childhood mortality. Am J Prev Med, 2011. 41(6 Suppl 4): p. S398–S405.

[36] Elmariah, H., et al., Factors associated with survival in a contemporary adult sickle cell disease cohort. Am J Hematol, 2014. 89(5): p. 530–535.

[37] Quinn, C.T., et al., Improved survival of children and adolescents with sickle cell disease. Blood, 2010. 115(17): p. 3447–3452.

[38] Wierenga, K.J., Hambleton, I.R. and Lewis, N.A., Survival estimates for patients with homozygous sickle-cell disease in Jamaica: a clinic-based population study. Lancet, 2001. 357(9257): p. 680–683.

[39] Lee, A., et al., Improved survival in homozygous sickle cell disease: lessons from a cohort study. BMJ, 1995. 311(7020): p. 1600–1602.

[40] Telfer, P., et al., Clinical outcomes in children with sickle cell disease living in England: a neonatal cohort in East London. Haematologica, 2007. 92(7): p. 905–912.

[41] Lobitz, S., et al., Incidence of sickle cell disease in an unselected cohort of neonates born in Berlin, Germany. Eur J Hum Genet, 2014. 22(8): p. 1051–1053.

[42] Frommel, C., et al., Newborn screening for sickle cell disease: technical and legal aspects of a German pilot study with 38,220 participants. Biomed Res Int, 2014. 2014: p. 695828.

[43] Kunz, J.B., et al., Significant prevalence of sickle cell disease in Southwest Germany: results from a birth cohort study indicate the necessity for newborn screening. Ann Hematol, 2016. 95(3): p. 397–402.

[44] Grosse, R., et al., The prevalence of sickle cell disease and its implication for newborn screening in Germany (Hamburg metropolitan area). Pediatr Blood Cancer, 2016. 63(1): p. 168–170.

[45] Kohne, E. and Kleihauer, E., Hemoglobinopathies: a longitudinal study over four decades. Dtsch Arztebl Int, 2010. 107(5): p. 65–71.